T0269916

Praise for
Smart but Scattered

"A revolutionary guide for parents. The second edition offers fresh perspectives on important issues like the impact of technology on developing minds. *Smart but Scattered* gives parents skills and confidence to enhance their child's success—with strategies that take just 5 to 10 minutes a day."
—Julie Gettman, PhD, NCSP, ABSNP, Executive Director,
School Neuropsychology Institute

"As a pediatric neuropsychologist, I have recommended *Smart but Scattered* to hundreds—if not thousands—of parents. I didn't think it was possible to improve on a classic, but the authors have done just that! With deep insight and empathy, the book provides abundant ideas and activities to increase executive function skills. Information about technology—a distraction for most 'scattered' kids—is a wonderful addition to the second edition. I love this book."
—Ellen Braaten, PhD, author of *Bright Kids Who Can't Keep Up*

"The second edition improves on the original masterpiece! The authors empower you to foster your child's self-awareness and growth—even if executive skills aren't your own strong suit. What sets this book apart is its user-friendly format, combining scientific insights with actionable advice. The questionnaires alone make the book worthwhile, providing crucial insights into your child's strengths and weaknesses. This is an invaluable resource for anyone dedicated to nurturing a child's potential."
—Michael Delman, MEd, Founder and CEO, Beyond BookSmart

"This masterfully written book is an indispensable resource. It is packed with practical, evidence-based strategies that you can readily implement to support your child's development. I cannot recommend this book highly enough!"
—Lynn Meltzer, PhD, President and Director, Research Institute
for Learning and Development, Lexington, Massachusetts

"Groundbreaking.... Comprehensive, accessible, and hopeful.... Dawson and Guare's work should be considered essential. (starred review)."
—*Library Journal*

Smart but Scattered

Also Available

FOR GENERAL READERS

Smart but Scattered—and Stalled:
10 Steps to Help Young Adults Use Their Executive Skills
to Set Goals, Make a Plan, and Successfully Leave the Nest
Richard Guare, Colin Guare, and Peg Dawson

Smart but Scattered Teens:
The "Executive Skills" Program for Helping Teens Reach
Their Potential
Richard Guare, Peg Dawson, and Colin Guare

The Smart but Scattered Guide to Success:
How to Use Your Brain's Executive Skills to Keep Up, Stay Calm,
and Get Organized at Work and at Home
Peg Dawson and Richard Guare

The Work-Smart Academic Planner:
Write It Down, Get It Done, Revised Edition
Peg Dawson and Richard Guare

FOR PROFESSIONALS

Coaching Students with Executive Skills Challenges, Second Edition
Peg Dawson and Richard Guare

Conducting School-Based Functional Behavioral Assessments:
A Practitioner's Guide, Third Edition
*Mark W. Steege, Jamie L. Pratt, Garry Wickerd, Richard Guare,
and T. Steuart Watson*

Executive Skills in Children and Adolescents:
A Practical Guide to Assessment and Intervention, Third Edition
Peg Dawson and Richard Guare

Smart but Scattered

The Revolutionary Executive Skills Approach to Helping Kids Reach Their Potential

SECOND EDITION

Peg Dawson, EdD
Richard Guare, PhD
Colin Guare, MS

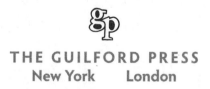

THE GUILFORD PRESS
New York   London

Copyright © 2025 The Guilford Press
A Division of Guilford Publications, Inc.
www.guilford.com

All rights reserved

The information in this volume is not intended as a substitute for consultation with healthcare professionals. Each individual's health concerns should be evaluated by a qualified professional.

Purchasers of this book have permission to copy worksheets, where indicated by footnotes, for personal use or use with clients. These worksheets may be copied from the book or accessed directly from the publisher's website, but may not be stored on or distributed from intranet sites, internet sites, or file-sharing sites, or made available for resale. No other part of this book may be reproduced, translated, stored in a retrieval system, or transmitted, in any form or by any means, electronic, mechanical, photocopying, microfilming, recording, or otherwise, without written permission from the publisher.

Printed in the United States of America

This book is printed on acid-free paper.

Last digit is print number: 9   8   7   6   5   4   3   2   1

Library of Congress Cataloging-in-Publication Data

Names: Dawson, Peg, author. | Guare, Richard, author. | Guare, Colin, author.
Title: Smart but scattered : the revolutionary executive skills approach to helping kids reach their potential / Peg Dawson, EdD, Richard Guare, PhD, Colin Guare.
Description: Second edition. | New York : The Guilford Press, [2025] | Includes bibliographical references and index.
Identifiers: LCCN 2024036456 | ISBN 9781462555741 (hardcover) | ISBN 9781462554591 (paperback)
Subjects: LCSH: Parenting. | Executive ability in children. | Children—Life skills guides. | Child development. | Parent and child.
Classification: LCC HQ755.8 .D39 2025 | DDC 649/.1526—dc23/eng/20240911
LC record available at *https://lccn.loc.gov/2024036456*

Authors' Note: In this book, we alternate among masculine, feminine, and plural pronouns when referring to a single individual to represent as many readers as possible as our language continues to evolve. We sincerely hope that all will feel included. All illustrations of individuals are composites or thoroughly disguised to protect individuals' privacy.

Contents

PART III
Putting It All Together

Purchasers of this book can download and print worksheets at
www.guilford.com/dawson4-forms for personal use
or use with clients (see copyright page for details).

Introduction

When we wrote the first edition of *Smart but Scattered*, we had some reservations. Not about the general topic—executive skills—nor about the audience we wanted to reach—parents. Having already written a book for a professional audience that had been well received, we were convinced that helping people understand how these skills play such an important role in development was a worthwhile endeavor. We were also pretty sure that we could explain all this to a lay audience using easily understood language and concepts—because we'd been presenting to parents for a while on the topic and our presentations were always well-received. *And* we were convinced that we knew intervention strategies that parents could use to help their children strengthen their executive skills. After all, we helped parents in our clinical practice use these strategies with the children they brought to us for help, and we'd used many of the same tools with our own children.

What we weren't sure about was whether a parent, just by reading a book, would be able to translate our suggestions from the written word into action that would result in observable benefits for their children, and for the parents themselves. We knew that the self-help section of every bookstore is packed with books offering advice on every topic imaginable. We just weren't sure whether those books did much more than give their authors a royalty check a couple of times a year.

But we crossed our fingers and hoped, and thanks in part to the great title suggested to us by our brilliant editors (Kitty Moore and Chris Benton), the book began to sell and to reach a pretty wide audience. And then we began hearing from parents. One mother mentioned to us in a workshop that she'd helped her daughter come up with a bedroom-cleaning routine based on our suggestions. She said she hovered in the bedroom to supervise her daughter until the point where her daughter turned to her and said, "Mom, you don't have to watch me. I have the checklist!" And a dad told us that after reading *Smart but Scattered* his relationship with his son improved significantly, not because he used a particular technique or routine, but because he understood his son a whole lot better and was less critical of him as a result. And any number of parents have told us that their favorite part of the book is the chapter where they assess their own executive skills profile because it gave them insight into both themselves and how their kids are not carbon copies of them, which was confirmed when they completed the survey that allowed them to determine their child's executive skills profile.

Since the first edition of *Smart but Scattered* was published, a lot has happened! We've lived through a pandemic, which hopefully is now behind us, as well as a technological revolution, which promises to continue to evolve and to impact children in ways we could not have anticipated even a decade ago and may not be fully able to anticipate going forward. On a personal note, our children have grown up and we are now grandparents, which gives us the opportunity to watch executive skills develop in a new generation of children. Our understanding of executive skills has deepened because of these experiences, and this second edition reflects that.

We've also come to believe, even more than we did before, that if we want to help children develop strong executive skills, we need to partner with them rather than direct them, collaborate rather than compel. We know these skills take a minimum of 25 years to reach full maturation, but from a surprisingly early age we can engage children in conversations that enable them to fully participate in a process of discovery and problem solving. This process not only helps them learn about themselves and what they're capable of, but also expands their capabilities as they try out new skills with the support and encouragement of their parents.

About This Book

As we have worked with other children—and watched our own children grow up—we've found that all kinds of children may struggle with executive skill challenges and that what you can do to help will vary depending on the age and developmental level of the child, as well as on your own strengths and challenges and which problems are causing all of you the most trouble. If you can target the right behavior and choose the right strategy, you can have a positive, significant, and long-lasting impact on your children's ability to develop executive skills. Helping you figure out where your child needs help and the best angles of attack for strengthening those executive skills is the main goal of Part I of this book.

Chapters 1–3 provide an overview of executive skills, how they develop, how they show themselves in common developmental tasks, and how you and the environment can contribute to the development of strong executive skills. Different scientists and clinicians have categorized and labeled executive skills in various ways, but all of us in this field agree that these are the cognitive processes required to (1) plan and direct activities, including getting started and seeing them through, and (2) regulate behavior—to inhibit impulses, make good choices, change tactics when what you're doing now isn't working, and manage emotions and behavior to achieve long-term goals. If you look at the brain as organizing input and organizing output, executive skills help us manage the output functions. That is, they help us take all the data the brain has collected from our sensory organs, muscles, nerve endings, and so forth, and choose how to respond.

In Chapter 1 you'll not only learn more about the specific functions of executive skills but also a little about how the brain develops, and, more specifically, how executive skills develop in children, beginning at birth. This understanding should give you an idea of how far-reaching the functions of executive skills are and why challenges or deficits can limit a child's daily life in so many ways.

To be able to identify your child's particular executive skill strengths and challenges, of course, you have to know when the various skills are expected to develop—just like you did for motor skills like sitting, standing, and walking when your child was a baby and a toddler. Most parents already have an intuitive sense of the developmental trajectory for executive skills. We, and our children's teachers, naturally adjust our expectations to fit each child's growing capacity for independence, even though we probably don't consciously label these milestones as the acquisition of various executive skills. Chapter 2 will give you a closer look at this trajectory, listing the common developmental tasks that require the use of executive skills at different childhood stages. We'll also show you how executive skill strengths and challenges tend to follow certain patterns in individuals, although it's also true that the skills overall may be better developed in some people than in others. You'll begin to form a picture of your child's strengths and challenges with a set of brief tests, and you can assess your own profile in Chapter 3. This picture will help you start identifying possible targets for the interventions offered in Parts II and III.

The first chapter in Part II (Chapter 4) gives you a set of principles to follow when deciding the best angle of attack for a particular problem task or executive skill your child needs. Three of these form the framework for all the work you're going to do, and each of these is described in the chapters that follow (Chapters 5–7): (1) make adjustments in the environment to improve the goodness-of-fit between the child and the task; (2) teach the child how to do the tasks that require executive skills; or (3) motivate the child to use the executive skills already within his repertoire. We generally recommend a combination of these three approaches be used to ensure success. To get started, you can decide whether you'd like to adopt some of the scaffolding techniques in Part II to boost your child's executive skills in a seamless fashion during the course of the day.

You'll also want to target certain problem situations that are causing lots of aggravation for all and/or certain executive skills that are causing your child problems across all the domains of her life. Part III starts with principles that underlie all the strategies in this book, so we recommend reading Chapter 8 before using any strategy with your child. Chapter 9 offers teaching routines aimed at the problems most commonly reported by parents of the children we see in our clinical practice. These routines give you a set of procedures, and in some cases a script, that will help your child learn to manage activities of daily living with less effort and turmoil, whether it's following a bedtime routine, handling changes in plans, or learning to manage feelings and impulses more effectively. Many parents find it easiest to begin with these routines because they directly address a task that's a source of conflict every day and because we've supplied all the steps and tools you need. You may find this the best way to get used to executive-skill-building work and the shortest route to observable results. Parents need motivation too, and there's nothing like success to keep you going. These routines tell you how to adapt the routine for your child's age. They also identify the executive skills needed to perform that task, so if you find that the same skills are needed for the tasks causing your child the most trouble, you may decide to read and work on those skills in the corresponding chapters that follow.

Chapters 10 through 20 take up each executive skill individually. We describe the typical developmental progression of the skill and give you a brief rating scale you can use to determine whether your child is on target or lagging with respect to skill development. If you feel your child's skills are generally adequate but could use some tweaking, you can follow the general principles we list for how to do this. If you recognize that problems are more pronounced, however, you can create your own intervention based on the models we provide for a couple of more intensive interventions, focusing on those problem areas that arise most frequently in our clinical practice. These interventions incorporate elements of all three methods described in Part II.

We're confident that, given all these different choices, you'll find a way to help your child build weak executive skills into stronger ones. But we live in an imperfect world, so Chapter 21 includes troubleshooting suggestions for those times when you run into a brick wall, including questions you should ask yourself about the interventions you have tried, as well as guidance for how and when to seek professional help.

Since we wrote the first edition, it has become evident that how children interact with technology (phones, tablets, and laptops) has become considerably more complicated. In our parent presentations, one of the most common questions we are asked is about technology. What effect is it having on development—and not just executive skill development but cognitive development more generally and social development—and even physical development? And what guidelines can we recommend for managing that technology? There are whole books written on this topic, but Chapter 22 is an addition to this book that outlines the key considerations parents need to take into account when making decisions about access to and use of technology by their children.

As parents, you can help your children use strong executive skills to get homework done and form good study habits, but you can't follow them into the classroom. Most scattered children encounter problems in school as well as at home. In fact, it may very well be your child's first teachers who have made you aware of your child's executive skill challenges. Chapter 23 describes how schools typically support executive skill development, and it offers suggestions for how to work with teachers and the school to make sure your child gets the necessary help and support in school as well as at home. This includes suggestions for how to avoid adversarial relationships with teachers as well as how to access additional support, such as 504 Plans or special education, if needed.

In our parent presentations, there is invariably someone in the audience who raises their hand and says, often with considerable hesitation, "Everything you suggest sounds great, but I have executive skill challenges myself. How can I ever help my kid when I'm struggling with many of the same issues?"

We've addressed this in this book, but despite our assurances and our recommendation that you start small and go slowly, you may find yourself feeling the same way as you read *Smart but Scattered*. So before you begin reading the book, we'll share with you "the perfect intervention to support executive skill development" that we provide those overwhelmed parents in our trainings. Here it is: the perfect intervention to support executive skill development is one (1) that takes no more than 5 or 10 minutes a day and (2) that you're willing to do forever (or as long as it takes).

When we first started sharing this advice, we thought we were being a bit whimsical. Can you really improve executive skills in 5-minute increments? And then parents started sharing with us examples of how this really worked. What we've learned from this is that the two parts of that intervention go hand in hand. If it took more than 5 or 10 minutes a day, you couldn't keep it up long enough for it to "stick." We've also learned that it won't take forever—but it may well take longer than you expected it to.

As you read this book, you may want to return to this question: What's one thing I could do with my child that would take no more than 5 minutes a day? We think this book will help you answer that question.

PART I

What Makes Your Child Smart but Scattered

1

How Did Such a Smart Kid End Up So Scattered?

"Hey, Mom, Mom, can I watch my show?"

"Hmmmm, yes, for like 10 minutes. We need to stop at the store on the way to pick up your brother."

"OK! . . . Hey, Mom, can I have my tablet?"

"I don't have your tablet, sweetheart."

"Oh . . . Where *is* my tablet?"

"I have no idea, Clem. On the couch? Maybe *in* the couch? Listen, I have to finish some work before we leave. Please have your shoes on. Is everything else ready? Clem? Hellooo?"

* * *

"It wasn't on, or in, *or* under the couch, Mom."

"Is everything *else* ready? Like did you fill the water dishes?"

"What? Oh, um, yeah, yeah . . . Mom, do you think Booster took—"

"OK, well, then it's somewhere else. No, Clem, Booster has no thumbs; Booster is a dog. He doesn't watch *Rocketeer*. I can't help you right now; we are leaving in"—she taps her phone—"seven minutes. I love you very much. Now go somewhere else."

I checked the couch, but did I really check the couch? I've found things looking in the same place twice before. No, definitely not there, and no tablets allowed in bedrooms, so definitely not there. On top of the toilet, in Mom's bag, under a book on the skinny table in the hallway, the shelf in the kitchen cabinet where I put it down while I open snacks, slid in between boots in the closet when I put my shoes on, back to the couch because, just maybe,

9

under my sweatshirt on one of the dining table chairs, that little place right by the door opposite the dog's dishes where I leave it before going outside—water dishes! Run back to the kitchen, check under the sink for the tablet (why not?), fill cup, bring the cup back, fill the dish. Check dog bed, couch one more time, where. is. it.

"Clem! Time to go!"

"Mommy, I looked everywhere; the tablet is gone! What the heck! You said I could watch my show for 10 minutes. I was supposed to be able to watch my show!"

"Well, that is just so, so sad. But! We need to leave. Where are your socks, Clem? I asked if *everything* was ready, and you said yes, yes? We made a list this morning, and on that list was taking your clean clothes to your room and putting them away, and I know there are socks in that basket. Go, run, I don't care if they match—I don't even care if one is actually a glove—just hurry."

As it turns out, the tablet was in the laundry basket, and, much to Mom's dismay, the couch cushions were on the floor, cabinets and closet doors were open at random, a trail of water ran from the kitchen sink to the dog's dish, and the clean clothes were still very much not put away.

It would surprise us if there were parents out there who had *not* had experiences like the one just described. Children are an endless source of love, joy, comfort, pride, humor, and fascination for their parents. Caring for them, teaching them, and seeing them grow and learn is among the most fulfilling things we do. It even gives us a chance to glimpse into the past and see day to day the plethora of experiences, trials and errors, and bits of learning that gradually transform us from infants to adults.

We call these precious years, undoubtedly. But we, and Clem's mom in the story above, would never call them easy. A morning where everything seems to go awry, where our child seems to *always* be in the wrong place, at the wrong time, doing the wrong thing. Clem's story from this one morning is not particularly unusual. But what about yesterday, or tomorrow, or later that afternoon? All kids space out, get sidetracked, blow their tops, and run out of time. But some kids do it more than others, and some much more, to the point where it's mornings like the one in the story that are "normal." For those parents who have stories like Clem and her Mom's from time to time, we recommend this book as a way to explore and understand more about executive skills and why they matter in our children's lives and ours.

For those parents who say *I live this story all the time* or *This story is a near daily occurrence* or *This happens so often that it's a real source of stress, not only for me but for my child,* we are here to say that your experience is real, your child's well-being and your relationship with them are clearly very important to you, and we think the concepts and tools in this book can help. The *kinds* of things we are talking about are universal. *How often* it happens is less typical. You are a committed parent raising a bright child endowed with tons of skills. Some focused work in the area of executive skills may help you experience fewer mornings like the one just described and give your child a better chance to use all their traits to their advantage.

What Are Executive Skills?

Executive skills are the cognitive processes that allow us to attend to events in our environment, plan and initiate actions, control our emotions, and manage time. They have been compared to the conductor of an orchestra, an air traffic controller, or a project manager. Simply stated, they are the skills that enable us to regulate our behavior, direct our actions, and achieve our goals. Over the course of their development, they are the skills that empower our children to become independent and self-sufficient adults.

What do executive skills look like? Let's take something as simple as two 8-year-olds who are watching a favorite TV program and decide to get a snack. Both are described as "good kids" by their parents.

Child A
- Decides on popcorn and apple juice
- Waits for a commercial, goes to the kitchen, discovers there is no popcorn
- Scans the other snacks and quickly chooses Goldfish
- Gets the juice out, pours a glass, puts juice away
- Puts some Goldfish in a bowl, puts the Goldfish back, and returns to TV room
- Finishes the show and takes her bowl and glass to the sink
- Goes out to play

Child B
- Decides on popcorn and apple juice
- Doesn't want to leave show; asks mother to get snack, but mother is busy
- Stands in the middle of the living room waiting for a commercial, goes to the kitchen, discovers there is no popcorn
- Complains loudly to mother that her brother ate all the popcorn
- Scans snacks but can't decide what to have; finally settles on Goldfish
- In a hurry now, gets juice out, spills some on counter while pouring, leaves juice out
- Takes the bag of Goldfish to the TV room
- Finishes the show, leaves glass and Goldfish in TV room, and goes out to play
- Mother, surveying kitchen and TV room, calls child back to house to clean up
- Child complains that mother ruined her playtime

In this example two children with the same intention produce quite different outcomes, for themselves and their parents. In so doing, they give us a window into their different executive skills.

As parents we have a central goal for our children: that they grow up to be independent, self-sufficient members of a community with satisfying interpersonal relationships and work. Executive skills are fundamental to that goal since they underlie the decisions and behaviors our children engage in.

Our Model

In the mid- to late 1980s clinicians and researchers recognized that the frontal lobes of the brain, particularly the prefrontal cortex, were *especially* susceptible to damage from traumatic brain injury. Those injuries caused deficits in sustained attention, response inhibition, working memory, emotional control, and self-awareness among others. This group of skills became known as *executive functions* because they play a major role in a person's ability to successfully execute or manage their behaviors. Our initial work in executive skills dates to this time period. We worked with many children and adults who had sustained a traumatic brain injury, and as part of that process we evaluated their cognitive and behavioral difficulties. In time we learned that executive skills deficits were a common denominator in many of the challenges they faced as a result of a brain injury. We also noted less severe but similar types of problems in children with significant attention disorders. This connection was the beginning of our investigation into the development of executive skills across a range of children and adults, and we realized they are essential skills for all of us. While there are other systems of executive skills (the Resources include references for these systems), our model is designed specifically to help parents and educators develop strategies that promote the development of executive skills.

We base our model on two premises:

1. *Most individuals have an array of executive skill strengths as well as executive skill challenges.* There also appear to be common, predictable patterns of strengths and challenges. Our goal is a model that enables people to identify those patterns, so that kids could be encouraged to draw on their strengths and work to enhance or accommodate their challenges to improve overall functioning. It also makes sense for parents to identify their *own* strengths and challenges; parents with a good understanding of their own skill profile provide more empathic and effective support to their children.

2. *Identifying areas of challenge enables us to design and implement interventions to address those areas.* We want to help children build the skills they need or manipulate the environment to mitigate the problems associated with the skill challenges. The more discrete the skills are, the easier it is to develop specific definitions of them. When the skills can be operationalized, clearly described, it's easier to create interventions to improve those operations. For example, let's take the term *scattered*. It's great for a book title because, as a parent, you read the word and know immediately that it describes your child. But *scattered* could mean forgetful or disorganized, lacking persistence, or distracted. Each one of those problems suggests a different solution. The more specific we can be in our problem definition, the more likely we are to come up with a strategy that solves the problem.

Our scheme consists of 11 skills:

- Response inhibition
- Working memory
- Emotional control
- Flexibility
- Sustained attention
- Task initiation
- Planning/prioritizing
- Organization
- Time management
- Goal-directed persistence
- Metacognition

We can group or order executive skills chronologically, by the order in which they develop. Knowing the order in which the skills emerge during infancy, toddlerhood, and beyond gives us a general understanding of what to expect from a child (or what *not* to expect) at a particular age, and therefore what kinds of *experiences* are most suited to help to grow these skills. We don't *expect* an 18-month-old to have the same emotional control as a 5-year-old, so it makes sense that the situations we use to help them practice this skill will also be different. The table on pages 14–15 lists the skills in order of emergence, defines each skill, and provides examples of what the skill looks like in younger and older children.

The Development of Executive Skills in the Brain: Biology and Experience

As is the case with many of the child's abilities, there are two main contributors to the development of executive skills—biology and experience. In terms of the biological or neurological contribution, the *potential* for executive skills is already a part of the brain's wiring at birth, similar to its potential for language. Of course at birth, executive skills, like language, exist only as potential; no baby is born with a mental library of words sourced from their genes, just as no baby is born with "preloaded" executive skills. The child's brain has within it the basic neurological equipment for these skills to develop. Every ball—a tennis ball, soccer ball, ball of yarn—has "hardwired" physical properties that will affect how it rolls, bounces, or holds its shape. At the same time, whether it actually *does* any of these things depends greatly on how it is hit or kicked or bowled. Just as a ball will "change" its path as a result of outside forces, a child's brain, including executive skills, shapes and refines itself based on what it encounters out in the world.

Genes play a major role, and your genes likely have some impact on your child's skills. If you don't have good organization, time management, attention, or other skills, there's a reasonable chance that your child can also evidence these challenges. However, **heritable does not mean unchangeable**! Your interactions with your child and their experiences that you facilitate can both positively impact executive skills.

Developmental Progression of Executive Skills

Executive skill	Definition	Examples
Response inhibition	The capacity to think before you act—this ability to resist the urge to say or do something allows your child the time to evaluate a situation and how his or her behavior might impact it.	A young child can wait for a short period without being disruptive. An adolescent can accept a referee's call without an argument.
Working memory	The ability to hold information in memory while performing complex tasks. It incorporates the ability to draw on past learning or experience to apply to the situation at hand or to project into the future.	A young child can hold in mind and follow one- or two-step directions. The middle school child can remember the expectations of multiple teachers.
Emotional control	The ability to manage emotions to achieve goals, complete tasks, or control and direct behavior.	A young child with this skill can recover from a disappointment in a short time. A teenager can manage the anxiety of a game or test and still perform.
Flexibility	The ability to revise plans in the face of obstacles, setbacks, new information, or mistakes. It relates to an adaptability to changing conditions.	A young child can adjust to a change in plans without major distress. A teenager can accept an alternative such as a different job when the first choice is not available.
Sustained attention	The capacity to keep paying attention to a situation or task in spite of distractibility, fatigue, or boredom.	Completing a 5-minute chore with occasional supervision is an example of sustained attention in the younger child. A teenager can pay attention to homework, with short breaks, for 1 to 2 hours.
Task initiation	The ability to begin projects without undue procrastination, in an efficient or timely fashion.	A young child is able to start a chore or assignment right after instructions are given. A teenager does not wait until the last minute to begin a project.
Planning/ prioritizing	The ability to create a roadmap to reach a goal or to complete a task. It also involves being able to make decisions about what's important to focus on and what's not important.	A young child, with coaching, can think of options to settle a peer conflict. A teenager can formulate a plan to get a job.

Executive skill	Definition	Examples
Organization	The ability to create and maintain systems to keep track of information or materials.	A young child can, with a reminder, put toys in a designated place. A teenager can organize and locate sports equipment.
Time management	The capacity to estimate how much time one has, how to allocate it, and how to stay within time limits and deadlines. It also involves a sense that time is important.	A young child can complete a short job within a time limit set by an adult. A teenager can establish a schedule to meet task deadlines.
Goal-directed persistence	The capacity to have a goal, follow through to the completion of the goal, and not be put off by or distracted by competing interests.	A first grader can complete a job to get to recess. A teenager can earn and save money over time to buy something of importance.
Metacognition	The ability to stand back and take a bird's-eye view of yourself in a situation, to observe how you problem solve. It also includes self-monitoring and self-evaluative skills (for example, asking yourself, "How am I doing?" or "How did I do?").	A young child can change behavior in response to feedback from an adult. A teenager can monitor and critique her performance and improve it by observing others who are more skilled.

As for other factors, any type of trauma or physical insult to the brain, particularly one involving the frontal lobes, will adversely affect executive skill development, as will exposure to lead, toxic chemicals, and drugs. Adverse environmental factors include poverty; chronic, significant stress; and parental anxiety and depression. Unfortunately, these factors not only affect how well a child's skills can grow, but can also temporarily or permanently suppress a skill (for example, a person experiencing stress will exhibit worse executive skills than they would normally). However, assuming reasonably typical biological equipment and the absence of significant genetic anomalies or environmental traumas, brain development can proceed as it's supposed to.

Neurology: Growth and Development + Experience = Executive Skills

Before we consider the developmental sequence, however, we need to look briefly at the way executive skills relate to the brain and brain development. At birth, the child's brain weighs about 370 grams (13 ounces). By late adolescence this has *tripled* to 1,300–1,400 grams, or about 3 pounds. Several changes in the brain account for this significant growth. Typical brain growth occurs through the generation of nerve cells (neurons) and their supporting cells (neuroglia). These cells are the building blocks of the nervous system. In order for nerve cells to "talk" with each other, they develop branches, called axons and dendrites, which allow them to send and receive signals from other cells.

When we talk about the material that makes up the brain—neurons, dendrites, axons, and so forth—we can think about this in terms of shadings of the brain—that is, gray and white matter. White matter is bundles of axons that connect different brain regions so they can communicate, and it's white due to a process called *myelination*. Myelin is a fatty sheath that forms around the axon and provides insulation that helps to increase speed of transmission of nerve signals. Myelination makes the "conversations" between neurons more efficient. Myelination begins in the earliest stages of development, and in the frontal lobes it continues well into young adulthood. This is one of the key features of frontal lobe development and mirrors the development of executive skills, which extends to nearly the third decade of life.

Gray matter is made up of nerve cells or neurons, dendrites, and the connections between them called *synapses*. Typically, as in a game of telephone, dendrites get a message (in the form of chemicals called *neurotransmitters*) from another neuron and pass it to the body (soma) of their neuron. If the neuron gets the right combination of messages at the same time, it will send out its own message. The neuron starts the message, the axons transmit the message (usually made up of chemicals) across a tiny gap (a synapse) to dendrites of another cell, where the process starts again. Unlike the myelination process that epitomizes white matter, the development of gray matter is a bit more . . . well, gray.

An adult brain has about eighty-six billion neurons, and on average each neuron has 7,000 connections (synapses) with other neurons. Most of the neurons are present at birth; the number of connections (synapses) between cells starts small (about 2,500) and grows. But contrary to what you might expect, in early childhood (2 years), the number of synapses (connections between neurons) is *50 percent greater than* the number in the adult brain! So the number of synapses explodes during the first few years of life, peaks before age 5, and then declines over time (with a couple minor exceptions, discussed below) all the way into adulthood. Why? If some is good, isn't more better?

The answer is that we have evolved to account for the fact that the environment contains many unknowns. Imagine planning out a town but only being able to build roads, without knowing where anything else would go. Building the roads early is easier to do now than later, and if you aren't sure which ones you'll need, then one simple solution is to build a ton of roads. The town becomes populated, and you eventually see that some roads are used constantly, some get traffic here and there, and others are never or rarely used. The empty roads are a problem: they take up space, they cost money to maintain, and they don't really go anywhere. Nobody would be worse off if they weren't around. So what's the solution? Demolish the extra roads of course! Roughly speaking, this is the same process our brains undergo during pruning. We encounter a wide variety of environments and conditions, and adapting to them is an important and very effective skill. Our genes can't predict the future environment and build us accordingly, so instead it is programmed to build a ton of junctions (synapses) and connecting roads (dendrites, axons). The initial increase occurs during a period of rapid learning and experience in early childhood. As the pruning process consolidates these connections (and therefore also our skills), the gray matter (synapses, dendrites) and white matter (axons) that are not needed or used drop away. This consolidation continues until a second period of significant development that begins around age 11 or 12 that also corresponds to a phase of rapid learning and development. After this time, there are no more "blooms" of new synapses, only another 10 to 15 years of gradual pruning (minor fluctuations occur over the course of everyone's life; this particular, universal process will end for most people in their mid- to late twenties). The diagram below shows the human brain with the approximate location of major functions, including executive skills, in the prefrontal cortex.

Research indicates that this growth spurt in the brain during early childhood and again prior to adolescence occurs primarily in the frontal lobes and particularly in the prefrontal cortex. Thus, it is as if the brain is preparing itself both for the development of executive skills and for the significant demands that will be made on executive skills during adolescence. We don't mean to oversimplify. The brain is a very complex organ, and evidence from brain-imaging studies continues to suggest that areas other than the prefrontal cortex are involved in the development of executive skills. But the prefrontal systems are among the last areas of the brain to develop fully, in young adulthood, and are the final, common pathway for managing information and deciding how we will

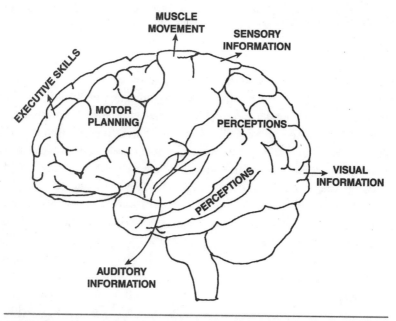

The human brain, with the approximate location of major functions.

behave. When you consider the critical functions of the frontal lobes, it's easy to see how important these brain structures must be to the development of executive skills.

Neuroscientists at the National Institute of Mental Health have suggested that a "use it or lose it" process may be occurring in the frontal lobes during this time. Connections that are used (the "busy roads") are retained, while those that are not exercised are pruned. If this is the case, then practicing using these skills is important not only for learning self-management, but also for the development of brain structures and pathways that will support these skills into later adolescence and adulthood. During this period, parents and teachers can play a critical role in the learning and development of executive skills.

To summarize, we are not born with executive skills that are developed or available for immediate use. In the period immediately following birth, while the basic elements of the neurological substrate that will support these skills is available, they will only become behaviorally evident as the infant develops and interacts with her environment. Executive skills and language share this circumstance. Assembled, but not yet programmed (that is, adaptable), at birth, they need input from the outside world to develop their unique characteristics and patterns.

As the skeletal structure of skills emerge, they're influenced by the genes that we inherit and the biological and social environments in which we live. Barring the unexpected, executive skills will begin to develop and present themselves in the infants' behaviors soon after birth in a slow developmental process that extends into adulthood.

Sequence of Executive Skill Development

Early infancy is a time of great learning, adjustment, and effort for parents, but in the context of executive skills it is paradoxically the least complicated. At birth, children are completely reliant on us for their care and safety. In fact, at the beginning, we *are* their executive skills. *Frontal lobe surrogacy* is a term we often use to describe all the ways in which parents donate, lend, and deploy their own executive skills on behalf of their children. There are no debates, no gray areas, no ambiguity about *whose* skills to rely on because newborns are totally dependent; their needs are big in quantity but small in scope. Parents have *all* the responsibility, but it is limited to the constant provision of a few basic needs. In "exchange" parents are also free to make every decision and take complete control over both the environment and how the newborn interacts with it. We design and organize their environment, establish feeding and sleep schedules, and initiate when and how we interact with them. Newborns have very few behaviors beyond crying and sleeping with which to manage their world. When they cry, we attend to and respond to their distress and do our best to determine the cause and remedy it. They live completely in the present and in the first few months respond only to what they can see, hear, touch, or taste, right now, in this place right here. Within a few months, however, infants become more active, evidencing social smiles, turning their head to voice or sound, making eye contact, cooing, and grasping at objects. From here, development of executive skills begins to accelerate.

Research indicates rudimentary executive skills emerge at about 6 months of age. For example, attention and task initiation are evident in the infant's attempt to reach for and grasp an object. Researchers have shown that it's around this time that infants follow an object of interest and can resist looking away from it even when a distraction is presented. Studies also have documented the emergence of visual working memory in infants. This provides infants with the ability to hold, in working memory, objects, people, and locations that they cannot immediately sense.

Sustained attention, response initiation/inhibition, and working memory provide the infant with the early capacity to direct their own behavior. Emotional expression, emerging at about 6–8 months, adds another significant component to this capacity for self-direction. While smiles come first and represent an expression of pleasure or happiness, negative emotions (such as fear) also start to appear.

The 8-month-old infant can now direct her behavior toward or away from objects, people, and locations in her environment. The development of emotional responses underlies the eventual development of emotional control. This quartet of fledgling skills, plus physical developments like crawling and then walking, form the basis of approach-avoidance behavior. The infant increasingly selects the situations in their environment that they choose to move toward or away from. The beginnings of cognitive flexibility and task persistence appear around 12 months and organization at 18–24 months. Emotional control, metacognition, planning, and time management come a little later, ranging from preschool to early elementary school.

Beginning with this period of development, children use their natural curiosity to explore the world, try out their skills, and make decisions based on the results. They are little scientists, gradually building a mental model of the world, making predictions, assessing the results, and making changes. Children want to understand their world and manage their own behavior. Trial and error is a crucial part of this process; our kids want to test their skills and interact with us in a way that they feel our encouragement and support as they explore.

Experience and practice play a key role in the development of these skills, both at a behavioral level and in the underlying brain structures that support these skills. We know from our own experience and from watching our children that practice improves skill learning. Research shows that practice and learning also result in changes to neurons, synapses, and the development of myelin along nerve transmission pathways.

So where does biology leave your child? We know that executive skills are critical to independent living, which is among the most fundamental and important goals of parenting. As we have said, at birth executive skills exist only as potential; the newborn has no actual executive skills. The frontal lobes and associated areas, and therefore executive skills, will require approximately 25 years to develop. Given these factors, children cannot rely solely on their own frontal brain systems to regulate behavior.

What's the solution? We *lend* them our frontal lobes while theirs are getting up to speed. This is where you—and your child's teachers—come in. Clearly childhood offers parents and teachers a critical opportunity to enhance the learning and development of executive skills in a child.

Experience: Lending Your Child Your Frontal Lobes

As we have said, in early infancy you simply *are* you infant's frontal lobes, with control of the environment and decision making completely in your hands. But within 6 months or so, when she can begin to remember people, events, or objects, even for short periods of time, your baby's world gets bigger, and she can have it with her whenever she's awake. This is the emergence of working memory. Over the next few months, her mobility and natural curiosity will combine with working memory to drive exploration. This is the beginning of our opportunity, as parents, to provide the experiences and interactions that will encourage the development of this skill and build a foundation for independence and decision making. Think about this, for example. If Dad or Mom leaves and does not come back immediately, the baby can look to the last place she saw them and cry. Dad or Mom might return. If this happens, the baby "understands" (remembers) at some level that "if Dad or Mom leaves and I want them back, they'll come if I cry." Or we repeatedly play "peek-a-boo" and the infant learns that we'll come back and also develops anticipatory excitement because when exactly we'll come back is a surprise. Each new experience becomes a stored memory that is activated when the situation is repeated. Remember a trip to the zoo or aquarium or supermarket? If the experience was enjoyable, each time the child goes again, he moves with more independence and better anticipation of what will happen. Equally important, this skill begins to transfer and generalize to other, similar situations. It's why, for example, as adults we are able to go to an unfamiliar supermarket and find our way around, albeit not as efficiently as in our neighborhood store.

Working memory allows the child to recall a past event, apply it to a present situation, and predict what might happen. This skill grows as experience grows; the more information we have to draw on, the better inferences we make about what is currently happening and what could come next. For example, suppose your child is now 11 years old. She might say to herself, "Last Saturday after I cleaned my room, Mom let me invite a friend over and took us out for pizza. I'll ask her if we can do that again after I help her with chores today." Or the 17-year-old could say, "If my friend asks me to go to the game tomorrow night, I need to say I can't. The last time I went out before a test I didn't leave enough time to study and got a lousy grade."

Obviously, in the early years you do much of the work. This includes providing the toys, games, activities, and social interactions your child engages with. With mobility and language, she becomes less dependent on you, and you don't have to be so close by. In fact, by incorporating some of your actions and words into working memory, she has begun to internalize some of your executive skills! This process continues throughout childhood, culminating in late adolescence/young adulthood. As development continues, other people—teachers, coaches, peers—will contribute to this repertoire of experiences.

This brings us to a second key skill that begins developing in the infant at a little later time than working memory: response inhibition. The ability to respond or not respond to a person or an event is at the heart of regulating behavior. We are all aware of the trouble our children can and do get into when they act before thinking. And we are impressed by the self-control of the child who can see a tempting object and not immediately touch or take it.

As with working memory, when an infant begins to develop this skill at around 10–12 months, we don't see dramatic, overnight changes. But from 12 months on, a baby's ability to inhibit a response grows significantly. You might see your 10- to 12-month-old crawling or walking toward his mom in the next room. Whereas two or so months earlier he might have been distracted by a toy along the way, now he moves right past the toy on his way to Mom. During the same period, you may notice that your baby can now withhold some kinds of emotional expression and show others depending on the situation. We've probably all had the experience of trying to engage a baby of this age, who then doesn't respond at all or even turns away. Feels like rejection, doesn't it? Even at this young age, a baby is beginning to learn the powerful effect of responding or not responding to a particular person or situation. The 3- or 4-year-old shows this skill by "using his words" instead of hitting a playmate who tries to grab his toy. The 9-year-old is using the same response inhibition skill when he looks before running into the street to get a ball. And the 17-year-old shows response inhibition by staying near the speed limit instead of responding to his friend's suggestion, "Let's see what this thing can do."

We all understand how critical a skill response inhibition is. Its absence can be dangerous and often leads to risky behavior or legal conflicts. For the very young child, risk taking often is inadvertent, driven by curiosity in the absence of experience. The result is their engaging in activities without understanding the potential consequences. Beginning in infancy and through the toddler and preschool years you loaned your child this ability by setting boundaries and limits for them, using gates, doors, and child-proof locks and simply putting a lot of hazardous articles out of reach. You also provided very close supervision. You undoubtedly try words—a sharp *"No!"* or *"Hot!"*—and in a few cases you may have allowed natural consequences to play a part—or you couldn't prevent them from playing a part, such as when your child suddenly reached out unexpectedly and touched something hot or fell off a couch or cushion. As the child develops and learns to negotiate the environment, some risks are diminished, such as the stairs once the child has the ability to navigate them safely. You feel less need to constantly be by their side or have eyes on them. This means there are more opportunities for the child to explore on their own but there also are more opportunities for risk.

If independence and self-management are the goals we have for our child, the key to this is opportunity to explore, test out their skills, make their own decisions and learn from their experience what works and what doesn't. That they share this goal becomes obvious once they can move on their own and even more so when they begin to speak and tell us "No!" or "I do it myself!" From this point forward as our children develop, our role will be to slowly cede control to them, commensurate with the self-control they display. In other words, as their executive skills develop the need for ours will fade. Perhaps you have witnessed this development: in the 3-year-old who tells himself, in a voice that interestingly sounds like your own, not to do something; or in the 8-year-old who manages her own snack and clean-up; or in the 11-year-old who remembers on her own the equipment she needs for soccer. This process continues throughout childhood, culminating in late adolescence/young adulthood. It might be useful to imagine a balance, or a seesaw. At the beginning, parents are on the low side, and the children are up high, the parents have all the control (and responsibility, the *weight*) of the executive skills. Soon, and with growing speed, the child acquires skills, and the adult lets go of the control (and responsibility) of the parts of life relevant to that skill.

Parenting from here on out entails a balancing act between freedom on one hand and supervision on the other. We know that freedom—to be curious, to explore, and to test skills via trial and error—is at the heart of your child's developing executive skills and self-control. And mistakes and risk taking are an essential (and inevitable) part of this process, hence the need for supervision. How much freedom? How much supervision? There is no one-size-fits-all for parents. Fortunately as parents we have our own executive skills as well as a variety of tools at our disposal to help guide the decisions our child makes. We'll describe a few tools here that we will discuss in more detail in later chapters.

Tools

The first is your own behavior, highlighted in the simple phrase *monkey see, monkey do*. The more technical term is *observational learning*. Children want to be like us, so they imitate or *model* our behavior, for better or worse. If we like to cook, they'll want to cook. If we are careful crossing a street, they'll be careful. If we like to read, they will want to read. If we like to swim, they'll want to swim. But that doesn't mean they are limited to our likes. If we're not comfortable swimming but take them to the pool and attend to and encourage them, they will model peers in a swim class. Also, imitation isn't limited to our preferred activities. Children watch how we treat other people, manage feelings, organize our belongings, and solve problems. When we model executive skills in our actions, they are more likely to model these skills.

Modeling sets the stage for the introduction of a second tool important for executive skills and self-regulation, the introduction of routines and schedules. Routines involve planning, organization, time management, task initiation, and goal attainment, among other skills. They are an important source of predictability, comfort, and safety for children. In their absence, children feel anxiety and stress. But let's be clear here. We are not talking about parents creating schedules and activity routines for everything a child does. There is ample evidence that this type of control undermines development of executive skills and self-control because it eliminates exploration and decision making. Typical early routines set by parents involve morning wake-up, meals, and bedtime. We advocate actively involving children as early as possible as participants in these routines (dressing, helping with meal prep, cleanup, and the like) as steps toward independent management and eventually deciding on their own routines.

A third tool is "serve and return," a phrase from Harvard University researchers describing a way to interact with our children that encourages exploration of their choices and interests. Essentially this means attending closely to what our children are doing and actively engaging with them on their terms. With toddlers and young children this might involve repeating their vocalizations or movements, asking them to describe what they are doing or looking at, or taking turns rolling a ball or playing catch with each other. With older children showing interest, reflecting on what they are doing, or asking them to show us how to do some activity all reflect our regard for what they value. By doing this, we learn what they are interested in and how to build on these interests.

Last but not least are boundaries, rules, and limits. For infants and toddlers there are the obvious ones in the form of gates, cabinet and door locks, car seats, and so on. As children get older, limits are set in the context of activities. Let us repeat that risks and mistakes are an essential and inevitable aspect of learning. How do we manage this? One important option is to teach and encourage alternative behaviors (petting the dog instead of pulling its tail, using words instead of grabbing or hitting). By providing error feedback and suggesting (or having the child suggest) alternatives, a child learns that mistakes can be corrected and they are capable of progress. Simply punishing a mistake tells a child what not to do but not what to do instead. Another option is implementing rules and limits. This involves framing things as an incentive rather than a negative consequence (when you finish brushing your teeth, we can read a book). Research indicates that positively framed rules are consistently more effective than those that are negatively framed (if you don't brush your teeth, we won't read a book).

If we are reasonably consistent in the behaviors we model; the routines, rules, and consequences we set; and the interest we show in their interests and activities, our children will gradually internalize them as the inner voice to guide their actions. In so doing, our own role as "surrogate" frontal lobes will gradually decrease.

So Why Does *Your* Child Have Executive Skill Challenges?

While there is no single or simple answer to this question, research, particularly over the past 10–15 years, has helped to clarify the factors that impact executive skills. We've noted that genes play a role in a child's executive skills. As with other skills and characteristics, our children inherit executive skills from the genes we pass on. But, as we have also learned, heritable is not synonymous with unchangeable.

We've also noted that physical trauma such as head injury or through exposure to toxic substances, including lead, heavy metals, drugs, alcohol, and cigarette smoke, also negatively impacts executive skills. Research has also now documented the adverse effects of poverty, chronic stress, and family depression and anxiety on these skills.

What if children haven't experienced some type of physical or environmental trauma? It's important to know that children can and do vary in the development of these and other executive skills without exposure to adverse events. As is the case with almost any set of skills, children (and adults) have strengths and challenges that fall along a continuum. There are certainly children for whom time seems irrelevant. And who among us has not known a little "absent-minded professor" who cannot keep track of her belongings? Patterns of strengths and challenges like these can be perfectly normal developmental variations.

Beyond these factors, another possibility is a diagnosis of attention-deficit/hyperactivity disorder (ADHD). Current estimates put the prevalence of ADHD in the 5–10 percent range. The prototypical "scattered child" is one with this disorder, and there is a consensus among researchers that ADHD is fundamentally a disorder of executive skills. Russell Barkley, for example, sees the disorder as one of reduced ability to self-regulate. While a number of executive skills can be affected, chief among these are response inhibition, sustained attention, working memory, time management, task initiation, and goal-directed persistence. If a child has this cluster of executive skill weaknesses, ADHD should be considered.

Executive skill challenges have also been identified in children with autism spectrum disorder (ASD). The prevalence rate for ASD in the United States is approximately 2 percent. Children with ASD evidence challenges with cognitive flexibility, working memory, and response inhibition.

Regardless of the source, if executive skill struggles are affecting your child's performance in school, at home, socially, athletically, or in any domain where you naturally want to see your child thrive, it is important to address them. Executive skills are increasingly critical for success in our complex world, so if your child resembles Clem from the beginning of this chapter or seems scattered in other ways, it's worth your time—and will ultimately save you time and distress—to do what you can to give your child's executive skills a boost.

2

Identifying Your Child's Executive Skill Strengths and Challenges

In Chapter 1 we gave you definitions for the 11 executive skills that comprise our model, and we provided examples of what each skill looks like in young children and how each skill might display itself in teenagers.

To truly understand how executive skills affect our children, though, we need to be able translate the skills into observable behaviors. See if you can figure out what executive skills are on display in each of the following vignettes.

- Marin encounters frequent homework challenges, particularly with math. She often forgets the instructions and gets angry when her mother suggests a process that doesn't match the one she was taught at school.

- Tayshawn's parents expect him to do chores on the weekend. Cleaning his bedroom is one chore that's always on the list, but there are other chores like sweeping the kitchen floor, changing the kitty litter, raking leaves, or putting laundry away. He has figured out that if he gets through his chores early in the day, he can spend the rest of the day doing all the fun things he's planned for the weekend. He's developed a routine of starting right after breakfast, rewarding himself with small breaks after he's finished each chore, and getting back to work promptly after each break by reminding himself that the sooner he finishes his work, the sooner he gets to play.

- Lydia likes having a clean bedroom and a clear workspace for doing homework. She usually puts away each toy after she finishes playing with it, but if that doesn't happen, she makes sure before she goes to bed each night that everything is in its designated spot in the bedroom. And when she finishes working on a project on her desk, she returns the arts and crafts materials to the bin she set aside for this purpose. She looks at her clear desktop and smiles, knowing that when she decides to do another art project, she has a space to work and can gather her materials quickly.

● Mark has a hard time with mealtimes. He has two older brothers, and everybody at the table has something they want to talk about. When a thought pops into Mark's head, he has to share it right away, otherwise the conversation will move on without him. And ideas pop into his head frequently, so the rest of the family gets mad at him for interrupting them. He gets bored listening to others talk, and he'll remember he was right in the middle of building a cool LEGO construction, so he wanders off to work on that before he's finished eating his vegetables. His mom may say, "Where do you think you're going?" and he calls out over his shoulder, "I just thought of something. I'll be right back."

● Grant wants a new controller for his Xbox—the elite kind that comes with all sorts of features that his standard controller lacks. But it's expensive, and he knows that even if he saved up all his weekly allowance, it would take him a long time to earn enough money. So he goes to his parents with a proposal: "If I do extra chores each week, do you think you could pay me for them?" His parents offer a couple of options, but they're not willing to pay him very much for the added work. Then he remembers that his next-door neighbor is pretty old, and he suspects, based on what his lawn looks like, that keeping up with lawn mowing is hard for him. So he talks with Mr. Riley, explaining that he's trying to save up money for something and asking whether Mr. Riley would be willing to pay him to mow his lawn every week. Mr. Riley likes the idea, but he's worried about Grant's following through. Grant creates a weekly schedule and a work contract, and he tells Mr. Riley that he's willing to keep mowing the lawn even after he's saved up all the money he needs.

Were you able to spot Marin's executive skill challenges? Clearly, working memory is an issue because she can't remember how to do the math homework. The fact that she loses her temper when her mother tries to help her indicates that emotional control—at least in some situations—is hard for her. And finally, the fact that she struggles when her mother tries to show her a different way to do the work suggests that flexibility is an issue.

Tayshawn, on the other hand, is exhibiting a number of executive skill strengths. Task initiation is clearly a strength, and the fact that he's figured out a way to manage his attention (building in breaks at reasonable intervals) suggests he's good at sustained attention. He's also developing good planning and time management skills, by setting up routines to follow that will get him to his end goal (having the rest of the day free). And since he's set a goal for himself, he's beginning to strengthen goal-directed persistence.

What about Lydia? Organization is clearly her strong point. Not only has she set up her bedroom and workspace the way she wants them, but she also recognizes that there's some work involved in maintaining her organizational system. Being good at this skill means not only being able to design effective organizational systems, but being able to maintain them over time. Lydia is clearly able to do that.

You probably figured out that Mark struggles with response inhibition. Not only does he interrupt others frequently during dinner, but if something occurs to him (like getting back to that LEGO project), he runs off to act on that thought without stopping to think about what he was supposed to be doing when the idea came to him. Very often children who struggle with response inhibition also have trouble with emotional control, but this is not true in Mark's case: he doesn't blow up when his mom prompts him to return to the table, but he can't help doing one small thing with his LEGOs before he comes back to finish his dinner.

And now let's look at Grant. He's got some impressive executive skill strengths, the most obvious one being goal-directed persistence. But equally strong is metacognition, which is the executive skill that's integral to problem solving. Grant was able to set a goal, but he was also able to think about the obstacles that might get in the way of his achieving his goal. He had observed his next-door neighbor's lawn and concluded that lawn mowing might be hard for him. So he "connected the dots" (a great metacognitive skill) and figured out how to solve a neighbor's problem while at the same time solving his own problem. In addition to goal-directed persistence and metacognition, though, Grant is pretty good at planning and time management—two additional skills he'll need to achieve his goal (and you can bet he will achieve his goal!).

As you can see with these examples, executive skills play a role in children's behavior every day—and probably all day long. Sit back and watch how your child spends their spare time, navigates social relationships, manages homework or chores, and deals with obstacles or disappointments. Can you identify which executive skills your child is drawing on when successful—and which ones the child is struggling with when they hit roadblocks? By understanding what executive skills your child is strong in, you can find ways to reinforce those strengths ("I love the way you didn't just ask us for money to buy that remote but figured out a way to earn the money to buy it on your own"). And by looking for patterns suggestive of executive skill challenges, you can begin to think about how to intervene to help your child strengthen those skills.

How Can You Tell
Where Your Child's Executive Skills Are?

The place to start with this assessment process is understanding what's developmentally appropriate at any given age. There are a number of ways to assess whether your child's development is on target with respect to executive skills.

Is Your Child Generally Meeting Expectations at School?

First of all, if your child is generally successful in school—earning reasonable grades but also fulfilling the kinds of responsibilities schools demand, such as homework management—chances are their executive skills are progressing nicely. Of course there's a chance that your child does fine in school and not as well at home, and that may be why you're reading this book. This can occur for any number of reasons. Schools have reliable routines and schedules, explicit, regularly reviewed expectations and rules, and peer models for expected behavior. In other words, the school environment serves as a surrogate frontal lobe. Parents play this role also, but home is naturally less structured than school, and schedules and expectations can change often. There may be more stressors at home (for example, siblings who get on each other's nerves), or the expectations for executive functioning may be out of sync with your child's development or skill set (either too high or too low). Your own executive skill weaknesses could even make home a more challenging place for your child—see Chapter 3 on the goodness of fit between parents and children.

To figure out where your child stands, you need to be aware of the kinds of tasks and responsibilities that are typically expected of children at different ages. The table on pages 29–30 lists the kinds of tasks that require executive skills that children at different ages are usually capable of performing, either on their own or with cueing or supervision from an adult.

Observing Your Child in the Context of Friends and Peers

It can be helpful to look at your child's behavior in the presence of same-age friends or peers as one indicator of strengths and challenges. Does she interact easily with peers, take turns, or demand her own way? When something doesn't go her way, does she take it in stride or have a meltdown? Does she seem able to follow the rules of an age-appropriate game or confused about what is expected? Does she think before she acts or engage in impulsive, risk-taking behaviors? Keep in mind, though, that there is a *range* of normal development. Just as we don't expect all children to begin walking at 12 months on the dot or combining words at 18 months, it's normal for children to vary around an average point.

If you feel your child might be delayed in terms of executive skill development, particularly with regard to peers, you may want to have a conversation with your child's classroom teacher. This offers another viewpoint from someone who knows your child and can provide some objective feedback. Teachers also have a built-in norm group to compare your child to—especially when they have several years of experience teaching at the same grade level. You may also find it helpful to talk to your child's pediatrician, especially if you think the executive skill weaknesses may be associated with an attention disorder.

Is There a Discernible Pattern to Your Child's Executive Skill Strengths and Challenges?

While some children's executive skills are delayed across the board, it's common for children (and for adults, as you'll see in the next chapter) to be strong in some skills and struggle in others. We've seen certain skill challenges (and strengths) cluster together in individuals. Frequently, for instance, children who struggle with response inhibition also struggle with weak emotional control. These are children who act and emote before

Developmental Tasks Requiring Executive Skills

Age range	Developmental task
Preschool/ kindergarten	Run simple errands (for example, "Get your shoes from the bedroom")
	Tidy bedroom or playroom with assistance
	Perform simple chores and self-help tasks with reminders (for example, clear dishes from table, brush teeth, get dressed)
	Inhibit behaviors: don't touch a hot stove, run into the street, grab a toy from another child, hit, bite, push, and so on
Grades 1–3	Run errands (two- to three-step directions)
	Tidy bedroom or playroom
	Perform simple chores, self-help tasks; may need reminders (for example, make bed)
	Bring papers to and from school
	Complete homework assignments (20-minute maximum)
	Decide how to spend money (allowance)
	Inhibit behaviors: follow safety rules, don't swear, raise hand before speaking in class, keep hands to self
Grades 4–5	Run errands (may involve time delay or greater distance, such as going to a nearby store or remembering to do something after school)
	Tidy bedroom or playroom (may include vacuuming, dusting, and so on)
	Perform chores that take 15–30 minutes (for example, clean up after dinner, rake leaves)
	Bring books, papers, assignments home and take them back to school
	Keep track of belongings when away from home
	Complete homework assignments (1-hour maximum)
	Plan simple school project such as book reports (select book, read book, write report)
	Keep track of changing daily schedule (for example, different activities after school)
	Save money for desired objects, plan how to earn money
	Inhibit/self-regulate: behave when teacher is out of the classroom; refrain from rude comments, temper tantrums, bad manners

(continued)

Age range	Developmental task
Grades 6–8	Help out with chores around the home, including daily responsibilities and occasional tasks (for example, emptying dishwasher, raking leaves, shoveling snow); tasks may take 60–90 minutes to complete
	Babysit younger siblings or other kids for pay
	Use system for organizing schoolwork, including assignment book, notebooks, and so on
	Follow complex school schedule involving changing teachers and changing schedules
	Plan and carry out long-term projects, including tasks to be accomplished and reasonable timeline to follow; may require planning multiple large projects simultaneously
	Plan time, including after-school activities, homework, family responsibilities; estimate how long it takes to complete individual tasks and adjust schedule to fit
	Inhibit rule breaking in the absence of visible authority

thinking—they're as likely to say something foolish as to fly into a meltdown at the least provocation. Children who are inflexible also tend to struggle with emotional control—a change in plans they weren't expecting leads to a tantrum. Sometimes children struggle in all three executive skills together (response inhibition, emotional control, flexibility); if your child falls into this category, you know how challenging it can be for you to keep your cool when trying to manage the daily trials and tribulations that seem to define your child's life.

Some other combinations we see frequently are these: youngsters with challenges in task initiation also often struggle with sustained attention—not only are they slow to get started on homework or chores, but they also are likely to quit before it's done. These children generally have weak goal-directed persistence. However, we've found that if goal-directed persistence is a relative strength, we can encourage the child to use that skill to override their weaknesses in task initiation and sustained attention. These are the kids we can spur on to get their homework handed in consistently if we tell them that they can earn points for handing in homework on time and, once they have enough points, they can buy that video game they've been hounding us about.

Another common combination is time management and planning/prioritizing. Kids who have these as strengths seldom have difficulty handling long-term projects. If these are challenges, however, they not only don't know where to begin a long-term project; they also don't know *when* to begin it.

Finally, we often see a relationship between working memory and organization. Sometimes kids use a strength in one skill to offset a challenge in another (it doesn't matter how messy your bedroom is if you can remember exactly where you put your shin guards)—unfortunately, some children who struggle with working memory also struggle with organizational skills. These are the kids for whom parents need to build in extra time to get ready for soccer games—you'll need it to search through the mess to find the sports equipment!

Jess is 13. They've always been a conscientious student—they keep their notebooks organized, write down all their assignments, start their homework when they get home from school and keep at it until it's done. When given a long-term project, Jess gets nervous if they don't at least start it the day it's assigned. While this all sounds good, managing their nerves is challenging. If they misplace a study guide or forget to bring home a book they need to study for a test the next day, they're likely to have a meltdown. And they just hate creative writing assignments: they can never think of anything to write about, and when they finally get an idea, they still can't think of what to say beyond the obvious. They ask Mom to help and then are likely to bite her head off if they don't like her ideas or if she attempts to get them to do more thinking on their own.

Jess's 11-year-old brother, Jason, has a whole different way of operating. He views homework as a burden to be put off as long as possible and completed as quickly as possible. His backpack is a mess because he just throws in papers and books at the end of the day, thinking he'll sort things out at a later time (that never seems to come). His mother is constantly on his case in the morning about getting ready for school on time and at night about his homework. While the drudgery of daily math and spelling homework drives him nuts, he loves the freedom that more open-ended assignments give him. He has a lively imagination and can talk for hours about how fantasy fiction differs from science fiction. Science projects that require him to figure out how to make something work or work better are so much fun he doesn't even think of them as homework. He can't understand why his brother gets so worked up over things. Jess, on the other hand, hates the way Jason keeps their dad waiting every morning as he ambles through his morning routine, oblivious to the fact that they risk being late for school.

Jess's best developed executive skills—task initiation, sustained attention, and time management—seem to be their brother's most challenging skills. On the other hand, Jason's strengths—flexibility, metacognition, and emotional control—are in short supply for Jess. When planning ways to help children, it's helpful to understand how executive skills often form a cluster of strengths and challenges. Strategies to address one struggle often help bolster another. If we can help Jess handle difficult situations more flexibly, we may end up helping them manage their emotions more effectively as well. And if we can improve Jason's ability to begin tedious tasks without undue procrastination, we may find he has more time—or more energy—to finish them.

Using Rating Scales to Find Your Child's Strengths and Challenges

By now you may be familiar enough with the individual executive skills to describe your own child's strengths and challenges pretty accurately. You can confirm your assessment by completing one of the rating scales on your child (see pages 33–40). Because well-developed executive skills look different at different ages, we've created four question-naires, representing four age groups (preschool, lower elementary, upper elementary, and middle school). Select the scale that fits your child.

While some of the items on these scales are quite explicit (for example, "Can complete a chore that takes 15–20 minutes"), others will require some judgment on your part (for example, "Adjusts easily to unplanned-for situations"). When you're not sure how to rate an item, think about other children the same age as your child, or think about what an older sibling was like at the same age.

Capitalizing on Strengths

How can you use this information to help your child? Look at your child's executive skill strengths. These should be skills that you can take advantage of to help the child function effectively in daily activities. We gave you an example earlier of using goal-directed persistence to override problems with task initiation and sustained attention. Another example would be using your child's metacognitive strengths to help them solve problems that arise from challenges in other executive skills ("Andre, I know you're good at solving problems. What's something we could do to help you keep track of your sports equipment, so you don't have to run around like a madman before every game?"). You can also build on your child's executive skill strengths by communicating that they are particularly good at this skill and reinforcing them for using it effectively. For instance, if your daughter is pretty good at task initiation, she can become even better if she is praised for using this skill. "I like the way you get started on homework before dinner," you might tell her, or "I like it that I don't have to tell you more than once when it's time to feed your rabbits."

Perhaps your child's strongest skills are still not particularly effective (an average score of 9 or less would suggest this is the case). Nonetheless, you can build on this skill by noting those times when your child does manage to use the skill effectively and praise him for doing so. If response inhibition falls a little short, then praising your son for "holding his fire" when his younger brother messed up his LEGO creation may help him improve this skill.

Praising children for using executive skills need not be reserved for the areas of comparative strength. *Any time* you see your child making good use of any skill, the effective use of praise can help build that skill. This may be the most underused strategy that parents and teachers have to help children build skills and appropriate behavior. We will discuss this in greater detail in Chapter 7.

Addressing Challenges

Now look at your child's executive skill challenges. Chances are, when you think about the kinds of things your children do that get them in trouble or get you particularly annoyed, they align with or more of their executive skill challenges. Maybe it drives you

Executive Skills Questionnaire for Children
Preschool/Kindergarten Version

Read each item below and then rate that item based on how well it describes your child. Then add the three scores in each section. Find the three highest and three lowest scores.

Strongly agree	Agree	Neutral	Disagree	Strongly disagree
5	4	3	2	1

Score

1. Acts appropriately in some situations where danger is obvious (e.g., avoiding hot stove). ☐
2. Can share toys without grabbing. ☐
3. Can wait for a short period of time when instructed by an adult. ☐

Total score: _____

4. Runs simple errands (e.g., gets shoes from bedroom when asked). ☐
5. Remembers instructions just given. ☐
6. Follows two steps of a routine with only one prompt per step. ☐

Total score: _____

7. Can recover fairly quickly from a disappointment or change in plans. ☐
8. Is able to use nonphysical solutions when another child takes toy away. ☐
9. Can play in a group without becoming overly excited. ☐

Total score: _____

10. Is able to adjust to change in plans or routines (may need warning). ☐
11. Recovers quickly when something doesn't go as expected. ☐
12. Is willing to share toys with others. ☐

Total score: _____

13. Can complete a 5-minute chore (may need supervision). ☐
14. Can sit through preschool "circle time" (15–20 minutes). ☐
15. Can listen to one to two stories at a sitting. ☐

Total score: _____

16. Will follow an adult directive right after it is given. ☐
17. Will stop playing to follow an adult instruction when directed. ☐
18. Is able to start getting ready for bed at set time with one reminder. ☐

Total score: _____

(continued)

From *Smart but Scattered, Second Edition*, by Peg Dawson, Richard Guare, and Colin Guare. Copyright © 2025 The Guilford Press. Permission to photocopy this material, or to download enlarged printable versions (*www.guilford.com/dawson4-forms*), is granted to purchasers of this book for personal use; see copyright page for details.

Score

19. Can finish one task or activity before beginning another. ☐
20. Is able to follow a brief routine or plan developed by someone else (with model or demo). ☐
21. Can complete a simple art project with more than one step. ☐

Total score: _____

22. Hangs up coat in appropriate place (may need one reminder). ☐
23. Puts toys in proper locations (with reminders). ☐
24. Clears off place setting after eating (may need one reminder). ☐

Total score: _____

25. Can complete daily routines without dawdling (with some cues/reminders). ☐
26. Can speed up and finish something more quickly when given a reason to do so. ☐
27. Can finish a small chore within time limits (e.g., make bed before turning on TV). ☐

Total score: _____

28. Will direct other children in play or pretend play activities. ☐
29. Will seek assistance in conflict resolution for a desired item. ☐
30. Will try more than one solution to get to a simple goal. ☐

Total score: _____

31. Can make minor adjustment in construction project or puzzle when first attempt fails. ☐
32. Can find novel (but simple) use of a tool to solve a problem. ☐
33. Makes suggestions to another child for how to fix something. ☐

Total score: _____

KEY					
Items	**Executive skill**	**Items**	**Executive skill**	**Items**	**Executive skill**
1–3	Response inhibition	13–15	Sustained attention	25–27	Time management
4–6	Working memory	16–18	Task initiation	28–30	Goal-directed persistence
7–9	Emotional control	19–21	Planning/prioritizing	31–33	Metacognition
10–12	Flexibility	22–24	Organization		

Your child's executive skill strengths (highest scores)

_____

_____

_____

Your child's executive skill weaknesses (lowest scores)

_____

_____

_____

Executive Skills Questionnaire for Children
Lower Elementary Version (Grades 1–3)

Read each item below and then rate that item based on how well it describes your child. Then add the three scores in each section. Find the three highest and three lowest scores.

Strongly agree	Agree	Neutral	Disagree	Strongly disagree
5	4	3	2	1

Score

1. Can follow simple classroom rules. ☐
2. Can be in close proximity to another child without need for physical contact ☐
3. Can wait until parent gets off phone before telling him/her something (may need one reminder). ☐

Total score: _____

4. Is able to run errands with two to three steps. ☐
5. Remembers instructions given a couple of minutes earlier. ☐
6. Follows two steps of a routine with one prompt. ☐

Total score: _____

7. Can tolerate criticism from an adult. ☐
8. Can deal with perceived "unfairness" without undue upset. ☐
9. Is able to adjust behavior quickly in new situation (e.g., calming down after recess). ☐

Total score: _____

10. Plays well with others (doesn't need to be in charge, can share, etc.). ☐
11. Tolerates redirection by teacher when not following instructions. ☐
12. Adjusts easily to unplanned-for situations (e.g., substitute teacher). ☐

Total score: _____

13. Can spend 20–30 minutes on homework assignments. ☐
14. Can complete a chore that takes 15–20 minutes. ☐
15. Can sit through a meal of normal duration. ☐

Total score: _____

16. Can remember and follow simple one- to two-step routines (such as brushing teeth and combing hair after breakfast). ☐
17. Can get right to work on classroom assignment following teacher instruction to begin. ☐
18. Will start homework at established time (with one reminder). ☐

Total score: _____

(continued)

From *Smart but Scattered, Second Edition*, by Peg Dawson, Richard Guare, and Colin Guare. Copyright © 2025 The Guilford Press. Permission to photocopy this material, or to download enlarged printable versions (*www.guilford.com/dawson4-forms*), is granted to purchasers of this book for personal use; see copyright page for details.

Score

19. Can carry out a two- to three-step project of own design (e.g., arts and crafts, construction). □

20. Can figure out how to earn/save money for an inexpensive toy. □

21. Can carry out two- to three-step homework assignment with support (e.g., book report). □

Total score: _____

22. Puts coat, winter gear, sports equipment in proper locations (may need reminder). □

23. Has specific places in bedroom for belongings. □

24. Doesn't lose permission slips, notices from school. □

Total score: _____

25. Can complete a short task within time limits set by an adult. □

26. Can build in appropriate amount of time to complete a chore before a deadline (may need assistance). □

27. Can complete a morning routine within time limits (may need practice). □

Total score: _____

28. Will stick with challenging task to achieve desired goal (e.g., building difficult LEGO construct). □

29. Will come back to a task later if interrupted. □

30. Will work on a desired project for several hours or over several days. □

Total score: _____

31. Can adjust behavior in response to feedback from parent or teacher. □

32. Can watch what happens to others and change behavior accordingly. □

33. Can verbalize more than one solution to a problem and make the best choice. □

Total score: _____

KEY					
Items	**Executive skill**	**Items**	**Executive skill**	**Items**	**Executive skill**
1–3	Response inhibition	13–15	Sustained attention	25–27	Time management
4–6	Working memory	16–18	Task initiation	28–30	Goal-directed persistence
7–9	Emotional control	19–21	Planning/prioritizing	31–33	Metacognition
10–12	Flexibility	22–24	Organization		

Your child's executive skill strengths
(highest scores)

Your child's executive skill weaknesses
(lowest scores)

_____   _____

_____   _____

_____   _____

Executive Skills Questionnaire for Children
Upper Elementary Version (Grades 4–5)

Read each item below and then rate that item based on how well it describes your child. Then add the three scores in each section. Find the three highest and three lowest scores.

Strongly agree	Agree	Neutral	Disagree	Strongly disagree
5	4	3	2	1

Score

1. Handles conflict with peers without getting into physical fight (may lose temper). ☐
2. Follows home or school rules in the absence of an adult's immediate presence. ☐
3. Can calm down or de-escalate quickly from an emotionally charged situation when prompted by an adult. ☐

Total score: _____

4. Remembers to follow a routine chore after school without reminders. ☐
5. Brings books, papers, assignments to and from school. ☐
6. Keeps track of changing daily schedule (e.g., different activities after school). ☐

Total score: _____

7. Doesn't overreact to losing a game or not being selected for an award. ☐
8. Can accept not getting what he/she wants when working/playing in a group. ☐
9. Acts with restraint in response to teasing. ☐

Total score: _____

10. Doesn't "get stuck" on things (e.g., disappointments, slights). ☐
11. Can "shift gears" when plans have to change due to unforeseen circumstances. ☐
12. Can do "open-ended" homework assignments (may need assistance). ☐

Total score: _____

13. Can spend 30–60 minutes on homework assignments. ☐
14. Can complete a chore that takes 30–60 minutes (may need a break). ☐
15. Is able to attend sports practice, church service, etc., for 60–90 minutes. ☐

Total score: _____

16. Is able to follow a three- to four-step routine that has been practiced. ☐
17. Can complete three to four classroom assignments in a row. ☐
18. Can follow established homework schedule (may need reminder to get started). ☐

Total score: _____

(continued)

From *Smart but Scattered, Second Edition,* by Peg Dawson, Richard Guare, and Colin Guare. Copyright © 2025 The Guilford Press. Permission to photocopy this material, or to download enlarged printable versions (*www.guilford.com/dawson4-forms*), is granted to purchasers of this book for personal use; see copyright page for details.

Score

19. Can make plans to do something special with a friend (e.g., go to movies). ☐
20. Can figure out how to earn/save money for a more expensive purchase. ☐
21. Can carry out long-term projects for school, with most steps broken down by someone else. ☐

Total score: _____

22. Can put belongings in appropriate places in bedroom or other locations in house. ☐
23. Brings in toys from outdoors after use or at end of day (may need reminder). ☐
24. Keeps track of homework materials and assignments. ☐

Total score: _____

25. Can complete daily routines within reasonable time limits without assistance. ☐
26. Can adjust homework schedule to allow for other activities (e.g., starting early if there's an evening Scout meeting). ☐
27. Is able to start long-term projects enough in advance to reduce time crunch (may need help with this). ☐

Total score: _____

28. Can save allowance for 3–4 weeks to make a desired purchase. ☐
29. Is able to follow a practice schedule to get better at a desired skill (sport, instrument); may need reminders. ☐
30. Can maintain a hobby over several months. ☐

Total score: _____

31. Is able to anticipate in advance the result of a course of action and make adjustments accordingly (e.g., to avoid getting in trouble). ☐
32. Can articulate several solutions to problems and explain the best one. ☐
33. Enjoys the problem-solving component of school assignments or video games. ☐

Total score: _____

KEY					
Items	Executive skill	Items	Executive skill	Items	Executive skill
1–3	Response inhibition	13–15	Sustained attention	25–27	Time management
4–6	Working memory	16–18	Task initiation	28–30	Goal-directed persistence
7–9	Emotional control	19–21	Planning/prioritizing	31–33	Metacognition
10–12	Flexibility	22–24	Organization		

Your child's executive skill strengths (highest scores)

_____
_____
_____

Your child's executive skill weaknesses (lowest scores)

_____
_____
_____

Executive Skills Questionnaire for Children
Middle School Version (Grades 6–8)

Read each item below and then rate that item based on how well it describes your child. Then add the three scores in each section. Find the three highest and three lowest scores.

Strongly agree	Agree	Neutral	Disagree	Strongly disagree
5	4	3	2	1

Score

1. Is able to walk away from confrontation or provocation by a peer.
2. Can say no to a fun activity if other plans have already been made.
3. Resists saying hurtful things when with a group of friends.

Total score: _____

4. Able to keep track of assignments and classroom rules of multiple teachers.
5. Remembers events or responsibilities that deviate from the norm (e.g., special instructions for field trips, extracurricular activities).
6. Remembers multistep directions, given sufficient time and practice

Total score: _____

7. Is able to "read" reactions from friends and adjust behavior accordingly.
8. Can accept not getting what he/she wants when working/playing in a group.
9. Can be appropriately assertive (e.g., asking teacher for help, inviting someone to dance at a school dance).

Total score: _____

10. Is able to adjust to different teachers, classroom rules, and routines.
11. Is willing to adjust in a group situation when a peer is behaving inflexibly.
12. Is willing to adjust to or accept a younger sibling's agenda (e.g., allowing someone else to select a family movie).

Total score: _____

13. Can spend 60–90 minutes on homework (may need one or more breaks).
14. Can tolerate family gatherings without complaining of boredom or getting in trouble.
15. Can complete chores that take up to 2 hours (may need breaks).

Total score: _____

16. Can make and follow nightly homework schedule without undue procrastination.
17. Can start chores at agreed-upon time (e.g., right after school; may need written reminder).
18. Can set aside fun activity when he/she remembers a promised obligation.

Total score: _____

(continued)

From *Smart but Scattered, Second Edition,* by Peg Dawson, Richard Guare, and Colin Guare. Copyright © 2025 The Guilford Press. Permission to photocopy this material, or to download enlarged printable versions (*www.guilford.com/dawson4-forms*), is granted to purchasers of this book for personal use; see copyright page for details.

Score

19. Can do research on the Internet either for school or to learn something of interest. ☐
20. Can make plans for extracurricular activities or summertime activities. ☐
21. Can carry out a long-term project for school with little or no support from adults. ☐

Total score: _____

22. Can maintain notebooks as required for school. ☐
23. Doesn't lose sports equipment/personal electronics. ☐
24. Keeps study area at home reasonably tidy. ☐

Total score: _____

25. Can usually finish homework before bedtime. ☐
26. Can make good decisions about priorities when time is limited (e.g., coming home from school to finish project rather than playing with friends). ☐
27. Can spread out a long-term project over several days. ☐

Total score: _____

28. Is able to increase effort to improve performance (e.g., change study strategies to earn a higher grade on a test or bring up report card grades). ☐
29. Willing to engage in effortful tasks to earn money. ☐
30. Willing to practice without reminders to improve a skill. ☐

Total score: _____

31. Can accurately evaluate own performance (e.g., in sports event or school performance). ☐
32. Is able to see impact of behavior on peers and make adjustments (e.g., to fit in with a group or avoid being teased). ☐
33. Can perform tasks requiring more abstract reasoning. ☐

Total score: _____

KEY

Items	Executive skill	Items	Executive skill	Items	Executive skill
1–3	Response inhibition	13–15	Sustained attention	25–27	Time management
4–6	Working memory	16–18	Task initiation	28–30	Goal-directed persistence
7–9	Emotional control	19–21	Planning/prioritizing	31–33	Metacognition
10–12	Flexibility	22–24	Organization		

Your child's executive skill strengths
(highest scores)

_____

_____

_____

Your child's executive skill weaknesses
(lowest scores)

_____

_____

_____

nuts that your son consistently forgets to bring home the books he needs for homework or leaves expensive sports equipment on the playing field or at his friend's house. It's likely that working memory is one of his areas of challenge. If your daughter's messy bedroom is a bone of contention between you, and if it seems like she's always frantically looking through her backpack for missing papers or study guides, then organization is likely a significant challenge for her.

So what do you do about these areas of challenge? Part III of the book will take up each executive skill in turn and outline intervention strategies that can either minimize the negative impact of the challenge or help children improve their ability to use the skill. You may be tempted to jump ahead and read the chapters that address your child's struggles—especially if you have problems with response inhibition yourself, something we'll help you discover in the next chapter. However, we encourage you to read through (or at least scan!) all the chapters in this book in order before getting down to work because we lay a foundation that we think will help you identify the most effective interventions given your child's developmental level and the nature of his or her difficulties. Before you get to Part III, we have a little more information to offer on what you're dealing with and then, in Part II, some important general advice.

3

How Your Own Executive Skill Strengths and Challenges Matter

It's 8:30 in the morning, and Donna's 14-year-old son, Jim, left for school over an hour ago. Now it's time for Donna to get to work, but when she checks to make sure her cell phone is in her purse, she finds it's missing. She remembers that Jim borrowed it yesterday when he was at a baseball game with a friend and used it to call her for a ride home. Would he have put it in his sports bag, his jacket, or his jeans after he called her? This is why she finds herself in his bedroom rummaging through the rubble for any sign of her phone. Usually she just closes the door to his room, so she doesn't have to look at the mess. This is her latest strategy for coping with this problem that has caused tension in their relationship for years. Donna, according to her son, is a "neat freak"—someone who won't leave a single dirty dish in the sink, who hates it when her kids leave the top off the toothpaste tube, and who stacks magazines neatly on the coffee table in the living room, carefully recycling any issues more than a month old. Jim, in his mother's words, is a "total slob"—it would never occur to him to throw out old candy wrappers, let alone keep important things like cell phones in a consistent place. Chances are he knows exactly where it is, but she has no way of contacting him. With a cursory glance at the mess in his bedroom, Donna gives up. She hopes there's no emergency when she's on the road at work for which she'll regret not having her phone.

Ten-year-old Mindy's dance practice ended 25 minutes ago, and all the rest of the students have been picked up by their parents and are on their way home, while her father is nowhere to be seen. Mindy paces back and forth in the hall outside the classroom, looking out the window and stopping to check each time a car enters the busy community center parking lot, hoping it's her father. Her fists are clenched, and her face looks like a storm cloud. When it's her mother's turn to pick her up, she can count on her being early. She and her mom are time conscious. Mindy gets ready for school with at least 15 minutes to spare before she has to go to the bus stop. She knows exactly how long it will take her to do her homework, and she makes sure she finishes it before dinner every night. Her dad, though, seems to have no notion of time. He's chronically late, always tries to do "just one more thing" before leaving for work in the morning or shutting his office door at night. And if he gets stopped on the way to his car by a colleague with a question after work . . . well, forget it; that's a 10-minute conversation at least, even if he knows he's promised his wife he'll be home at a certain time. Whenever her dad's late, Mindy always starts imagining something bad happening to him. Maybe he got in a car accident on the way over—or maybe he forgot about her and scheduled a late afternoon meeting! When she sees her dad's car pull up right outside the community center, she's out the door before he can open the car door. "Where *were* you?!" she says, an edge of panic in her voice. "Hey," her dad says, stepping out of the car and taking her in his arms. "You knew I wouldn't forget you," he says soothingly. "I just had a phone call that went on longer than I thought it would."

Sound familiar? If your son's or daughter's executive skill challenges drive you crazy, there's a good chance that it's because you're strong in those executive skills. You probably know how this goes just like Donna does: Your son needs to be prodded repeatedly to get ready for school on time; you haven't been late to work in 5 years. Your daughter plunges into histrionics at the slightest change in plans; you like nothing better than to be surprised. Your child never seems to start his homework without being threatened with the loss of every privilege he has or to finish it unless you're standing over him throughout; you always get your chores and errands out of the way first thing, so they're not hanging over your head. Donna can't fathom how her son can stand to be so disorganized. But that's because she doesn't have the strong working memory that Jim relies on and doesn't understand how it can substitute to a great degree for the organizational skills that he lacks. Likewise, if you believe in starting unpleasant tasks right away and seem to know instinctively how to break down a large task into smaller subtasks, it may be doubly irritating to see your son put off long-term projects until the last minute and then not have any idea what to do first.

In our work with children with executive skill problems, we've found that the problems often seem more pronounced when those children have parents with a very different pattern of strengths and challenges. If Donna lacked organizational skills too, she might empathize with her son's deficiencies and more readily share how she has learned to compensate for them. Instead she sometimes feels her son must have come from another planet, and it's hard for her to bridge this gap and help him build the skills he lacks.

Mindy can't imagine why her dad doesn't see the importance of being on time, and she can't easily calm herself when his tardiness upsets her. Because he doesn't think being a little late is a big deal and rarely loses his cool, Mindy's father keeps showing up late to pick her up and keeps marveling at how she "overreacts." The two don't really understand each other, and Mindy's weakness in emotional control isn't addressed—at least not by her father.

When parents have one set of executive skill strengths and challenges and their children have another set, they're missing out on what we call "goodness of fit." Not only is the potential for conflict between parent and child over daily routines increased, but the stage isn't set for helping the child build the deficient skills. As you'll learn in Chapters 4–7, and then once you get into the interventions described in Part III, there are various ways that you can help a child compensate for and even eliminate challenges in executive skills. They all, to some degree, involve interacting differently with your child. Until you understand how your executive skill strengths and challenges dovetail—or don't—with your child's, it may be tough to know where to change your act. When you have a clearer understanding, about the nature of executive skills in general and about your own processing style specifically, you'll find it easier to understand your child and to identify intervention strategies that are a good match for your child's strengths.

Ironically, it's not just having the same strengths that helps you and your child work together toward getting things done effectively and helping the child practice executive skills to further their development. It can also be having the same challenges. But only if you're aware of this fit. If you really don't start from the understanding that you both lack, say, the ability to sustain attention, you can end up terribly frustrated when you try to complete a big chore, like cleaning out the garage, together. A lot of blame can be flung back and forth as you both face the fact that an unpleasant task is being dragged out longer and longer. It's easier to see that your child isn't paying attention than it is to see the same weakness in yourself. This is why it's so important to identify your own executive skill strengths and challenges in this chapter. When you go into projects and routines knowing that you and your child face the same challenges, you can find ways to work through them together with humor and cooperation.

When you discover your own executive skill patterns, you might also find another way that you and your child actually have goodness of fit that you wouldn't expect. You may have a strength that is a natural complement to your child's weakness. Mindy's dad, for example, is highly flexible. Once he recognizes this as a strength, he might be able to strategize how he could show Mindy that flexibility can help her deal with situations where her expectations aren't going to be met. Maybe she can learn that there are options that would prevent her from simply getting upset and out of control. For example, he might explain that he is not as good at keeping track of time as she is and that she should build in an extra 20–30 minutes before she starts worrying about him. Or he might suggest they make a game of estimating how late he will be—she could write down her estimate on a piece of paper, and if it matches the time he arrives, she earns a gold star. Both these ideas have the added benefit of helping Mindy understand that she and her father are different. Life is full of people being late, and if Mindy can learn to accept her father's tardiness—who knows?—it may help her be tolerant of her own partner when she finds herself living with someone just like "dear old Dad."

To help you understand your own executive skill strengths and challenges, take the brief questionnaire on pages 45–46.

Because this is a brief questionnaire and it includes a limited number of items for each executive skill, the results may not capture you perfectly, but they should give you

Executive Skills Questionnaire for Parents

Read each item below and then rate that item based on how well it describes you. Then add the three scores in each section. Find the three highest and three lowest scores.

Strongly disagree	Disagree	Tend to disagree	Neutral	Tend to agree	Agree	Strongly agree
1	2	3	4	5	6	7

Item   **Your score**

1. I don't jump to conclusions. ☐
2. I think before I speak. ☐
3. I don't take action without having all the facts. ☐

Your total score: _____

4. I have a good memory for facts, dates, and details. ☐
5. I am very good at remembering the things I have committed to doing. ☐
6. I seldom need reminders to complete tasks. ☐

Your total score: _____

7. My emotions seldom get in the way when performing on the job. ☐
8. Little things do not affect me emotionally or distract me from the task at hand. ☐
9. I can defer my personal feelings until after a task has been completed. ☐

Your total score: _____

10. I take unexpected events in stride. ☐
11. I easily adjust to changes in plans and priorities. ☐
12. I consider myself to be flexible and adaptive to change. ☐

Your total score: _____

13. I find it easy to stay focused on my work. ☐
14. Once I start an assignment, I work diligently until it's completed. ☐
15. Even when interrupted, I find it easy to get back and complete the job at hand. ☐

Your total score: _____

16. No matter what the task, I believe in getting started as soon as possible. ☐
17. Procrastination is usually not a problem for me. ☐
18. I seldom leave tasks to the last minute. ☐

Your total score: _____

19. When I plan out my day, I identify priorities and stick to them. ☐

(continued)

From *Smart but Scattered, Second Edition*, by Peg Dawson, Richard Guare, and Colin Guare. Copyright © 2025 The Guilford Press. Permission to photocopy this material, or to download enlarged printable versions (*www.guilford.com/dawson4-forms*), is granted to purchasers of this book for personal use; see copyright page for details.

Item	Your score
20. When I have a lot to do, I can easily focus on the most important things.	☐
21. I typically break big tasks down into subtasks and timelines.	☐

Your total score: _____

22. I am an organized person.	☐
23. It is natural for me to keep my work area neat and organized.	☐
24. I am good at maintaining systems for organizing my work.	☐

Your total score: _____

25. At the end of the day, I've usually finished what I set out to do.	☐
26. I am good at estimating how long it takes to do something.	☐
27. I am usually on time for appointments and activities.	☐

Your total score: _____

28. I think of myself as being driven to meet my goals.	☐
29. I easily give up immediate pleasures to work on long-term goals.	☐
30. I believe in setting and achieving high levels of performance.	☐

Your total score: _____

31. I routinely evaluate my performance and devise methods for personal improvement.	☐
32. I am able to step back from a situation in order to make objective decisions.	☐
33. I "read" situations well and can adjust my behavior based on the reactions of others.	☐

Your total score: _____

KEY					
Items	**Executive skill**	**Items**	**Executive skill**	**Items**	**Executive skill**
1–3	Response inhibition	13–15	Sustained attention	25–27	Time management
4–6	Working memory	16–18	Task initiation	28–30	Goal-directed persistence
7–9	Emotional control	19–21	Planning/prioritizing	31–33	Metacognition
10–12	Flexibility	22–24	Organization		

Strongest skills   Weakest skills

_____   _____

_____   _____

_____   _____

an idea of the executive skills that come most easily to you as well as those with which you struggle the most.

If you're not sure about your executive skills profile, go through the strengths and challenges one by one and ask yourself whether you remember having the same strengths and challenges as a child. If so, these are likely true inherent executive skill strengths and challenges. As a child, for instance (this is Peg speaking), I can remember my mother harping on me to clean my room. It wasn't that I didn't like a clean bedroom—it's just that it took *so much effort* to keep my bedroom tidy. Even now, as an adult, I continue to struggle with that. In contrast, I remember always being keenly aware of time—how long it takes to do things, how much time it takes to get someplace—and today I have excellent time management skills. I see the same strengths and challenges in my children—both my adult sons struggle with tidiness, but they're always on time for any appointment. However, they seem to have inherited their ability to manage their emotions from their father, and to this day they tease me when I panic over misplaced car keys or other minor or temporary inconveniences.

Of course you may be reminded by this exercise, as one of our workshop participants is occasionally, that where you once had a weakness, you now have a strength. This may be because a parent helped you learn an executive skill by reinforcing it. Reviewing your childhood memories about executive skill strengths and challenges and comparing your skills to those of your own parents and those of your children will hone your ability to see how parents and children can have similar or different executive skills. This exercise may help you learn more about yourself but also about the fit between you and your child.

In the case of the second pattern—when your challenges coincide with your child's—tensions often arise because your child lacks the capacity to "pick up the slack" or to counteract the negative effect of your own challenges. For instance, if you and

---

Flexibility: The Antidote to a Parent–Child Mismatch

Did your questionnaire scores show a strength in flexibility? If so, you're in luck if you and your child have opposite patterns of executive skills. Flexibility means you're probably pretty adaptable, and that makes you less likely to be irritated or annoyed by your child's executive skill weaknesses, whatever they are.

- Use your awareness of this gift to make a special promise to stay loose in those situations where your child's executive skill weaknesses *do* tend to drive you crazy.

- On the downside, you may find it hard to put in place an intervention to address an area of weakness in your child and stick with it long enough for it to work. But let's stick with the positive for now, OK?

your daughter have weak working memory and lousy organizational skills, then keeping track of things like field trip permission slips, report cards that need signatures, or sports equipment will be very difficult. We might also add that spouses who have different executive skill profiles often run into trouble with each other for the same reasons. In fact, in our clinical practice we often find that when one spouse's executive skill strengths match the challenges of their partner, this often signals tension points in the relationship—which may then become material to address in marriage counseling.

If, as you read this chapter, you decide you'd like to know more about how to manage your own executive skill challenges, you may want to take a look at our book *The Smart but Scattered Guide to Success*. We wrote that after realizing that a lot of the strategies that work with kids can be tweaked to work with adults.

Compensating for a Fit That's Not So Good

So what to do when these patterns emerge? Here are some tips that might make things go a little more smoothly:

When your strengths coincide with your child's challenges:

• *See if you and your child can come to some agreement that your child will accept your help where he's weak and you're strong, so his challenges don't get him in trouble.* For instance, if you're good at time management and your son is not, he may accept your help in estimating how long it will take to finish writing the first draft of his book report and can plan his time accordingly. We hasten to add, however, that some—perhaps many—children will resist this kind of advice or assistance from their parents, particularly as adolescence kicks in and they have no interest in listening to their parents' advice on *any* matter, let alone something where their parents seem to feel their own skills exceed those of their children.

• *Be creative in using your strengths to help your child enhance skills.* If you have good organizational skills, for instance, you are more likely to be able to help your child develop effective organizational systems (described in more detail in Chapter 17) than if this is a weakness for you too. But as we just said, your child may not be that open to this kind of help from you, so you might have to be innovative and subtle about it. Let's say your daughter is highly artistic and visual. You know that having containers that help you organize materials is an easy way to stay on top of regular tasks. Maybe your daughter will be open to using these tools if you take her on a shopping trip to buy bright-colored trays and compartmentalized storage pieces along with stickers and markers for decorating them. As you read earlier, Mindy's dad used his strength in flexibility to come up with a humorous way to help his daughter handle her emotions. A parent who's good at planning might help her child learn how to carry out a complex task by writing down each step on a separate index card, then shuffle the cards and have her child put them in a logical sequence.

• *Make a point of identifying where you are weak and your child is strong.* If you understand that the source of some of your frustration lies in the fact that your skills profile is very different from your child's, you may feel less irritated and frustrated when you see the weakness coming out in your child. But don't stop there; remind yourself—and your child—of where the child has a strength that you lack. This will really keep up morale when you need it most. Perhaps response inhibition is a strength of yours and a weakness of your son's. You may be able to put that in some perspective by acknowledging that flexibility, an equally important executive skill, is a strong suit for your son but not for you: "Remember the last time we went to the movies together and the movie I wanted to see was sold out? I was ready to walk out and go home in a huff, and you just said, 'Hey, maybe there's another movie we can see.' And when it turned out there was nothing we wanted to watch, you were the one who suggested we play a round of miniature golf and get back to the theater really early for the next showing. You bounce back much better than I do!"

When you and your child share the same challenges:

• *Work at it, so you can laugh about shared challenges rather than weep about them.* "Honey, you and I are both organizationally challenged," you might say, "so maybe we can help each other. It may feel like the blind leading the blind, but it's all we've got!"

• *Since neither of you can claim superiority, you may be able to brainstorm solutions to common problems with your child.* Perhaps you notice that you can't have a discussion with your 13-year-old without emotions escalating quickly on both sides. Maybe you can put your heads together to come up with ways you can help each other talk about emotionally charged topics without either of you losing control.

• *Before you throw up your arms in exasperation over something your child does, remind yourself that you grew up with the same challenges and yet somehow made it to adulthood OK.* Tell yourself your child may work out OK too, despite the system's glitch. Perhaps you can think of a story from your own childhood to share with your child. I remember (this is Peg talking) my mother telling me about how her brothers had to drag her back to hear her mother read the end of *Hansel and Gretel,* so she would know it turned out OK in the end. As a child who struggled with emotional control myself, I found it comforting to hear how the same problem affected my mother when she was a girl.

• *Consider taking a more systematic approach to address your weak executive skill at the same time you work on the same skill in your child.* The steps you would take to do this are:

1. Identify your child's weak skills by filling out the appropriate questionnaire in Chapter 2.
2. Identify your own weak skills by completing the questionnaire in this chapter.

Make sure you're honest! It will help to complete the questionnaire with the assistance of your partner or someone else who knows you well.

3. Identify two to three recurring or repeating behaviors that your child shows that are indications of an executive skill weakness that you want to work on that matches your weak area.
4. Do the same for yourself. Identify situations where your weakness in the same executive skill interferes with effective daily functioning.
5. For yourself, identify the one place where this behavior most annoys people and identify a strategy you can use to address the problem in that situation.
6. Talk to your child about his/her specific behaviors and the situations in which they occur. Explain how you have a similar problem and talk about how you intend to work on it.
7. Together, agree on a solution to the child's problem and a cueing strategy to remind your child to use the solution.
8. Watch the behavior and apply the strategy.

We recommend this process for several reasons. First, completing the questionnaires for yourself and your child confirms that there are executive skill challenges you share. Second, identifying situations that cause problems for both of you helps you better understand the skill and how it affects you and your child. This may make it a little easier to empathize with your child when before you may have felt only irritation. Third, designing an intervention strategy for yourself may make it easier to identify potential strategies your child can use.

Let's walk through this process using an example of a parent and child who have weak organizational skills. Lucia sees how this problem in her 13-year-old daughter, Amanda, frequently creates tension in the family. Amanda loses her assignment book and then has no place to keep track of her homework. She leaves homework on her cluttered desk at home because when she's done for the evening, she doesn't put everything back in her backpack to make sure it gets to school in the morning. And she can't find favorite clothes or belongings because of the mess in her bedroom. As to herself, Lucia realizes that at least once or twice a week she sets down her cell phone in a random place that makes it difficult for her to find as well as hard for her to remember that she wants to have it with her when she leaves for work in the morning. She also keeps forgetting to recharge the phone, so even when she has it with her, the battery is often too low to use.

Lucia first decides on a strategy to help her keep track of her cell phone. Her phone allows her to program it with daily reminders, so she sets a reminder that causes the phone to ring shortly after she gets home from work. This reminds her to place the phone on the charging dock. She also sets an alarm for the morning, just before she leaves for work, that reminds her to take the phone with her.

Now she sits down with Amanda to talk about her organizational problems. She describes how she will handle her own organizational problem and asks Amanda to identify one problem situation that she wants to tackle in a similar fashion. Amanda chooses to work first on keeping track of her assignment book. She decides that every morning when she wakes up she'll place a large neon sign on her bed that says, "Is your assignment book in your backpack?" At night she'll see the sign when she turns down the covers to go to bed. At that point she'll carry the sign over to her backpack, make sure the assignment book is in the backpack, and then lay the sign on top of the backpack, so she'll remember to put it back on her bed before leaving for school in the morning.

When Overload Widens the Gap

We all know that when we're under stress, our ability to cope deteriorates. The most obvious example: if you have a "short fuse" (weak emotional control) under the best of circumstances, you know you're likely to erupt more quickly and more intensely on a bad day. A day like this: You were up in the middle of the night tending to your sick pre-schooler, then your second-grade daughter threw a fit right as the school bus was arriving at the door because she lost the toy she'd been planning to take to show-and-tell for a week, and you'd barely finished dealing with that crisis when your spouse announced his car was due for a service appointment and he needed you to drop him off at work on your way to your office. When you got to work, your boss told you that a client would be making an unexpected visit to the office to find out the status of his account and you knew you were behind schedule. If you were able to contain your emotions with your boss, your poor assistant might end up suffering the brunt of your frustrations.

Through years of working with executive skill strengths and challenges, we've found that in situations of stress or overload, your ability to call on your executive skills may decline in general, but those skills that are most susceptible to impairment are those that were weakest to start with. We sometimes call this the "weak organ theory" (in any illness, organs that are weakest to start with are most susceptible to further breakdown). Dick has learned, for instance, to recognize that I'm under particular stress (this is Peg again) when he asks me an innocuous question and I answer him between clenched teeth. Emotional control is not my strong point. And I know when I walk into his office and find his conference table piled high with papers, folders, and books that Dick has probably overcommitted himself and his organizational skills are breaking down still further.

When your weakest executive skills seem to suffer a setback, this is a good clue that your stress level is rising. Knowing this about yourself, you may be able to put systems in place to reduce the stress or to cope with your decline in executive functioning. This could mean asking a spouse, friend, or even your child to help out in ways they might not normally, or it could mean putting goals or projects on hold while you deal with the stressful situation. Postponed projects may very well include the work you're doing with your child to improve his executive skills. Periods when you're coping with an illness in the family, financial setbacks, or marital conflicts may not be the best time to try to teach your child to clean up his bedroom. Behavior change—yours or your child's—is hard work and is most likely to be successful when undertaken in periods of calm.

Even when you're not having to manage major stressors, you should be attuned to daily situations that might impact your ability to follow through effectively with any plan you've come up with to help your child improve executive functioning. A stressful day at the office, not getting enough sleep last night, or having to fast in preparation for a medical procedure the following day can shorten your fuse or increase your impatience with your child. When these events occur, you may be able to prepare yourself by recognizing that it will take extra work on your part to remain cool, stay the course, or follow through with consequences. This will be particularly important in situations where consistency is essential. If you're working with your child to be able to take no for an answer, it's better for you to make the extra effort to hold the line than to give in and decide to try again tomorrow.

Sometimes, though, it may make sense to set aside the plan briefly. If you and your child have made a pact that today is the day you two were going to plan out their science project, you may make the decision that, due to unforeseen circumstances, it's not a good day to do this. You may present the issue as having two possible solutions: "Sam, I'm feeling a little under the weather, and I know I promised to help you with your science project, but I don't think I can today. Would you like to work on it a little by yourself and go till you get stuck, or would you rather wait until tomorrow, when I'll be able to give you more help?" Sometimes these unforeseen circumstances lead children to rise to the occasion in ways that parents might not anticipate.

It's not just your stress level that can affect an intervention; it's also the stress your child may be feeling. What are some events that are likely to cause your child to feel stressed? In general, they're probably the same things that cause you to feel stressed— having too much to do with too little time to do it, being expected to do something they don't feel capable of doing, feeling that they're being criticized unfairly (particularly if it's for something over which they feel they have no control), or having relationship problems in general. In a child's life, this might mean having homework piled on by several teachers or being given an open-ended homework assignment that requires "thinking outside the box." Or maybe your child comes home and reports that their science teacher accused them of copying off another child's test and wouldn't listen to their explanation. Or your child tells you that they overheard kids talking about them in the restroom and laughing at them for being so short and skinny in the eighth grade.

Any of these events can interfere with performance. Just *how* they may interfere with performance depends in part on what the child's profile of executive skill strengths and challenges are. The way you help your child cope may vary depending on the child's executive skills profile, although in general we recommend you acknowledge how the problem makes your child feel (what psychologists call *reflective listening*—"You must be feeling overwhelmed by the homework load," or "It must make you feel kind of powerless when you see that a teacher is not listening to your side of the story").

The good news is that if you recognize the problems for what they are—system overloads that particularly tax skills that are weak to begin with—you can intervene either before, during, or after the problem arises to minimize the fallout.

Being aware of stressors that overload the system and widen the executive skill gap is one important way to start paying attention to the fit between your child and the environment when you're trying to help your child build or enhance executive skills. Parents and teachers alter the environment to ensure a good fit all the time so that kids have the best possible chance to build competence. Modifying the environment when the task before your child taps directly into his executive skill challenges is particularly important. Sometimes your child can opt out of a task that is just a terrible fit for his executive skills. Other times you have to find a way to manipulate the environment, including aspects of the task itself, to make the task a good fit for your son or daughter. We'll discuss this in more detail in upcoming chapters.

PART II

Laying a Foundation
That Can Help

4

Nine Principles for Improving Your Child's Executive Skills

At this point, you probably have a reasonably good idea about what executive skills are and the essential role they play in the ability of your child to learn, problem solve, and successfully manage the challenges the child will encounter throughout life. In viewing your child through an executive skills lens, you likely also are developing a picture of their strengths and challenges and beginning to understand why they easily manage some tasks and struggle with others. And perhaps you are thinking about how to address the child's challenges and capitalize on strengths.

In this chapter we introduce nine principles that will guide your efforts in helping your child develop executive skills. They constitute a set of "rules" that form the foundation of interventions for executive skills, in both addressing challenges and enhancing strengths. We encourage you to keep them in mind as you adapt the strategies in Part III to your child's unique needs or develop your own strategies. In the remainder of Part II, you'll read more about the application of the most important principles.

1. Intentionally promote the development of executive skills rather than expecting the child to acquire them simply through maturation.

We've noted that in the first 12 months, infants develop a fledging core of executive skills including attention, task initiation, working memory, and emotional expression. Research is clear that from this point on your child's experiences play an essential role in the development of executive skills and that children who struggle with these skills do not simply "outgrow" the difficulty. That means that as a parent, through the interactions you have and the experiences you provide, you have an ideal opportunity to help develop your child's executive skills. There's a good chance that you are already engaging in many of the behaviors that will enhance your child's skills even though you may not think of your actions in these terms. For example, in Chapter 1 we introduced the notion of your being a "surrogate frontal lobe" for your child and how this slowly changes over time. Simply by virtue of watching you, your child has learned to imitate and internalize some of your skills—where to find objects, use tools, greet people. She has learned a sense of time and organization when you've established schedules and routines. When she needed help to complete a task or manage a situation, you helped her by providing prompts and then fading your support once you saw she could succeed. Being intentional or deliberate in supporting the growth of executive skills in your child involves the following on your part:

- Understanding what your child's strengths and challenges are. The question-naires in Chapter 2 are a starting point, but over time you'll develop an intuitive sense about these skills as you observe your child in different situations.
- Appreciating the importance of your style of interacting with your child as a way to maintain and encourage their readiness to learn and desire to discover their world.
- Knowing what strategies and tools are available to enhance these skills and the instructional methods you can use when your child is struggling with a task or situation because of an executive skill challenge.

We will touch on these topics in the following principles and address them in detail in the remaining chapters.

2. Encourage rather than fight your child's innate drive for mastery and control.

As most parents know, the "terrible twos" is a catchphrase that signals in earnest the beginnings of their child's desire for control and independence. "No" and "I do it myself" are common responses to a parent's directive to do something or offer to help. The strength of the child's drive to manage himself is reflected in both positive and negative behaviors. As parents we delight in our child's persistent efforts to master tasks—walking, building a LEGO structure, riding a bike, or writing a story. On the flip side, we are frustrated by his behavior, tantrums, or task refusal when his desire is denied or he doesn't follow a direction. The reality is that as our children become more independent, they will sometimes set agendas for themselves that will conflict with our agendas for them. How then do we balance support for their independence with the skills they will need and the values we want them to have? The following are ways to manage both:

- Create and post schedules and routines as your way to set the agendas for recur-ring daily activities that will continue to be important in your child's life. These include morning and bedtime tasks and rituals, mealtimes, chores, and after-school routines such as homework. For younger children picture schedules are effective, and as children get older you can move to daily and weekly calendars. Consistent routines and expectations provide a sense of predictability and comfort for your child and help her develop planning, organization, and time management skills. They also are key to preventing conflicts. If you haven't set an agenda for your child, she will create *her* own agenda. If you then come along and "surprise" her with a different plan for her time, she will be upset. Putting your agenda out first lets your child know what is coming and preempts her from staking a claim to that time. We will cover routines and schedules in detail in Chapter 9.

• If possible, start early and practice new tasks in small steps, increasing the challenge and the time demand only gradually. If you have young children, setting behavioral expectations and building habits will help to avoid many of the later conflicts over task completion that parents often face. When we say "early," we mean anytime from toddlerhood on. Children want to feel a sense of control and competence, and doing things like picking up crayons, putting toys away, and wiping the table off develops these feelings. But regardless of your child's age, the important thing is to start. Just keep these rules in mind: start small so that the task requires limited time and effort; model/demonstrate the task; have the child do it and encourage their effort; don't expect perfection!

• Present alternatives. The goal here is to move away from the "automatic no" that often triggers a protest from the child. We're not suggesting that you never say "no" or refrain from limit-setting. There are plenty of situations (hot stoves, objects in outlets, property destruction) where an immediate *"No!"* is the response called for. However, in other situations an alternative option creates a path for the child to get to her "want to" by first passing through your "have to." Known as "Grandma's law," or simply "first—then," it is an effective way to have children complete a less-preferred activity (like a chore) to get to a more preferred activity (such as watching a video). "First—then" fits nicely with schedules and routines.

• Build in choices as a way to encourage decision making and give your child a sense of control. Choices also open the door to negotiation. Limit choices to two or three options and think through the choices you will offer to ensure that you can live with the option your child chooses.

• Use negotiation. Negotiation is an opportunity to have a discussion with your child and come to a mutually acceptable agreement. It is an important step in children's learning that they have a voice, that you're willing to listen, and that they can advocate for themselves. It's also a way for them to learn how to listen to another's point of view. Not everything is a negotiation, and sometimes a rule needs to be followed. But sometimes kids have reasons for their choices that we haven't considered and that justify their position.

3. Consider your child's developmental level.

You wouldn't expect 4-year-olds to ready themselves for daycare, 8-year-olds to plan and cook meals, or 14-year-olds to live in their own apartment. Yet in our work we meet a lot of parents who hold expectations well beyond their child's level of development. We once worked with a parent, for instance, who expected her 8-year-old daughter to remember all on her own to take her asthma medication each morning, something most children need help remembering at least through the upper elementary grades, if not longer. And we routinely work with parents of high school freshmen who are frustrated because their children do not have a clear plan for the college they want to go to after they graduate and understand what they need to do to get into that college. They assume their children have the same future orientation they have. However, it is not unusual for even high school seniors to need assistance with this process from parents, school counselors, or both.

By the same token, we have also worked with parents who do things for their children that the children are capable of doing for themselves. If we want our children to build a sense of competence and self-control, giving them the opportunity to master tasks and solve problems is essential. Our role is to provide enough support and encouragement so that they persist in their efforts. That also means that we accept mistakes and failures as a natural part of this process and do not punish or criticize them when mistakes occur.

Understanding what's normal at any given age so that you don't expect too much or too little from your child is the first step in addressing executive skill. We included a table in Chapter 2 that lists the typical ages at which we expect children to perform tasks that involve executive skills. We have also included more detailed checklists in Part III that you can use to identify where your child stands in terms of developing specific executive skills.

But knowing what's typical for *any* given child at a certain age is only part of the process. The more important question is what's typical for *your* child. For example, it might be normal for the average 11-year-old to clean his room independently with a schedule and a reminder or two. That might not be the norm for your child, particularly if organization is a challenge. When your child struggles with a task like this, you'll need to step in and intervene at whatever level he is functioning at now. You will need to match the task demands to your child's actual developmental level if that's different from his peers or from what you would like it to be. Understanding your child's executive skills as well as the skills involved in a particular task will help you appreciate why some tasks are a struggle and how to manage them.

4. Move from the external to the internal.

This principle is the starting point for creating a good fit between your child's abilities and task demands. As we've mentioned, you acted largely as your child's frontal lobes when your child was really small. Executive skills training typically begins with something *outside* the child. Before your child knew how to safely cross a road, you modeled the behavior, holding his hand when the two of you reached a street corner. Eventually, because you did this and repeated the rule *Look both ways before crossing*, your child began to internalize the rule, and you gradually decreased your active role until you were satisfied that he was safe. In all kinds of ways, you organize and structure your child's environment to compensate for the executive skills your child has not yet developed. When you decide to help your child develop more effective executive skills, begin by using your executive skills and fading your support as your child learns the skill. Some examples:

- Cueing a child to brush their teeth before they go to bed rather than expecting them to remember to do this on their own.
- Keeping tasks very brief rather than expecting a young child to work for a long time to complete a chore.
- Keeping birthday parties small to avoid overstimulating a child who struggles with emotional control.
- Having a toddler or preschooler hold your hand when walking through a busy parking lot.

Remember that the external includes changes you can make in the environment, the task, or the way you interact with your child. Consider all three possibilities whenever you're going to try to modify something external to the child to make a task manageable and encourage the development of executive skills. You can make minor changes in the physical or social environment. This can be something as simple as having a child with ADHD do her homework in the kitchen, where she can be monitored and given reminders and encouragement to stay on track. For a child who struggles with emotional control, it might mean finding younger playmates or limiting play dates to one child at a time or having a parent or babysitter on hand to supervise beyond the age when this is typically done for kids. Finally, you can change the way you (or other adults, like teachers) interact with your child. You may already be doing some of the last now that you know how your executive skills compare with your child's, but there are more specific ideas for interacting differently, as well as modifying the environment or the task, in Chapter 5.

5. Modify tasks to match your child's executive skills and capacity for effort.

Some tasks require more effort than others. This is as true for adults as it is for children. Think of that task at your office that you keep putting off—you know, the one that doesn't get done because you can think of a million things you have to do that are more pressing than that one. Or think of that chore you've been hounding your spouse about for weeks. It's not that they—or you, for that matter—*can't* do it.

In fact, though, there are two kinds of effortful tasks: ones that you're not very good at and ones that you are very capable of doing but just don't like to do. The same is true for children, and different strategies apply depending on which kind of task is under consideration.

If we're talking about tasks the child is not very good at, we're also likely talking about tasks that involve executive skills that are a challenge for your child. Take getting dressed independently in the morning, a typical task for 8- to 9-year-olds. Planning, organization, time management, and attention all come into play. If it's a struggle, you handle the task by breaking it down into small steps and starting with either the first step and proceeding forward or the last step and proceeding backward, and you don't proceed to the next step until the child has mastered the previous step. With dressing, beginning at the end would involve prompting the child for the entire task except the last step (putting on socks and shoes). Starting at the beginning might mean having the child simply straighten the top sheet when learning to make the bed. You encourage the child for doing a good job and limit the child's responsibility to that last or first step until that step becomes second nature or so easy the child can do it with her eyes closed, and then you move back or on to the next step. Where you start depends on what steps, if any, your child can already do.

But really, it's the second kind of effortful task that parents tend to be frustrated about. These are the ones where you think your children avoid a task "just because they don't like it." If a task has become a battleground between you and your child, it's best to change the nature of the battle. The goal is then to teach your child to exert effort by getting them to override the desire to quit or do anything else that's preferable. The way to do this is to make the first step *easy enough* so that it doesn't feel particularly hard to the child. Continue with just that step until it becomes routine and then add the next step. Encourage the child with positive feedback about their efforts. Often this gradual approach will solve the problem. But if you still get pushback, see the next principle about incentives.

When we work with parents of children who resist tasks that take effort, we've found it helpful to have them use a scale, say, from 1 to 10, when gauging how hard the task feels to the child. Ten on this scale is a task the child can do but that feels *very, very hard*, while 1 on this scale is something that requires *virtually no effort at all*. The goal is to design or modify the task so it feels like a 3.

You can help your child use this scale to plot how to do the work that needs to get done. Let's say the one job you expect your 13-year-old to do steadily throughout the summer is mow the lawn. And let's say you find yourself hounding him week after week to get it done. You finally realize that he avoids it because he finds it incredibly boring and time-consuming (and therefore requiring a lot of effort). You may find it helpful to explain the 10-point scale to him, ask him to rate lawn mowing, and then ask him what could be done to lower lawn mowing from a 10 to a 3. For example, you might get him to identify how much time spent mowing the lawn might feel like a 3 to him. If so, adjust your expectation. Over time, the effortfulness will decrease and very gradual increases can keep the task at a 3.

This scale can also be applied to aversive homework assignments. You could get your child to begin homework planning by rating each assignment in terms of how hard it feels. Then the child could decide on the order in which to do the assignments based on that rating—and you might encourage them to build in small breaks for the ones with higher ratings (or even switch off between easy and difficult tasks).

6. Use incentives and rewards, if necessary, to get your child started.

An incentive is anything that motivates your child to perform an activity, and a reward is the payoff for successfully completing that activity. So the real issue here is what motivates our children (and us) to engage in a behavior. There are two types of motivation—intrinsic and extrinsic. Intrinsic motivation means doing an activity for the enjoyment and challenge it presents, while extrinsic motivation means doing the activity for the promise or payoff of a tangible reward (video game, snack, money, and the like).

The research is clear about two things: competence, self-control, and a desire for relatedness are powerful intrinsic motivators; and intrinsic motivators are superior to extrinsic motivators in producing lasting behavior change. Solving problems and overcoming challenges are naturally motivating. Most children want to master things like learning to climb stairs, ride a bike, or drive a car. For a lot of children this also extends to doing "grownup" things like helping to cook, clean up, and fix things. In addition to building a sense of competence, these tasks are an opportunity to spend time with a person they love. As we noted, tasks that are a "good fit" for a child, challenging but within their capacity, are often intrinsically motivating.

But as we explained in Principle 5, other factors come into play. Like adults, children find some tasks more effortful or tedious than others. In addition, when they're engaged in an activity they're interested in, putting that aside to do a nonpreferred task can be a struggle. Incentives have the effect of making a task seem less effortful because they give the child something to look forward to once the task is done. For "have-to" or "must-do" tasks, incentives are a way to enlist cooperation and learn habits. Whenever possible, the "first—then" incentive approach is preferable because it capitalizes on activities that the child already enjoys, such as playing with a friend or watching a video. To implement this type of incentive, completion of the less preferred or nonpreferred task is a condition for getting to the preferred activity. "As soon as you do _____, you can do _____." The incentive is there to ensure that there's a payoff for the child for expending the effort it takes to complete the task. As noted above, if the task involves a high degree of effort for the child (it has multiple steps or takes a long time, like room cleaning or homework), this approach is most effective if you initially reduce the task demand. Practice improves proficiency and reduces perceived effort. By very gradually increasing the task demand, proficiency increases at each step without the task feeling more effortful. Over time this approach also helps children learn the strategy of completing the "have-tos" before getting to the "want-tos" or learning to delay gratification. We will have much more to say about this and other incentive systems in Chapter 7.

7. Provide just enough support for the child to be on a path toward success.

This appears to be so simple as to be self-evident, but in fact the implementation of this principle may be trickier than it appears. The principle includes two components that are of equal weight—(1) *just enough support* (2) *for the child to be on a path to success.* Parents and other adults who work with children tend to err in one of two directions. They either provide too much support, which means the child is successful but fails to develop the ability to perform the task independently, or they provide too little support, so the child fails repeatedly—and, again, doesn't develop the ability to perform the task independently.

Here's a simple example: When children are ready to learn to open doors by themselves, we stop doing it for them but stand by, ready to intervene at the first point where the child stops succeeding. Maybe the child can put his hand on the doorknob but doesn't know how to turn it. You, his mother or father, then put your hand gently over his and turn his hand and the doorknob until it opens. The next time the child encounters a closed door, maybe he can begin to turn it, but he can't turn the knob far enough to make it open. Again, you put your hand on his, but only after he's attempted to turn the handle unsuccessfully. Through repetitions, the child eventually can open the door on his own. If, however, you insisted on continuing to pull the door open for your child, he wouldn't learn to do it on his own. If you stood there and let your child's frustration mount as he tried to no avail to open the door, he'd learn nothing about opening the door—except maybe that this was an unpleasant effort to avoid.

The same principle applies with any task you want your child to master. Determine how far she can get in the task on her own and then intervene—don't do the task for her, though; just offer her enough support (physical, verbal, modeling depending on the task) to get her on the path toward success. The goal is to leave a degree of challenge for your child and encourage her progress and efforts to persist. Trial and error is an important and necessary part of the learning process. This may take some practice, and it certainly takes close observation, but you'll get the hang of it.

8. Keep supports and supervision in place until the child is moving toward success.

We see parents who know how to break down tasks, teach skills, and reinforce progress, and yet their children still fail to acquire the skills they want them to gain. More often than not, this is because of a failure to apply this principle and/or the next one. These parents set up a process or a procedure, see that it's working, and then back out of the picture, expecting the child to keep succeeding independently. One of the more common examples we see is the system that parents put in place to help their children get organized. They may walk them through a process of cleaning their desk, for instance, or they may buy them the notebooks or binders they need to organize their schoolwork, and even help them decide how they will use those notebooks, but they are too quick to expect their children to maintain the organizing scheme on their own.

Research indicates that it can take weeks to months for adults to establish a routine or change a behavior. Not surprisingly, this varies depending on the routine and the value to the person. For children, especially if executive skills are involved, the timeline is longer because as children grow, the demands of the routine change and already learned behaviors are resistant to change.

We routinely encourage parents to be alert for small signs of progress. The more precisely you define the problem to begin with, the more likely you are to see that progress. Before you begin to implement any of the interventions described in this book, or even one you come up with on your own, you may want to take a few minutes to write down exactly what the problem looks like—or sounds like (as in the case of temper tantrums)—right now. Describe the behavior in precise terms (for example, *forgets to hand in homework assignments; cries whenever there's an unexpected change in plans*), and either estimate or count how often it happens or how long it lasts. If it's a behavior that involves intensity (like a temper tantrum), you can rate it on a scale from *mild* to *severe*. Periodically (that is, every few weeks), you may want to pull out what you wrote and see if the progress is visible. We provide a worksheet to help you monitor improvement at the end of this chapter.

We should point out, however, that in the very early stages of attempting to change a behavior, it can sometimes get worse before it gets better. If your child cries at bedtime unless you agree to lie down with him until he falls asleep, and you decide to try to extinguish that behavior, you will likely find that the crying increases in duration or intensity before it begins to decline. Any behavioral intervention designed to address problems with emotional control or response inhibition—particularly if your strategy involves ignoring one set of behaviors while trying to teach replacement behaviors—is particularly likely to result in an increase in the problem before improvement becomes evident.

The more carefully you design (and measure) the intervention, the sooner you are likely to see progress. In our experience some parents are better able to implement precise interventions and record-keeping than others. For those who are not so precise, using periodic "check-ups" should help you see that progress is indeed occurring.

9. When you do stop the supports, supervision, and incentives, fade them gradually, never abruptly.

Even if you stick with the supports you put in place long enough to allow your child to learn to do the task or use the skill independently, you may be tempted to cut them off all at once. Instead, you need to fade them so that the child can achieve gradual independence with the skill. Let's consider a bike-riding analogy. If you've ever taught a child to ride a bike, you know that you start out holding on to the back of the bike to keep it upright. Every once in a while as your child practices, you let go for a second or two to test whether the child can keep the bike going without too much wobbling. If so, you gradually let go for longer and longer. You don't hold on to the back constantly and then suddenly just let 'er fly and expect the child and bike to keep going without a crash.

Remember from Principle 7 to *provide just enough support for the child to be on the path to success.* Don't keep cueing or prompting a child who doesn't need you to do that. But don't go from everything to nothing either!

We'll talk more about the fading process in the next three chapters, and in Part III you'll see the process in action in detailed illustrations. You should be able to rely on these principles whenever you're deciding how to tackle a problem task with your child or whenever you want to hone an overall skill. In fact, you might find it helpful to review these principles anytime you find yourself stumped or stalled while using the strategies in Part III. Sometimes we forget how important it is to stick to the ground rules when life and its demands—on us and our kids—get complicated.

Three Ways to Instill Executive Skills

Embedded in these principles is a way to view any behavior you want to change, including the acquisition and use of executive skills. Behavior management experts often call this the ABC model. A in this model stands for *antecedent,* B for *behavior,* and C for *consequences.* The idea is that there are three opportunities to take measures to elicit or change the behavior as desired: by changing what comes before it (the external factors, or environment), by aiming directly at the behavior itself (through teaching), and by imposing consequences (incentives or penalties). In Chapter 5 we'll talk about modifying the environment to reduce problems with executive skills, by focusing on the antecedents to behavior—those external conditions that make executive skill problems either better or worse. In Chapter 6 we turn to the behavior itself and show you how to work with your children to acquire executive skills. (The form on the facing page provides a framework to log and keep track of specific behaviors.) Finally, in Chapter 7 we talk about using motivation to encourage children to use executive skills. Once you've read those chapters, you'll have what you need to design your own interventions to improve your child's executive functioning—or a solid base of understanding that will help you make the most of the interventions we've created for you and present in Part III.

How Much Progress Are We Making?

Date	Executive skill	Precise description of behavior (What does it look like/ sound like?)	Frequency (How often does the behavior occur?— times per day, per week, etc.)	Duration (How long does it last?)	Intensity (On a scale of 1 to 5, how intense is the behavior?)
Follow-up date		Does the behavior still look/sound the same?	How often does it happen now?	How long does it last now?	How intense is it now?
Follow-up 2					

From *Smart but Scattered, Second Edition*, by Peg Dawson, Richard Guare, and Colin Guare. Copyright © 2025 The Guilford Press. Permission to photocopy this material, or to download enlarged printable versions (*www.guilford.com/dawson4-forms*), is granted to purchasers of this book for personal use; see copyright page for details.

5

Modifying the Environment

A *Is for* Antecedent

As we said at the end of Chapter 4, modifying the environment is the first of three ways to change a behavior that requires executive skills. As you'll discover later in this chapter, there are a number of ways to alter the environment so your child can do a task successfully. But first you have to figure out what the fit between that task and your child is.

Matching the Task with the Child

It's Friday afternoon, and 9-year-old Caleb is excited about his friend coming for a sleepover tonight. His room, however, is a train wreck, and the deal with his parents is that he will pick up his room first—or no sleepover. He's playing a video game, and his mom reminds him that his room needs to be clean before dinner, which gives him a little over an hour to finish. Caleb continues with the game until his mother tells him he either start on his room now or call his friend to cancel the sleepover. He grudgingly heads to his room, complaining that this task will take "forever." He is greeted by books, sports equipment, and toys, a partially built LEGO structure and clothes, dirty and clean, on the floor. He gets the LEGO container and starts to pick up the pieces on the floor but decides to finish one section of the structure before putting it away. A half hour later his mother comes in to check on him and he's still building. "Caleb! Nothing's done, and you've only got a half hour to finish!" His mother is frustrated but not surprised. Room cleaning has been a consistent struggle, but she thought the sleepover deal would get him past it this time. "Please help me, Mom?" Reluctantly she agrees to supervise his efforts, and in 20 minutes the room is passable. "Caleb, if you had done this in the first place, you could have been done with plenty of time to spare! We need to find a better solution." "Yeah, I know. Thanks, Mom."

After his friend leaves on Saturday, his mom and dad propose they talk on Sunday to discuss room cleaning, and Caleb picks 11:00 A.M. to meet in his room. "What do you think would make this easier?" asks Dad. "If you or Mom helped me?" Mom smiles. "That's probably true, but we'd like to find a way for you to manage this on your own." "I don't know then. All this stuff—it takes forever!" "Well, when I saw your room Friday there were books, toys, sports stuff, and clothes. What would be the quickest to pick up?" "Clothes I guess; just throw them in the basket." "How long will it take?" "I don't know!" "Can we try it now?" "Now?" "Yeah, I'll spread your dirty clothes around the room, and you can time yourself using my phone while Mom and I wait in the hall. Holler when you're done." "Weird, but OK, I guess." Dad scatters clothes on the floor, shows him how to use the timer, and they leave. In a few minutes he hollers, "Done!" "How long?" "3 minutes, 21 seconds!" "Wow, quick pick-up! How about we start with just this, twice a week. You pick the days and times, and we'll get you a timer and help you make a schedule." "That's all?" "Yeah, for now. Let's just see how it goes."

That's not the end of the story or the final solution for Caleb and room cleaning. We'll come back to that in a bit. For now you might ask yourself, *Why not impose the consequence, cancel the sleepover? Wouldn't that solve the problem?* It could if knowing the expectation and being motivated were the only elements necessary to meet a goal. But think about this for a minute. Let's say you have a goal, like a resolution to exercise more or eat healthier. You know what you need to do, and presumably you're motivated if you set the goal. What else is needed? You need to be able to get started, resist temptations, ignore distractions, keep the goal in mind, and persist—in short, you need executive skills. For Caleb, task initiation, planning/prioritizing, and sustained attention are challenges, particularly for open-ended, less structured tasks. On the face of it, Caleb's mother saw this as a manageable task for him. Unlike him, she has good task initiation, planning/prioritizing, and sustained attention skills as well as plenty of practice with tasks like this. Mother's reaction, frustration but not surprise, suggests that she knows that this is a struggle for Caleb that motivation alone won't fix. What's the solution? Improve the fit between the task and the child's skills.

Think of the tasks and activities that children encounter during development— morning and evening routines, room cleaning, snack and meal prep, sports, artistic and musical activities, classroom performance, homework, and social interactions, to name a few. The demands vary, but independent, successful performance requires some combination of executive skills. As we've said, acquiring these skills takes time and practice. The good news is that our children want to explore, learn to master their environment, and we want that for them.

If their skills aren't quite up to the task, what do we do? We could abandon the task, but that eliminates the possibility of learning and skill development. We could wait, but time alone doesn't ensure skill development. We could let them try, which is, in fact, what we often do, and eventually they succeed. But when we do this, we observe their attempts, and if they appear to be making progress, we're comfortable with letting them persist. What if they fail over and over again? Ask yourself what happens if you fail at something over and over? More often than not, you abandon the effort and return only if you get help, change the task, or acquire the skill. For kids, if skill challenges lead to repetitive failures, then learning, and with it a sense of competence and self-control, suffers.

To use a swimming analogy, what we're looking for is some middle ground between just pushing them off the dock to see if they figure it out and wrapping them head to toe in floaties so that they never have to figure it out. We're used to doing this with our children for a variety of skills. We either help them, like by holding the bike seat, or we modify the task, by putting training wheels on, or both. With either approach, we're not expecting or demanding that our child learn the skill immediately. And we're not abandoning the task or activity because they can't independently succeed at it. Instead, we're modifying the task in some fashion so that it is a better match for where their skills are right now, and they can gradually master the task.

For some activities, like swimming or bike riding, the child's challenge is more obvious since it involves motor skills that are easily observed. With executive skills, the challenge isn't quite as obvious since we cannot as easily observe attention or planning or organization or task initiation. We infer them from our child's performance. And there is one additional complication. For some activities or tasks, our children seem to have the executive skills they need, and for others they don't. In our work we routinely hear this from parents: "How can he have an attention problem? He has no problem paying attention to video games!" The simple answer is that different tasks have different skill demands.

So how do we discover the task modification to improve its fit with our child's skills? By knowing our child's abilities, the task demands, and the environment where the task takes place. The following are considerations to help you clarify what the source of the mismatch is.

Identifying the Mismatch

1. *When you know your child's executive skill strengths and challenges, pay close attention to the child's behavioral and emotional responses to the task.* With the questionnaires in Chapter 2, you have a good start on understanding your child's executive skills. Combining this information with observations of how they react to various day-to-day activities will help fill out the picture of where and how they might struggle. Caleb was reluctant to start on his room and, when pressed by his mother, not only complained about the task but shared his feeling that it would take "forever." For her, the state of his room, zero progress, and the LEGO distraction, along with past history, confirmed the task–skill mismatch and convinced her of the need for a different solution.

2. *When your child seems to be avoiding a task, consider the possibility that the child's skills are not up to the task.* Children react to challenging tasks with a wide

variety of different emotional responses and behaviors that might not immediately signal that they *can't* do what they've been asked to do. For Caleb, it was avoidance, first
with the video game and then with LEGOs. When kids are reluctant to do a task, they,
like us, dawdle, find distractions, and do other tasks. They say the task is "stupid" or
"will take forever." Or they just don't do it and we take that as a sign of defiance. If this
happens repeatedly, consider they are doing this in lieu of saying, "I'm not sure how to
do this" or "This is too hard for me."

Of course some children do just this—say they don't know how to do the task—but
often the response from parents or teachers to that direct statement of truth is "Sure
you can, it's easy; all you need to do is this" followed by a couple of examples. We think
we're helping or encouraging them by saying this. In fact, it's discouraging and makes
them feel incompetent. From the parent's or teacher's perspective, the task does look
easy because they have the skill. Ask yourself, when you're struggling with a task, does
it make you feel more competent when someone says it's easy? We'd guess not. Assume
the same for your child and work with them to modify the task and develop the skill.

3. *Figure out what executive skills the task requires and ask yourself if these skills
match up with your child's skills.* Start with the task that's a struggle for your child.
Maybe it's getting ready in the morning, or bedtime routines, or room cleaning. Let's
take room cleaning as an example, something that most all parents expect of their kids.
Independent room cleaning, at a minimum, requires the following executive skills:

- Task initiation—the child starts the task without reminders or nagging.
- Sustained attention—the child needs to stick with the task long enough to get
  it done.
- Planning/prioritizing—the child needs a plan of attack and a priority of what to
  keep or throw away.
- Organization—the child has to have a specific place for everything.

When a task requires multiple executive skills, you may have observed or suspect a
specific stumbling block, like organization. You could address this by working with your
child to create specific, labeled containers or spaces. If you're not sure, you can address
each skill. Caleb and his parents started with simplifying the task to address planning
and attention, identified the laundry basket for organization, and suggested a schedule
of his choice for task initiation.

We understand that your child may be struggling with any number of different
tasks or activities. In Part III of this book, we've provided a host of different situations
to address these issues.

4. *Figure out whether some aspect of the environment is making the task difficult
for your child.* For children with newly emerging skills or with skill challenges, the presence of distractions can interfere with task completion, particularly if the distraction is
more interesting than the task. TV, video games, and phones come to mind, but a toy,
book, or any object that grabs a child's attention can interfere. More than once (this is
Dick talking) the fish tank in the kitchen interfered with my young son's getting to the

school bus on time. We're not suggesting you whitewash the environment but rather keep an eye out for recurring distractions.

Distraction also impacts how children respond to directions. If you feel like you're being ignored, ask yourself what your child was doing when you gave the direction. We've encountered many situations where parents gave a direction when the child was engaged in an activity of interest. If you expect them to understand and follow the direction, you need their undivided attention. Later in this chapter, we'll give you some ways to accomplish this without provoking frustration or a tantrum.

What about observing your child during the activity? Does that increase or decrease the likelihood of task success? That depends. If your child is trying to improve a skill (music practice, drawing, athletics) and you're in the habit of offering "constructive comments," then your presence and judgment can be an impediment. If you're not sure, ask them if they'd prefer to practice alone. On the other hand, if your child is susceptible to distractions or struggles with task initiation or planning, your presence may promote task focus or give them the opportunity to ask for help if they are stuck. This is often the case with homework.

For children with executive skill challenges, their interest in a task can have a significant effect on task performance. Maybe your child has no trouble remembering to take his musical instrument to school but routinely forgets his homework assignments. Or she remembers to get her sports equipment ready but forgets to feed the dog. That doesn't mean that working memory isn't a struggle for either child. It's a demonstration of the fact that motivation can have an energizing effect on executive skills and that low motivation hampers the activation of weaker executive skills. This is especially true for routines and repetitive tasks. That interest in a task affects performance probably comes as no surprise. Knowing that children can use executive skills more effectively when the motivation is sufficient, you may be able to find ways to link task performance to motivating factors that enhance your child's ability to effectively use executive skills that don't come easily to them. Chapter 7 will talk more about how to motivate children to use and reduce executive skill challenges.

5. **Observing that *your child can do a task sometimes but not all the time may mean you've identified an executive skill challenge*.** There is a big difference between being able to do a task and being able to do that task *consistently*. Those of us who are organizationally challenged (as I, Dick, am) understand this quite well; for me, it's obvious in the context of keeping my desk neat and tidy. Yes, I'm perfectly capable of cleaning off the desk. I *know how* to do this—what to keep on my desk, what to file, what to trash, and so on. Periodically (every few months) I used to do this, and it felt great. But I was still left with weeks of aggravation when I couldn't find something. My solution was to select one item type weekly (books, personal mail, and the like) and file those items. It's not perfect, but it's definitely better and at an effort level I can manage. This is what kids are often up against as they encounter tasks that tap their executive skill weaknesses: they may know what to do or how to do it, but to do it consistently, day in and day out, for as long as their parents or teachers expect them to do it is a whole other story!

In situations like this, you have a few options. For a child with organizational problems, you can simplify the task so it's quicker, and increase the frequency. Caleb's parents opted for just his clothes and twice a week as a starting point. If your child has a limited attention span, work with them to divide the task into parts with short breaks in between, such as with math homework problems.

While it's preferable to stick with routines and schedules, your flexibility is important. If your child has had a particularly busy or stressful day and is overtired or frustrated, one more demand can push them over the edge. It's OK to temporarily reduce the demand or change the schedule. Reducing the demand is preferable since it lets the child know the expectation is still in play. The operative word here is *temporarily*, and if you find that this is coming up more often, it's time to think about ways to address whatever triggers the fatigue or stress.

6. *If your child has handled the task some of the time, figure out what made success possible.* We're still talking about consistency here but from a different angle. Maybe there are inconsistencies in your child's performance because situational differences impacted performance. Did you do something that made the task easier for the child without even realizing you were doing so?

- Did you talk with your child about what he had to do before he got started (what we sometimes call "priming the pump")?
- Did you help your child break down the task?
- Did you suggest breaks after just 5–10 minutes of work?

I (Dick) worked with a girl who was routinely late for school on some days but not others. It took us a while to figure out that she was never late on days when there was band practice because she didn't want to be in detention and miss it.

If you or others feel confounded by your child's inconsistent ability to accomplish a certain task, look for differences in the two situations. List the situational factors involved in each in two columns and then compare to see where the keys to success might lie.

7. *If the child's executive skills seem a good fit for the task, is lack of confidence the reason for task avoidance?* Regardless of your child's skill level, if they lack confidence or anticipate failure, the task is a bad fit from their perspective. Children can lack confidence for a number of reasons:

- The task looks too big, and they can't see it as a set of smaller, more manageable steps. Caleb thought room cleaning would take "forever." This is especially likely to happen with more open-ended, less structured tasks.
- They have tried and failed repeatedly to meet adult expectations and assume that this will continue—so why try? This is especially true if their unsuccessful efforts have been met repeatedly with criticism or punishment.
- They have perfectionist tendencies (and/or may have parents with perfectionist tendencies). As a result they are particularly susceptible to low confidence since,

no matter how well they perform a task, it never quite meets either their expectations or those of others.

- Someone has always jumped in and rescued them as soon as they encounter an
obstacle, so they don't make mistakes or experience failure. They haven't learned
that they can overcome obstacles on their own (or with minimal assistance).
This can also occur if the child has no or few responsibilities and adults do most
everything for them.

- They struggle with flexibility. Children who are inflexible are more comfortable
when they know exactly what is expected or what will happen. New, unfamiliar
tasks can trigger uncertainty and anxiety about performance and lead to task
avoidance.

Fortunately there are a few steps you can take to address these issues. Repeated
failures, whether they come from executive skill challenges or expectations that exceed
a child's skill level, can be addressed with task modifications, as Caleb's parents did. If
task avoidance has developed as a result of criticism or punishment for errors in performance, changing the way adults communicate with a child about performance efforts
and error correction can increase their willingness to try. The goal is for children and
adults to see performance errors as an expected and necessary part of the learning process and as a natural path to improvement. This mindset is also the goal for children
and/or their parents who have perfectionist tendencies. The added component for them
is developing a tolerance for mistakes without a meltdown. For children who struggle
with flexibility, advance preparation is key since uncertainty is anxiety provoking. Pre-
viewing, schedules, and gradual exposure with support for new situations increases their
comfort level.

In all these situations, children are more likely to attempt and persist at a task if
they experience gradual progress and their efforts are met with words of encouragement
from adults. Research has demonstrated that children who are praised for their efforts
in the face of a challenging task rather than only for success are more likely to be persistent learners. The rest of this chapter describes specific ways to make environmental
modifications.

Three Ways to Modify the Environment

Consider the following situation: Tara, age 5, was a challenging child from birth. She
was colicky as an infant, had irregular sleep patterns, and was a fussy eater. As soon
as she could communicate a preference, she complained about tags and seams on her
clothing. Her parents found she fell apart at birthday parties and family gatherings and
predictably had meltdowns at these events. Temper tantrums routinely happened in
unfamiliar social situations and with changes in routine and transitions, especially if
she was tired or hungry. Meltdowns seemed to be the only way Tara knew to manage in

these situations. She seemed comfortable only with familiar, routine activities or when she knew in advance what would happen and with whom. Her parents talked with Tara about this and asked if she might be more comfortable if she knew in advance what would be happening. She wasn't sure but agreed to help them with a picture schedule for recurring activities—wake and sleep times, bedtime rituals, meals, and baths, all at roughly the same times daily. Television viewing was limited by time and program to avoid overstimulating content. With play dates, Tara agreed she did better with one child at a time, and they settled on 1½ hours max and planned structured activities such as craft projects or games that Tara chose. When they were invited to birthday parties, her parents contacted the host parent to find out the time frame and activities planned. They told Tara about these, so she could choose what she was comfortable with and gave her the option of arriving a little late and/or leaving little early—and said they would stay close at the party if she wanted to just observe an activity or leave. They did the same for family events. For any new activity they explained to her well in advance what would happen. As a result of these changes to their family patterns, Tara's tantrums and meltdowns diminished, and she gradually became more comfortable in social situations.

You may be familiar enough with the individual executive skills we've described to recognize that Tara has problems with flexibility and emotional control. The methods that Tara's parents put in place to help reduce her emotional outbursts fall neatly into the category of strategies that this chapter will discuss. Rather than starting with a direct effort to teach Tara how to manage her emotions, they worked together with her to structure the external factors (the antecedents) to reduce the likelihood that she would become overloaded. They knew it was unrealistic at such a young age to expect Tara to learn immediately how to manage her emotions, so they helped her structure her day so that she was less stressed and emotional outbursts were less likely. They paid attention to all the ways they could modify external factors (from Principle 4 on pages 60–61) but put a lot of emphasis on the social and physical environment.

The principle of starting with external modifications is so important—and so effective—because it reduces the demand on challenged executive skills. We don't ask our children to manage a situation that they're not yet equipped to handle, but we also don't eliminate the opportunity. Instead we work with them to change the situation just enough for them to manage the challenge and improve their skills. You'll probably find this approach familiar because you're already used to making environmental modifications as a way to create a path for learning. You provide water wings or life vests for swimming, training wheels or your hand support for bike riding, and hand holding for crossing streets. You help your child manage time and activities by creating schedules for meals, morning and evening routines, and playtime. Now you're going to learn how to address executive skill challenges in a similar way.

As we've explained, frontal lobe development involves two interactive processes, maturation of the brain over time and learning experiences. Remember the seesaw analogy from Chapter 1? During a good part of your child's development, your frontal lobes, in the form of executive skills, will carry more weight. How quickly the shift takes place depends on the skills your child brings to the table and the opportunities to learn that the child has. The skills they bring to the table are a function of maturation and their profile of executive skills. By understanding your child's profile, strengths and challenges, and observing their behavior, you'll learn which executive skills need support and in what situations. Thus, at any given point in time, if your child's executive skills are not sufficiently developed to manage the situation, the best immediate option is to modify the task or situation. This will give you the opportunity over time to work with your child on developing skills and gradually reducing the supports.

Back to Tara: Her parents helped her address emotional control issues with environmental changes. They built schedules and routines, modified television viewing, and reduced exposure to overstimulating events. These efforts were not designed to directly teach Tara to regulate her behavior or control her emotions. They were designed to create a path for her to successfully manage these challenging situations with the skills she had at that point.

The objective of environmental modifications is not to eliminate the challenges or create fail-safe situations. Rather, it is to reduce repeated failures that the child currently is not equipped to solve on their own and that could lead to task or situation avoidance. For Tara, they did reduce the likelihood of meltdowns so that she had the opportunity to learn about and enjoy these situations and they led to a more smoothly functioning family. As Tara acclimates to these situations, they also create options for her to increase her participation as well as to learn what she can tolerate and what she can do to cope or take herself away if needed. Over time, understanding her own behavior will allow Tara to begin to adapt the environment to meet her needs (for example, by leaving a noisy family party and going to her room to play). It will also help her learn how to cope with upsetting situations, such as by using self-soothing techniques or seeking an adult's help.

A wide variety of ways to modify or structure external factors to counteract the effect of weak or not-yet-developed executive skills is available to you, but they all fall into the three categories described below. You may find some of the following ideas familiar. Maybe you've used some of them without recognizing them as such. Or you've used them on and off but not consistently. We're going to give you ways to use these strategies systematically, help you pick up the particular practices you may not have been using so far, and show you how you can zero in more specifically on the methods that will target your child's particular executive skill deficits instead of randomly throwing the kitchen sink at them. For some kids, a more concerted effort to tweak the environment even in fairly basic ways is what's needed to give executive skill development a jump start. So please don't assume you've tried all this before and it hasn't been enough. You'll learn more about planning interventions for your child in Part III.

Change the Physical or Social Environment to Reduce Problems

To be effective, the types of changes need to be tailored to the executive skill challenge and the specific situation where the problem exists. The following are some of the ways that you can change the physical or social environment. Ideally the modifications you make allow the child to stay in the situation and meet the task demands, but if not, we'll give you some alternatives.

1. *Provide alternative activities.* For children with response inhibition challenges, waiting, for example in restaurants or cars, can be an issue. Having children select an activity to take with them (book, coloring book with crayons, handheld games, Etch A Sketch) fills in "wait time." These days, parents often use phones or tablets as an activity, which is fine as long as putting them away or surrendering them when directed is not an issue. If it's a problem, try other options.

2. *Limit access or add barriers.* In other situations, if technology is an issue, think about adding controls for cable TV and video games (cable providers, streaming services, Xbox, and PlayStation offer parental controls). Use passwords to limit access to computers and internet sites, and if you choose to let your children use social media like Snapchat, Instagram, or Facebook, know their passwords and let them know that you will regularly monitor their use.

Sometimes barriers are needed. For safety of younger children, we've noted gates for stairs and fences for yards. Barriers also apply to pools, fireplaces, wood stoves, and cabinets that contain medication or cleaning supplies. For older children who struggle with impulse control, if rules haven't worked, locks for parent workspaces and sibling rooms can help when you're not present to monitor.

3. *Reduce distractions.* Middle school kids tell us that distractions in the home can be a major barrier to homework completion. This includes siblings (or parents) watching TV, playing video games, or listening to loud music. Creating a "quiet time" and a homework space can increase your child's ability to focus on work and complete it efficiently. Working with your child to design a workspace that suits their needs saves you from guessing what's a good fit. Many young people use listening to music (for example with earbuds) to screen out distractions; white noise generators (such as some brands of headphones) are another way to block out distractions. Also, be mindful of the distractions that are present within a task situation, such as toys or books in a child's room when they are there to do a job like room cleaning or getting dressed for school.

4. *Provide organizational structures.* Remember that old expression "A *place for everything and everything in its place*"? It is certainly easier for children to develop organizational skills if organizational systems are in place. Providing coat racks and clearly labeled cubbies, storage bins for sports equipment and toys, and hampers in each bedroom for dirty clothes makes this a whole lot easier. And this is actually one example where, by prompting children to place belongings in their appropriate place, they will eventually internalize the concept of organization. You can also help shape organizational skills by letting kids know up front what level of organization is expected and how that expectation will be cued. For instance, take a photograph of what the final product should look like (as in a clean bedroom or playroom) so that you and your child together can compare their work to the photo. Work with your child to set up a schedule for

when/how often this will happen so that it becomes a routine. Middle school students may benefit from using apps (see the Resources) to help them organize tasks or plan their time. Remember also that kids learn by example. If your spaces and belongings are organized, your kids are more likely to follow your lead.

5. *Reduce the social complexity of a social activity or event.* Children who have problems with emotional control, flexibility, or response inhibition often struggle in complex social situations, such as when a lot of people are present or the event is unstructured. Simplifying means reducing the number of people and making the activity more structured. Keeping birthday parties small and ensuring there are carefully planned activities may make the difference between "a good time was had by all" and meltdowns. Open-ended social situations are particularly difficult for children who struggle with flexibility to manage. In this case, the burden on the child can be reduced by having them select the activity they are familiar with that will structure the social interaction (for example, watching a sporting event, movie or video, selecting familiar play activities, or visiting a museum or water park). Having clear rules for social situations and reminding children of the rules before the event begins can also help. House rules for play dates might include the following: take turns in games, snacks in the kitchen, rooms are off-limits, come get me if there's a problem, and both kids clean up at the end of the date. By reminding your child and their friend what the rules are at the beginning of the play date, you're placing those rules in working memory, so children are more likely to be able to retain and apply them.

6. *Change the social mix.* While learning to live and work with all kinds of people is an important life lesson for children, there are times when it makes sense for parents and children to alter the social dynamics. If conflicts with a particular playmate are more frequent, but your child wants to play with that child, play dates at your house where you can provide more supervision, structured activities, and time limits can help. Or maybe you've found that your son does great playing with more than one friend as long as one of those friends is not Joey (whom he does well with one on one). There's nothing wrong with structuring play dates or other social situations to manage the social dynamic. Where it's not possible to do this (such as at family parties), anticipate having to provide more supervision than usual to avoid problems. Also, work with your child in advance on default options. One option might be "If you're getting uncomfortable, tell me and we can decide what to do." Another might be "How about if I check in with you every so often to see if everything is OK?" And be sure to provide a bail-out like a menu of activities the child can do and a place the child can retreat to in the event that she needs a break.

Change the Nature of the Tasks Your Child Is Expected to Do

In the previous chapter we explained how important it is to match the child to the task. In this section we go into more detail about the kinds of task modifications that can help children use their developing executive skills more effectively.

Many youngsters with executive skill challenges do just fine as long as they're the ones deciding how to spend their time. They gravitate to activities that are intrinsically appealing to them and stick with them as long as the activities are interesting. When they stop being interesting, they shift to something else that *is* interesting. This explains why summer vacation tends to be less stressful than the school year—because the ratio of interesting to noninteresting activities is stacked in favor of preferred activities.

As parents, however, we all know that it's the rare individual indeed who gets to go through life doing only the interesting stuff. To help children prepare for the world of work and family responsibilities, we expect them to tackle tasks that are not particularly appealing to them—whether it's doing chores or homework, going to adult social events, or following schedules and routines. Many children can set aside their own preferences and do something they may not be particularly happy to do. Kids with executive skill challenges may not.

There are a wide variety of ways to ease the adjustment by working with them to modify the less preferred tasks:

1. *Make the task shorter.* For youngsters who struggle with task initiation and sustained attention, we generally say that when they begin the task *the end should be in sight.* These youngsters in particular are more likely to initiate and persist if the task looks short as opposed to one that looks like it will take "forever" (like raking the leaves if your yard looks to them like Sherwood Forest). Negotiate with them what they will do and for how long, keeping in mind the principle about keeping the effortfulness of the task lower as a starting point to build persistence.

2. *If a long task needs to be done in a timely manner (like by noon today), work with the child to build a task-break-task-break schedule that meets the deadline* rather than expecting, for example, the whole lawn done in one shot.

3. *Have the child select something to look forward to when the task is over.* We'll talk about this in more detail in Chapter 7 when we talk motivation but as we've noted incentives energize the use of executive skills, especially if those are skills the child struggles with. Keep in mind that the ratio of effort to incentive must be reasonable and shorter tasks are more likely to benefit from this approach.

4. *Make the steps more explicit.* Rather than sending your child to their bedroom with the assignment of "cleaning the whole room," work with him to break the task down into a series of subtasks. Caleb and his parents started with this when he chose "pick up my clothes." Whenever possible, let the child choose the order of pickup and offer to help them turn these into a written or visual checklist:

☐ Put my dirty clothes in laundry.
☐ Place clean clothes in dresser drawers or on hangers in closet.
☐ Put books on bookshelf.
☐ Put toys in toy chest.

A similar approach can be used for things like morning or bedtime routines or any other chore that involves more than one step. We offer a whole chapter of daily routines broken down this way in Chapter 9.

5. *Create a visual schedule with your child and let them choose where to post it.* This is similar to making checklists, but it can be applied more broadly to help the day go more smoothly. Building in set times in the day when things such as mealtimes, bedtimes, chores, and homework occur helps children remember what will happen and when they have free time. In addition, schedules help them internalize a sense of order and routine—prerequisite skills as well as a template for developing more sophisticated planning, organization, and time management skills later on. Keep in mind that schedule flexibility is key since family events, appointments, and after-school activities all may necessitate schedule changes.

6. *Build in choice or variety.* For some children, doing the same chore day in and day out is tedious. If chores are being built into a schedule, give children the option of choosing, from a chore menu, what they will do and revisit the schedule at set times (weekly, monthly) to ask if they want to change. Some parents also let the child choose when to do the chore, although this can be tricky since in most cases the parent will need to remember to prompt the child. Another option is to let the child make the time choice when initially building the schedule. We favor consistency since repetition aids habit-building.

7. *Make the task more appealing.* This might mean letting children complete the task with someone rather than alone or letting them listen to the radio or a favorite CD while they do the task. Some parents are very clever at turning chores into games. "See if you can pick up your toys before the timer goes off" can be a motivator, or "Let's place a bet—how many LEGO pieces do you think you can pick up in one minute on your bedroom floor? I bet 20—what's your bet?" Keep your number reasonably small, so your child has a good chance to win. Other ways to turn chores into games include:

- Challenge your child to pick up 10 things in 1 minute.
- Schedule "fast clean" sessions. A teacher we know holds 15-minute "fast clean sessions" to get her students to help her tidy the classroom. This is followed by 15 minutes of free play.
- Turn picking up the playroom into a game like musical chairs. Start the music and have children wander around the playroom. When the music stops, children "freeze" and then pick up items within reaching distance of where they are standing.
- Write down chores to be done on pieces of paper, which are folded and put in a jar. Children select one piece of paper and perform the chore written on it.

Change the Way You (or Other Adults) Interact with the Child

The more you understand executive skills and the role they play in helping children become independent, the more you'll see how you can alter the way you interact with your child to promote executive skill development. Specifically, there are ways you can interact with your child *before, during,* and *after* situations that involve executive functioning to increase the likelihood that the situation will go well either now or in the future.

What You Can Do before a Situation Comes Up

1. ***Rehearse with the child what will happen and how the child will handle it.*** Whenever Jaden's mom is on the phone, Jaden, age 7, tends to repeatedly interrupt in spite of her rule that he wait until she is done. She talks with Jaden and proposes that when she gets a call, he select a preferred activity that he can do independently from a short menu of options and play in the living room where they can see each other. They make up a picture menu of his choices (LEGOs, drawing, Play-Doh) and put these in containers in the living room. To practice this, she arranges for a friend to call her and explains why. When the call comes, she asks her friend to hang on for a minute and prompts Jaden to make his choice. He does, and at about 1-minute intervals she gives him a thumbs up for attending to his activity. She keeps the calls short at first (5 minutes) but over time gradually increases both the call length and the "thumbs up" recognition intervals as he is able to manage on his own. Actively rehearsing in advance can be used with any executive skill weakness, but it is particularly helpful with children who have problems with attention, flexibility, or response inhibition.

2. ***Work with your child to arrange visual and/or auditory prompts.*** Like most of the other interventions, giving children a choice in how and when they want reminders increases the likelihood that they will follow them. Reminder systems also increase a child's independence and help them learn a skill set that is increasingly important in an age of information overload. Options range from very simple such as a gym bag in front of the door or Post-it notes to more detailed such as picture and written lists and schedules. Phone- and tablet-based reminder and scheduling apps for kids are increasing available and popular, as are voice assistant devices in the home. All these options share a common purpose—helping your child manage a task or situation when you're not available and thus diminishing their reliance on you as a personal prompt. Youngsters who struggle with working memory, task initiation, time management, and planning can use these signaling systems to prompt themselves to do the tasks they need to do—chores, homework, appointments, telephone calls, or whatever else goes into managing the complex details of growing up in 21st-century America. If your child isn't familiar with the options, show her those you are comfortable with and explain that this is a way to eliminate your reminding or nagging and be in control of her own life. When she makes a choice, collaborate with her on how to develop or use it. For example, if it's a picture or word schedule, let her decide what pictures or words she wants to use. If it's an app or a voice assistant, model its use and then let her practice with it until she is comfortable.

3. ***Use verbal prompts or reminders.*** This is basically a shortened version of a rehearsal. "Remember what we talked about" will remind a child of a previous

conversation in which rules were laid down or a situation previewed. Other examples might be as follows: "What's the rule for playing in the front yard?" "What do you have to do before you get to call up Mike and invite him to come over?" "What do you have to do first as soon as you get home from school?" All these examples, by the way, have one common characteristic: *They help the child retrieve information.* If you're wondering, "What's the difference between telling my son he has to clean his room before he can call Mike and asking him what he has to do before calling Mike?" here's the difference: by asking your son to retrieve the information himself, you're increasing his ability to use his own executive skills, specifically *working memory and verbally rehearsing what he will do.* This brings him closer to independence. Of course, if he can't remember what he is supposed to do, you can help him out—but don't just say, "Clean your room." Rather, give him the minimal amount of information necessary for him to answer the question. You might give him some multiple-choice options or say, "It's about your room."

Ways You Can Interact with Your Child during an Activity or Situation

1. **Coach the child to elicit the rehearsed behavior.** A well-timed "Remember what we talked about" just before the situation is about to arise can make the difference for a child who struggles with working memory or impulse control. You may even want to take a quick break and step aside from the situation with your child to briefly go over that rehearsal again in a little more detail. We sometimes find it helpful to give kids "cue cards" that they can carry with them to remind them of the skill they're working on or how to carry out that skill. An example of a cue card for "listening" is shown on the facing page (it also includes space to record when the child uses the skill).

2. **Remind the child to check his list or schedule.** In the early phases of learning a routine or procedure, children may forget that there is a procedure that's been written down. A gentle reminder to them to check their list can get them back on track. And again, rather than telling them what step they're on and exactly what they have to do, prompting them to check the list aids the transfer of responsibility from parent to child.

3. **Monitor the situation to better understand the triggers and other factors that affect your child's ability to use executive skills successfully.** Even when you can't intervene quickly enough or there's nothing you can do at the time to avert a problem, you can use your observational skills to identify the factors that contribute to problems. Being present during a problem situation may enable you to see how a toy or game distracts your child from the task at hand, as did LEGOs for Caleb when cleaning his room. Or you can see how the pulling the cat's tail led to your daughter's getting scratched and crying. Of course, you can't always be there to see what causes problems to arise. But when you do happen to be present, you may be able to work with your child to modify the situation so that the outcome is different the next time.

Cue Card for Listening

Week of:	Monday	Tuesday	Wednesday	Thursday	Friday
Who? **When?**					
Face speaker					
Pay attention and show interest					
Keep body still					
Do not interrupt					
Overall rating of entire skill performance					

+ = independent/successful; h = with help; − = did not use skill or did incorrectly.

From *Smart but Scattered, Second Edition*, by Peg Dawson, Richard Guare, and Colin Guare. Copyright © 2025 The Guilford Press. Permission to photocopy this material, or to download enlarged printable versions (*www.guilford.com/dawson4-forms*), is granted to purchasers of this book for personal use; see copyright page for details.

What You Can Do Afterward to Improve the Situation in the Future

1. **Recognize your child's efforts to improve.** "You did a nice job looking at your schedule and starting to get dressed when you woke up," "Thank you for showing self-control and walking away when your brother teased you," and "I was impressed with the way you were able to set aside your video games without complaining when it was time for you to set the table" are all examples of ways you can reinforce effective use of executive skills. This will be discussed in more detail in Chapter 7.

2. **Debrief.** This means discussing the situation with your child to problem solve for a different outcome the next time. Start with getting your child's description and perspective on what happened, and if he left something out that you thought contributed to the problem, ask about that. For example, if he says, "I bumped into Tonya, and she dropped her snack; it was an accident," you might say, "OK, Dom, it was an accident. When you ran into the kitchen, do you think that might be why you bumped into her?" "I don't know, maybe." "Well, what's our rule when you're inside the house?" "Walk; don't run." "Yeah, so let's try to work on that to avoid accidents. Also, Tonya was pretty upset. Maybe if you accidentally bump into someone, you could say you're sorry and help them pick up?" "I guess so." "Good. Thanks for talking with me about this." In this case you've reviewed the problem, then listened to your child's view of it, and what might be done differently the next time. This strategy needs to be used judiciously. If emotions are running high right after the situation, debriefing should be done sometime after the incident when the involved parties are calm enough to hear and process the information. We've known parents concerned about their children's difficulty making friends who felt they needed to debrief after every social encounter. This had the effect of heightening their child's anxiety around social contacts rather than helping her learn ways of connecting with other kids. When it *is* used judiciously, however, debriefing can be "the teachable moment."

3. **Consult with others who are involved in the situation.** This might mean asking for feedback from a spouse who observed the event and might be able to offer useful insight into what happened. Or it might mean making a suggestion to a babysitter about how to handle the situation differently next time. In other words, consulting with others can give you the opportunity to change your own behavior or make suggestions to others for changing what they do to make things go more smoothly the next time.

4. **Respond constructively to errors and failure.** As we've said, errors and failures are an expected and necessary part of a child's learning and development. Children are naturally inclined to explore their environment, test out their skills, and manage their own behaviors. How we respond can encourage or discourage their learning. Sometimes parents try to protect their children by controlling the environment and trying to eliminate the chance of errors or failure, or by coming to the child's rescue so they don't fail. In so doing, they remove the opportunity for the child to bounce back on their own and learn from their mistakes. Sometimes parents criticize or punish their child for mistakes. Criticism and punishment alone tell the child they have done something wrong but

not how to change the behavior. Research indicates that criticism and punishment are not effective tools for lasting behavior change and can adversely affect your relationship with your child. They also can lead your child to avoid activities or to lie or hide problems they may need help with. We're not suggesting that there be no consequences for children's behaviors or that parents never react or get upset. What we are suggesting is that you work with your child to come up with a corrective action that addresses the current issue and that they can use in the future should the problem occur again. In the example in item 2 in this list, Dom's mother approached the problem in this way. Does it mean the problem won't happen again? Maybe not, but for both Dom and his mother it represents an opportunity to either prevent the problem or learn a corrective action. More about this in Chapter 7 when we discuss rules and consequences in detail.

As we said at the outset, modifying the environment does not require the child to instantly learn a new skill. However, many of the strategies we've described will, over time, help children internalize and use strategies that will aid the development of their own executive skills. In some cases, time and patience may be all that's needed. How do you decide? If there is evidence that your child is making steady progress and becoming more independent, it's reasonable to wait. If, on the other hand, your child continues to struggle in spite of modifications you have put in place, the next step is to combine skill instruction and motivational strategies with environmental modifications. You'll read about these interventions and their application starting in the next chapter and then throughout Part III.

6

Teaching Executive Skills Directly

B *Is for* Behavior

Laila, age 8, moved at a snail's pace in the morning. Getting ready on time required a litany of prompts from her mother at each step of the morning routine: "Laila, get dressed, finish your breakfast, brush your teeth, get your backpack." Sometimes it even took direct help with Mom picking out Laila's clothes and watching her till she was dressed. While she was working from home, her mother could afford the time to do this, although it was a source of frustration for both she and Laila. Recently, Laila's mother had taken a new job that required her to be in the office, so she no longer had the time to manage Laila's routine on top of her own. A series of ugly mornings brought things to a head, and she and Laila sat down one night after dinner. "Honey, I feel like mornings aren't working for either of us. Would you be willing to work with me on a plan to help mornings go better?" Laila said she would. "What do you think might help you get ready?" "I could make a list of what I need to do." "Great idea. "Do you want to use words or pictures or both?" "Both—can we take pictures of me?" "Sure, you can decide on the pictures."

They made a list, with Laila choosing the order of activities and pictures of herself doing each activity, which they finished with laminating sheets. Mom offered the option of a Velcro schedule with two columns—To Do and Done—so Laila could move the pictures after completing each activity, or a check box beside each picture. Laila chose the check box because it was more "grownup." Laila chose a place in her bedroom to post the schedule and put a second one in the kitchen. Her mom suggested that maybe they could pick out her clothes and get her backpack ready the night before since both could slow the process in the morning, and Laila agreed. On her own, Laila proposed an evening schedule with these two items plus tooth brushing and story time, so they made that schedule also. That left two issues in the morning, waking up and time management. Since getting up was not an issue for Laila, her mother agreed to keep waking her. For time management Laila suggested that her mom could tell her how much time she had left, but Mom said she wanted to avoid nagging, which neither of them liked. Mom suggested that maybe Laila could use her own timer to keep track. Laila wasn't sure, but when one of the options Mom offered was for Laila to use the Time Timer app on her mom's phone, Laila was on board. They downloaded the app, and Laila practiced setting it for each activity with her mom's help. It took a few days to get everything ready, and they did a couple of dry runs in the evening to work out any bugs. After a few days of reminders from her mom to check her schedule, Laila was off and running and feeling understandably proud of herself.

Chapter 5 focused on ways to modify the environment (the antecedents) to reduce the impact of executive skills challenges. That's often the easiest, first step to tackle the problems associated with executive skills. While they're particularly appropriate for the younger kids like Laila, they also can work well for older children. But not all environmental interventions are portable. For example, you can manage the social interaction environment in your own home or at some social events like parties, if you are present, as Tara's parents did. Or you can create schedules and prompts like Laila and her mother did. But at school, a friend's home, or social events without you, it's unlikely that the same modifications will be available. Since you can't ensure environmental modifications in all the situations your children will encounter outside the home, they will need their own repertoire of executive skills and strategies that are portable.

That means working together with your children to help them develop better-functioning executive skills. There are two different ways to help your child improve executive skills:

1. You can do so naturally and informally in the following ways:

   - Through activities of daily living—self-care, cooking, cleaning, shopping, banking, social events, and the like.
   - By providing children with experiences to explore and expand their interests—say, travel, or visits to playgrounds, zoos, museums, aquariums, and nature centers.
   - Through play, both free play as well as cards and board games, physical games, and sports, music, singing, and dance.

2. You can take a more targeted approach and work with your child on how to manage certain problematic tasks involving executive skills that you know your child lacks to some degree.

We'll explain how to use both approaches in this chapter. Many parents do in fact choose to do both. Research shows that participation in activities of daily living, play, and exploration of the environment have value in developing executive skills. As we've noted, children are intrinsically motivated by a desire for self-determination and the ability to make their own choices and manage their own behavior. Self-determination requires three elements—competence, autonomy, and connectedness. Participating in daily living activities, play, and exploration helps children build a sense of competence and autonomy and establish a sense of connectedness with parents and peers. At the same time, these activities enhance a range of executive skills including attention, inhibitory control, self-awareness, and working memory.

While informal approaches are an excellent tool for developing executive skills, they don't specifically address situations that may be troublesome for children (such as task initiation with room cleaning, emotional control with peers). These may require a more targeted approach that involves a specific intervention for that situation. We'll explain the steps in that approach following the informal learning discussion.

Developing Executive Skills Informally

Activities of Daily Living

What's the most effective way for children of all ages to acquire new skills? Through scaffolding. Scaffolding is a powerful instructional strategy in which parents (or teachers) provide support for children to enhance learning and mastery of new tasks. It is a bridge to independence. As such, it is a model for the role that parents will play throughout their child's development, gradually fading their support as their child demonstrates competence and mastery of new skills. In your parenting role, it's likely that you are already familiar with the practice of scaffolding, if not the term. When your child was learning to walk, you provided support, holding her hands as she took those first, unsteady steps. Over time, as she progressed in supporting her weight, you held one hand and then kept your hands inches away, eventually fading your support as she mastered walking and then running. You probably followed a similar process for climbing, bike riding, swimming, and other skills. While this was happening, your child was also watching all the other activities you were doing—cooking, cleaning, shopping, fixing things, interacting with people—and you noticed that in their own play they sometime imitated your actions and those of others. In these activities, learning new skills and imitating your actions, you see their desire for competence, mastery, and relatedness. Your child wants to be like you, able to do what you do, on their own.

Just as scaffolding has been an effective strategy in helping your child master physical skills, it has great value in helping your child learn and eventually master the multistep tasks of daily living. The payoff for you and your child is twofold. They practice and acquire the range of executive skills that are embedded in these tasks and gradually develop self-sufficiency in a set of life skills that they will need for independent living. Moreover, the executive skills your child develops can serve as a template that can be applied to accomplish other, real-world tasks.

There are a few important considerations to keep in mind if these activities are to be effective in promoting executive skills:

• *You have to be an active and available participant to model the skills, give directions or ask key questions, and encourage the child.* In other words, you need to be a good frontal lobe. Think of these as collaborative learning opportunities where you provide a degree of support that will decrease as your child becomes more skilled.

• *The child must have some legitimate choices and decision-making power in the activity.* That means that before you enlist your child's support, you should present choices that you can live with. For example, if it's cooking and your child gets to choose what she wants to cook, offer options you are comfortable with. If it's shopping and he gets to choose the snack foods, make sure the choices are snacks you want in the house. Depending on the task, you might also give her a choice of what part of the task she wants to do, like stirring, pouring, or putting ingredients in.

• *Be prepared to accurately gauge your child's interest, attention span, and endurance and provide enough support to enable him to be successful in and appreciated for whatever job he does.* To help with attention and interest, let your child know, a little in advance if possible, you would appreciate his help in deciding what to cook and put on the shopping list. Pick a time when your child is not already engaged in some other activity of interest and ask if it's a good time. For younger children especially, keep the activity short, the choices concrete, and at the first sign of fading attention or lack of interest, thank the child and end it. Later, when the choice has been acted on, acknowledge it to family, friends, or whoever else is around ("Ashley chose the dessert and helped make it!").

Let's take cooking as an example. This can be as simple as making a peanut butter sandwich or more involved like brownies or homemade pizza. The opportunity to do something with you and demonstrate the child's own competence and mastery is intrinsically motivating. Starting with foods that your child likes and that they can enjoy when the task is done provides additional motivation. Effective scaffolding for daily living tasks involves three components—modeling the physical aspects of the task, verbally describing what you are doing, and giving your child the opportunity to actively participate right away. They can be involved in helping you gather the ingredients and utensils needed, pouring, measuring, mixing, or any other option you are comfortable with. Over time you can move on to other foods as their skills improve. At more advanced stages, recipes become a form of scaffolding that increase independence. While other daily living tasks—self-care, cleaning, shopping—may not be quite as appealing as cooking, scaffolding can be equally effective since it capitalizes on the child's intrinsic desire for mastery, independence, and being "grownup" like you. Keep in mind also that tools we've already mentioned—picture and written schedules, checklists, timers—are scaffolding techniques that give your child ownership of the task. In Chapter 9 we provide scaffolding strategies for a variety of daily routines.

While scaffolding is well suited for daily living skills, it is applicable for any new activity or task that you introduce or that your child has an interest in learning. The strategy for new activities that have an action component remains the same—you model the action, describe what you are doing or sensing, and let your child try it. For younger children, you can use it for activities like painting, puzzles, dressing, building things, tooth brushing, and using playground equipment. It can be used as well as for activities that involve observation or sensory skills like looking at pictures or objects, tasting foods, listening to sounds, and touching objects. For older children, we use it to help children learn more complex skills like banking and money management, making appointments, babysitting, and eventually driving, among others.

Not all scaffolding involves physical demonstration. Verbal scaffolding enhances language development in children and is a primary means for them to acquire and remember information—facts, ideas, concepts, emotions, and experiences. Research shows that children whose parents employ "verbal scaffolding" with them at age 3 tend to have better problem-solving skills and goal-directed behavior (that is, executive skills) at age 6 than children whose parents don't use this technique.

What do we mean by *verbal scaffolding?* Providing explanations and guidance and asking questions at an appropriate developmental level for the child. It's actually another way of saying *provide just enough support necessary for the child to be on a path to success*, with an emphasis on helping children understand relationships, make connections between concepts, or connect new learning to prior knowledge. The more skillfully children can do all these things—see patterns, make connections, and draw on past knowledge—the easier it is for them to create plans or organizational schemes. Even more directly, these skills form the underpinning of *metacognition*, that more complex executive skill that involves using thought in the service of problem solving and self-appraisal. The more extensive the background knowledge children have and the more practice they've had building up that knowledge and connecting new information to known information, the easier it will be for them to access that information and use it for different purposes, including making plans, organizing material, and solving problems.

Verbal scaffolding is a strategy that parents often apply intuitively with younger children, perhaps because the rewards are so immediately evident. Seeing the pride on the face of a 2- or 3-year-old as she points to pictures of animals you name while you look at a book together or holds up the correct number of fingers when asked how old she is just naturally makes us want to use this type of scaffolding. However, as children become more independent and parents try to get more done in less time, verbal scaffolding can take a back seat, often to children's screen time with TV and computers. If you find yourself in that bind, keep in mind that verbal scaffolding can be used in a variety of contexts over the course of the day—when getting dressed in the morning, at the dinner table, remarking on things you see on the drive to school or daycare, when watching TV, and in the context of the kinds of play activities your child enjoys.

The more you can help children think about what they do and why—or think about the consequences associated with some actions and behaviors—the more they will be able to use that thinking in any problem-solving situation. Children who understand how certain events trigger certain feelings are more likely to gain control over their emotions or curtail their impulses. The more they understand a cause-and-effect sequence, the better they'll be able to plan a course of action. And when you explain why something is important, your children are more likely to remember that critical information when they need it. Of course, explanations alone are generally insufficient to help children acquire better-functioning executive skills—but instruction that lacks explanation is unlikely to be very effective.

Some other verbal scaffolding ways to infuse executive skill instruction into activities of daily living are as follows:

• *Explain instead of dictating.* Sometimes parents rely on direct commands and explicit instructions. We understand. Parents are busy, and there are situations when efficient movement by your child is what's needed. When you're trying to get kids out for school in the morning or get to an appointment on time, action, not explanation or negotiation, is the priority. When, "I need you to get your shoes on!" is met by "Why?" it's understandable that "Just do what I say!" or "Because I said so!" is your response. You feel you don't have the time or energy to craft an explanation, and even if you did, it is not a guarantee to action. And let's face it, sometimes "Why?" is a stall tactic. Situations that present inherent risks also prompt direct commands—hot stoves or objects, busy streets, jumping or falling from heights. While explicit directions or direct commands may seem more efficient or necessary in some situations, they are less likely to foster the development of executive skills than an approach that emphasizes the reason for something. The more your child understands about a given situation—cause and effect, why something is important, why something needs to be done in a certain way—the more likely he is to incorporate the information into his thinking and actions. Cause-and-effect explanations are a source of motivation if the child desires the outcome. "If you take your medication, your throat will feel better" or "If you put your bike in the garage, it will stay dry and won't rust." Explanations are essentially a verbal form of modeling. They also set the stage for helping children understand there are consequences for avoiding actions (sore throat, rusty bike). Explanations largely build the skill of metacognition, but they enhance working memory too. We remember things better when we have a reason for remembering.

• *Ask rather than tell.* Questions are a good way to get information about what a child understands as well as how they think about solving a problem. "Why do you think your sister was angry with you?" "What could you do to help her feel better?" "How do you think you could remember to give your teacher the permission slip?" If children are unable to propose solutions for these situations, you can provide scaffolding by offering a set of options and letting them choose one that fits. Questions encourage self-appraisal. "How do you think you did on your Scout project?" or "How did you do at soccer practice?" When children are going to engage in potentially challenging activities (like a presentation in class or a music recital) or when a planned event is changed (a friend cancels a play date), your questions, such as "How are you feeling about . . . ?" give you an understanding of your child's feelings as well as a chance to let her know you understand: "You're disappointed because you really wanted to play with Maya today."

Think about your questions and your child's responses as a way to understand and appreciate how they see their experiences. With their words, they are painting a picture of their view of the world.

Exploration in Community Settings

Learning opportunities that are self-directed, experiential in a hands-on way, and rich in content are known to enhance executive skills in children. That means that children's museums, nature centers, science museums, aquariums, libraries, and zoos, especially those that offer hands-on opportunities, are ideal environments for children to expand their interests and test out their skills. By actively participating with them, you can model and describe what to do if they are unsure as well as comment and ask questions about what they choose to do. In most cases, staff in these venues also are readily available to model and provide information. Equally significant in these settings is the ready availability of peers who present your child with opportunities for social interaction as well as learning new skills by observing and modeling the actions of other children.

A word about scaffolding and your role in these experiences, particularly with younger children: In Chapter 1 we discussed tools you can use to help your child develop executive skills. Modeling was one of them. Another was "serve and return," a way to interact with your children that encourages exploration of their choices and interests by attending closely to what your children are doing and actively engaging with them on their terms. The goal in these settings is self-directed learning. That doesn't mean you shouldn't suggest things for your child to see or try. What is does mean is that if they are not interested in your suggestion or have something they are more interested in, you should follow their lead and engage on their terms. This ensures that the experience is stimulating and enjoyable for them and that they will want to return and explore more.

Play

Extensive research shows that unstructured play enhances the development of executive skills. Unstructured play is defined as play that doesn't have a predetermined purpose or outcome and is not organized or structured by adults. When children engage in unstructured play, they are free to explore, create new experiences, and discover their world without preset rules, guidelines, and expectations. In addition to promoting social–emotional relationships, cognitive and language skills, physical development, and self-regulation, active play reduces toxic stress. Ideally, children would spend at least 2 hours each day in unstructured play and one of these hours in active outdoor play.

In fact, however, the trend for this generation of children has been in the opposite direction—that is, a decrease in unstructured play and more time in front of screens and in scheduled, structured activities. For example, it is estimated that American children, ages 5–7 years, average more than 3 hours of screen time per day and children 8–12 years average 5 or more hours of screen time per day. While screen time can have benefits (learning new information and skills), too much can lead to problems with socialization, sleep, behavior, and physical development, most notably obesity. For structured activities (sports, music, and dance lessons, for example) in children 3–12 years, it is estimated on average they spend 5 hours per week. It is worth noting that research indicates that neither screen time nor structured activities offer the same benefits for cognitive and social development and executive skills as does unstructured play.

We want to be clear here. Unstructured does not necessarily mean unsupervised. Depending on your child's age, their ability to follow limits, and the risks inherent in the setting—traffic, type of neighborhood, body of water, playground equipment—you may need to be outside to observe and ensure their safety. That said, your role is observation, not direction. If they want you to engage with them, the "serve and return" principle applies, where they lead and you follow. If your living situation limits the options for outdoor play, consider playgrounds (indoors and outdoors) as well as the community settings noted above as options for unstructured play.

Games

Games are another natural, informal way to help children develop executive skills. Classic games like checkers, Chinese checkers, and chess require planning, sustained attention, response inhibition, working memory, and metacognition, among others. The simplest of board games like Candyland require attention, response inhibition, and goal-directed persistence for young children, while games like Monopoly and Clue additionally involve planning and working memory. Battleship requires attention, planning, inhibition, and metacognition. Holding family game nights and encouraging your child to play such games with siblings and friends is always a good idea. You also can build executive skills with time-honored games like tic tac toe, hangman, and twenty questions when you're waiting in the doctor's office, taking a car trip, or waiting for your order at a restaurant.

Given the ever-present availability of computers, tablets, and smart phones, many kids find video games more appealing than the board games more familiar to parents and grandparents. In Chapter 22 we mention a few representative examples that help build executive skills. Most fall into some type of strategy/problem-solving category.

Direct Interventions for Teaching Executive Skills

All the informal approaches discussed so far can be very helpful to your child, but chances are, if you've picked up this book and read this far, you have a child with specific skill challenges that require a more direct intervention. What follows is an instructional sequence that can be used for addressing all kinds of behaviors (not just the ones we're focusing on in this book). It forms the framework for the interventions we've designed for specific routine tasks in Chapter 9 and for designing your own approaches aimed at particular executive skills in Chapters 10–20.

Step 1: Identify the Problem Behavior You Want to Work On

This may sound easier than it is. The more frustrated you are with your child, the more likely you are to refer to problem behaviors in global terms that do not describe specific actions. When we say a child is *messy, unmotivated, impulsive, distractible,* the words do communicate something about the child, but they really don't give us a starting point for addressing the issue. Helpful descriptions are those that depict specific behaviors that can be seen or heard and identify when or under what circumstances the behaviors occur. Here are some examples:

- Complains and procrastinates when it's time to do homework.
- Completes chores only when someone's there to repeatedly remind him.
- Leaves personal belongings all over the house.
- Tantrums whenever he loses a game.

Why is it important to define the problem behavior? Because it helps clarify, for you and your child, what you're going to address and where you're going to start. Teaching someone to be neat and tidy in life sounds like a huge undertaking. Teaching a child to pick up his personal belongings off the living room floor is a more achievable goal. Which brings us to the next step in the instructional sequence.

Step 2: Set a Goal

The goal, very often, is a positive restatement of the problem behavior. A goal says what the child is expected to do using terms that describe behaviors that can be seen or heard. Using the problem behaviors described above, the goals might be as follows:

- Starts homework without meltdown and requests help if stuck.
- Completes chores on time independently.
- Takes personal belongings out of living room before going to bed.
- Accepts outcome of game without a meltdown.

We have chosen these behaviors as examples because they are among those that parents have reported as sources of conflict with children. You may well have others— room cleaning, A.M. and P.M. routines, timely exits from home, and so forth. As you've have seen from examples already presented throughout this book, problem situations typically involve executive skill struggles of one kind or another. When a behavior is an ongoing source of frustration or conflict, a successful plan contributes to family harmony, encourages collaborative problem solving, and enhances executive skills.

Involve Your Child in Goal Setting

It's important to involve children in the goal-setting process from the outset rather than dictating to them what we expect them to do. This idea falls right in line with the scaffolding discussion earlier in this chapter: anything that encourages participation, decision making, and independent, critical thinking fosters executive skills. It also contributes to a collaborative relationship and increases the likelihood of buy-in from your child since they have ownership in the plan. In the scenario that began this chapter, Laila's mother sat down with her and discussed the problem. She enlisted her help in recognizing that the problem was real and keeping both of them from having a smooth start to the day. In their discussion, she let Laila take the lead and went along with some but not all of Laila's suggestions. In addressing a problem situation with your own child, be open-minded about their suggestions. If what they say is feasible, run with it, even if you think you have a better way. You can revisit parts that aren't working. But if you're not comfortable with some aspect, explain why and offer an alternative, as Laila's mother did with the suggestion that she be the timekeeper. Keep in mind that this is a process, and the eventual goal is the child independently handling the task.

Set Interim Goals

Determining the final outcome is important to the skill-learning process, but you won't always get there right away. So you may have to set and accept interim goals along the way. Completing the morning routine without reminders may be the final goal, but in the early stages you may need to start with a goal of completing the routine with no more than three reminders.

How do you know what a reasonable interim goal is? Ideally you take a baseline—you measure the current behavior and set as a first interim goal something that's a slight improvement on the current behavior. So if you find that it generally takes five or six reminders for your daughter to complete her morning routine, maybe getting started with no more than three or four reminders is a reasonable first step.

When we say "measure the current behavior," we really do mean *measure*. In the example above, we mean *count* the number of times the behavior occurs. Examples of ways to measure are listed here:

• **Time how long it takes between the time a child says she will start something and the time she actually starts** (as in "Sarah has agreed to start her homework every night at 7:00. Before putting in place an intervention, her mother times her for a week to see how much later than 7:00 she actually begins").

• **Time how long something lasts** (as in "Joey chose to play trumpet and says he will spend 20 minutes every day practicing. His mother's not sure about this, so she measures how long he actually practices so she has some data to point to when she talks with him about their agreement").

• **Count the number of times the behavior occurs.** This could either be positive behaviors (as in the number of days your child remembered to start homework at 7:00 P.M.) or problem behaviors (as in the number of meltdowns your 4-year-old has in the course of a day). If the number of behaviors is relatively small, you can count them all day long. If the behavior occurs frequently, then choose a part of the day to focus on (as in the number of complaints your child utters in the hour before dinner).

• *Count the number of reminders you need to give your child before she does what you've asked her to do.*

• *Create a 5-point scale and rate the severity of the problem behavior.* If your son has a problem managing stress or anxiety, a 5-point scale to measure his anxiety level that you and he could use might look like the following:

1—I'm doing fine.
2—I'm getting a little worried.
3—Now I'm nervous.
4—I'm feeling really upset.
5—I might lose control!

For further suggestions on how to use a 5-point scale, we recommend the book *The Incredible 5-Point Scale* by Kari Dunn Buron and Mitzi Curtis.

These kinds of baseline data are often most useful when you can display the results visually. An example of this can be seen in the graph below.

If taking a baseline and setting precise goals are more than you want to attempt, though, you should shoot for "some improvement" as an interim goal. As time goes on, if you think you're not getting that improvement, you may want to back up and consider taking some more precise measures, so you know for sure whether that's the case.

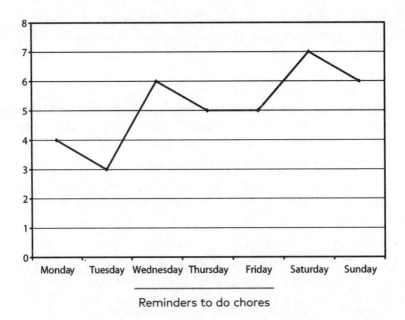

Reminders to do chores

Step 3: Outline the Steps the Child Needs to Follow to Reach the Goal

In Part III we provide lots of examples of this, using the kinds of problem situations that parents say are the most frustrating. But returning to Laila, she and her mother made a picture list of the different tasks she had to do before leaving the house to catch the school bus in the morning. Other skills, like learning to manage emotions, control impulses, or handle frustration, may be a little more challenging to think about using this procedure, but, again, we'll give you examples of how this might work in Part III.

Step 4: Turn the Steps into a List, a Checklist, or a Short Set of Rules to Follow

This accomplishes several things. First of all, it helps you and your child think clearly, logically, and succinctly about the skill she's trying to learn. Second, it creates a record of the instructional sequence that you and your child can refer to so she can remember the process. Third, by checking off each item in the list, your child has the satisfaction of recording progress toward a goal. Checking off items as they are completed provides intermediate reinforcers on the road to the larger goal (task completion or a reward that may come with task completion). Finally, it builds in self-accountability—it's a way of documenting that the child is actually successful in making progress toward or accomplishing his goal.

Laila and her mother made a picture schedule for Laila to follow, but another way to deal with helping children follow morning routines might be to create a checklist such as the one shown on the next page.

This checklist includes a column where you can tally how many reminders each step in the sequence required. This would be useful in situations where the biggest source of frustration to you is the number of reminders your child requires to get through her morning routine. After a week of using a checklist like this, progress will be readily apparent—as will the trouble spots (that is, which steps in the sequence require the greatest number of reminders). A copy of this checklist is included in Chapter 9. A blank general-purpose checklist is also included at the end of this chapter for those of you who want to create your own checklist to cover the particular skill sequence you want to teach.

Before we leave this step, let's talk about a different kind of skill we want to teach children. Let's say 12-year-old Arjun has a problem with emotional control. It shows up in lots of different situations, but what drives his dad crazy is how quickly he melts down when he encounters an obstacle during homework. It can happen for almost any kind of homework, but his dad has noticed that math seems to be the worst. He decides to talk to Arjun about better ways of managing his frustration around math. Arjun's father knows from experience that having this conversation in the middle of a meltdown is not likely to go well, so he waits until the end of a homework session that went smoothly for Arjun. He starts the conversation with his son by remarking on how well

Task	Number of reminders/ tally marks (////)	Done (✓)
Morning Routine Checklist		
Get up		
Get dressed		
Eat breakfast		
Put dishes in dishwasher		
Brush teeth		
Brush hair		
Get backpack ready for school		
Other:		
Other:		

From *Smart but Scattered, Second Edition*, by Peg Dawson, Richard Guare, and Colin Guare. Copyright © 2025 The Guilford Press. Permission to photocopy this material, or to download enlarged printable versions (*www.guilford.com/dawson4-forms*), is granted to purchasers of this book for personal use; see copyright page for details.

this session went compared to some others and asks Arjun why this might be. Arjun says, "Yeah, I knew exactly what to do. I remembered the way Mr. Frank told us how to do the homework. I get mad when I can't remember—or when I think I remember but it doesn't work out right."

Arjun's dad asks him if he knows before he even starts that the homework's going to be a problem or if it's only once he's started working. Arjun says, "Both—but what really makes me mad is when I thought I could do it but then I couldn't."

With a lot of sympathy and what psychologists call "reflective listening" (mirroring back the child's feelings, as in "That makes you so mad you want to throw your math book against the wall") Arjun's father was able to get Arjun to consider whether there were things he could do to help him manage the frustration more successfully. Arjun finally agreed that when he felt himself getting mad during math homework, he would do two things. First he would walk away from the problem for a few minutes. Quite literally—he agreed to get up from the desk in his bedroom and walk downstairs to the family room, where he was likely to find his dad working on his computer. If clearing his head didn't resolve the problem for him (and Arjun admitted that doing that sometimes helped him remember how to do the work), then Arjun agreed to ask his dad for help. The rules for managing math could be boiled down to two words: *walk* and *talk*. His dad took an index card and wrote on it:

```
┌─────────────────────────────────┐
│      Math Lifeline              │
│  1. Walk                        │
│  2. Talk (Ask for help)         │
└─────────────────────────────────┘
```

He taped the index card to Arjun's desk as a reminder.

If you or your child are not comfortable with your being the homework helper, there are a variety of homework helplines, many of them free, that provide homework help to students. In some situations, this may be preferable since it encourages choice and control by your child. In addition, it avoids potential conflict between you and your child about the effectiveness of your help.

Step 5: Rehearse and Support the Procedure with Your Child

Designing a procedure with your child that you both are comfortable with is an essential starting point. But it is just that—a starting point. You should expect that your child will need more than a single exposure to the steps involved to master the skill on her own. Children (like adults) require ongoing support and supervision as they learn a new skill. Expecting in advance that you'll need to provide support as a matter of course will help you have the patience to see the process through.

We recommend beginning this step by holding a practice session or two—what might be called a rehearsal or "dry run." Once Laila and her mom finished the preparation, her mom suggested that they try it out, and Laila agreed. She lay in bed as if sleeping, and her mother came in and said, "Laila, time to get up." Laila got up, went to her schedule, pretended to get dressed, and checked it off. Laila moved on to the remaining steps of breakfast and self-care. After this they also practiced the evening schedule of getting clothes and backpack ready. They agreed to do one more practice run the next night and then start. For the first week, her mom agreed to remind her about using the schedule. After 3 days, Laila wanted to manage it on her own and did so on her own going forward.

Arjun had no interest in a literal "walk-through" of the frustration management plan. On the edge of adolescence, Arjun thought that kind of role play was "dumb." He was, however, willing to do a mental rehearsal or "dry run" of the plan. His dad started: "OK, you're in your room starting your math homework problems and bang, you stop! What's the roadblock?" "I can't remember how to do the problem." "Then what usually happens?" "I get really ticked off, holler, maybe slam the book down." "Does it help you?" "Not really." His dad continued, "OK, same starting scenario but with your plan. When you look at the math problem, stop, and start to feel frustrated you . . . ?" "Walk downstairs to calm down, see if I think I can do it. If so, I go back to it. If not, I'll ask you for help." His dad asked if he wanted a reminder before he started homework. Arjun said maybe for a few days, so each night before homework for the first week his dad asked, "If you get stuck, what's the plan?" and Arjun told him. The first time he used the plan and it worked, he told his dad the mental run-through helped. After a few days Arjun waved off the reminders. They both noticed that he started using the same process for other frustrating homework.

Step 6: Fade the Supervision

This is basically a reiteration of the last two principles described in Chapter 4. You want to provide support for enough time to ensure that your child has acquired the skill or has reached a point that he no longer needs your support. The most effective way to accomplish that is to gradually fade the support as you see continued, independent progress. Your availability for support means that if your child stumbles, you can step back in long enough to help them resume momentum. It means you also can work with your child to modify steps that would improve the plan if you and your child are not getting the desired outcome.

Keep in mind that the work you've done in Steps 1–5 above can play a significant role in determining the amount of support you will need to provide on an ongoing basis. Ask yourself these questions:

- Is the goal specific, with limited, clearly defined steps?
- Are you and your child in agreement that the goal addresses a problem that involves both of you?
- Does your child have an active role in choices about how the plan is designed?
- Together, have you developed supports (checklists, schedules, cue cards, timers, and so on) that your child can use in your absence?
- Have you rehearsed the plan and worked out any bugs?

In the examples involving Laila and Arjun, both plans were front-end loaded to address these questions. The support needed from Laila's mom and Arjun's dad came in the form of reminders to initiate the plan, which both parents were able to fade over time. How do you know when to fade the reminders? There are a couple of options. If your child has had multiple days completing the plan with reminders, ask them if they would like to try it on their own. If they are not successful for a couple of days, resume the reminders. You can also fade reminders by moving from a statement (*Check your schedule.*) to a question (*What do you need to do?*). If the plan has multiple steps like Laila's, Mom may need to remind her at each new step. For some children the plan may need to be simplified, starting with a single step and adding each new step when the first is mastered. In Chapter 5 Caleb's parents did this to help him manage room cleaning. In the daily routines chapter (Chapter 9) and the individual skills chapters (Chapters 10–20), you'll see more fading examples.

Let's put the whole process together using as an example another very common childhood responsibility: room cleaning. Much as it takes time for language to develop in children, it also takes time for them to learn how to clean their rooms independently. In the beginning, parents who decide to work with their children on room cleaning use their own frontal lobes to help the child with a plan. And what do frontal lobes do?

- They help the child develop an organizational scheme and a plan.
- They provide options for the child to monitor performance.
- They provide encouragement/motivation and feedback about the success of the approach.
- They help the child problem solve when something doesn't work.
- They help the child determine when the task is completed.

Room cleaning typically starts with a place to store belongings. Chances are you have already created a basic organizational scheme (laundry basket, bookshelf, container for toys) in your child's room. If that step is covered, your role in the room-cleaning process depends in part on your child's age. The younger you start, the easier it will be for your child to build the habit and move toward independence over time.

Thus, stage 1 in teaching room cleaning is usually parent initiated and guided. Here are ways parents might approach the task with children of different ages:

- If you start with your toddler, you will take the lead using modeling and verbal scaffolding. While demonstrating, you say, "When we/you take your clothes off, we put them in the laundry basket like this." After modeling this behavior, you can give your child the next piece of clothing, walk with them to the laundry basket, and prompt them to put it in. Toddlers are good at modeling, so if you hand them the next piece of modeling, they may do it on their own or may need a prompt. If so, gradually fade the prompt and let them do more. Once they have this down, you can move on to toys and books.

- If your child is of preschool age (3–5), you can follow a similar procedure. It's likely a verbal prompt will be enough, but if not, you can model it. Another option is to give them a choice about what to start with (clothes, books, or toys?). With school-age children (like Caleb in Chapter 5), giving them as much control as possible through their choices is preferable—what to start with, where to store belongings, timers, and so on. Some children are particular about how to organize storage for particular toys (building materials, dolls, action figures, sports equipment), so this is another choice point for them. For children who struggle with executive skills involved in room cleaning, it's helpful to break the task into smaller steps and move on to the next as the child masters one step.

At stage 2 the same information is provided without the parent being the direct agent. Together the child and parent create a picture schedule, a list, or an audiotape as a prompt for the child. With younger children, toddler through preschool, picture schedules are preferred by them, particularly if pictures are taken of them carrying out the step. Parents prompt by saying, "Let's look at your schedule." It is also helpful if you take a picture of the room when the child has finished, so she has an example to work from.

At stage 3 parents step back a little more. Rather than tell the child to look at the schedule, they may say, "What do you need to do?" By asking rather than telling, and making the questions somewhat vague, they encourage the child to problem solve on his own (or at least retrieve from his own working memory what needs to happen next).

At stage 4 the transfer is now complete. The child may wake up on Saturday morning, look around his messy room, and say to himself, "What do I need to do?" Of course by now the child may actually be a teenager or a young adult! Sometimes it takes a long time for children to internalize this kind of process.

Take heart. Kids do learn—and the process may speed up (or at least stay on track) if they are motivated. That's the subject of the next chapter.

Steps for Designing a Direct Intervention to Teach Executive Skills

1. Identify the behavior issue you want to work on.

2. Together with your child, set a goal you both agree on, including interim goals if it needs to be broken down.

3. With your child, outline the steps to follow to reach the goal.

4. Turn the steps into a picture or written schedule, list, or whatever else your child prefers.

5. Monitor/supervise the procedure in the early stages to help problem solve or make changes.

6. Fade the supervision.

Checklist

Task	Number of reminders/ tally marks (////)	Done (✓)

From *Smart but Scattered, Second Edition*, by Peg Dawson, Richard Guare, and Colin Guare. Copyright © 2025 The Guilford Press. Permission to photocopy this material, or to download enlarged printable versions (*www.guilford.com/dawson4-forms*), is granted to purchasers of this book for personal use; see copyright page for details.

7

Motivating Your Child to Learn and Use Executive Skills

C *Is for* Consequence

Mara, age 5, likes to help her dad and is learning to set the table for dinner. He suggests that they start with one place setting and asks her which person she'd like to start with, and she decides to start with his. To scaffold the task, he says either he can take a picture of the place setting or Mara can trace out the finished setting on a paper placemat. She chooses to trace it. Dad models and verbally describes each step in the place setting. When the place setting is complete, Mara uses a crayon to trace each item. As she is doing this, her dad comments, "Mara, you're doing a nice job carefully tracing on your placemat." When she's finished, Dad puts the items away, and Mara does a practice run with prompts from her dad as needed. As she uses the placemat template to position each item, her dad says, "I can see you're working hard to put each object on your placemat drawing." After they finish, Dad laminates the placemat template, and they practice this routine each day for a few days before dinner. When Mara is successful without prompts, they gradually add each family member until in 2 weeks Mara is setting the table for the whole family.

The opportunity to play a musical instrument was introduced at school. Grady, age 8, tried a couple of different instruments and told his parents he wanted to play trumpet. They are happy to encourage his interest and explain that they are willing to rent an instrument and pay for lessons. Grady's part of the bargain is to commit to the practice schedule that his music teacher recommends. Grady readily agrees and starts lessons twice a week with 20-minute practice sessions four times a week at home. He and his parents agree on a practice schedule, and all is well for the first few weeks. Grady likes his teacher and looks forward to lessons. Consistent practice becomes a different issue, and Grady struggles with task initiation and persistence. His parents find that practice time is increasingly contentious. They wonder if he has lost interest in trumpet, but Grady insists he wants to continue. They discuss this with Grady and agree on a new arrangement. On his music schedule days, Grady will practice trumpet before he uses his 30 minutes of video game time, a "first—then" arrangement. His game time is a high priority, so even though he complains occasionally, he follows the agreement without major pushback.

Since starting middle school, Nia has had an increasing struggle with written assignments, particularly with planning of her work. Her parents have suggested a tutor in the past, but Nia insisted that she wanted to manage it on her own, and they knew that they shouldn't try to force the issue. This year, however, her struggles have increased, and Nia is frustrated to the point that she is avoiding assignments. Her parents and teacher have talked to her about getting extra help in school, but Nia is self-conscious about this, concerned that her friends will think she's "dumb." They again discuss a tutor, but Nia remains reluctant.

Nia has been lobbying for a smart phone for some time now, so her parents float the idea of a phone in exchange for her agreeing to work with a tutor. Nia is open to this idea if she can select the tutor and the phone. Her parents agree, provided Nia is open to parental controls on the phone, and she agrees. Together they identify three tutors in the area who specialize in working with student writing issues. Nia has a brief Zoom meeting with each of the three and selects one to work with. Nia and her parents meet together with the tutor, who outlines her expectations (practice exercises Nia will need to complete) as well as a schedule that she feels will meet Nia's needs. Nia agrees, and together they write a contract specifying the number of sessions she will attend and the expectations for each session. Based on this, they agree on a point value for each session and how many points she will need to earn for her phone. They design a 3-point scale that Nia and her tutor will complete independently at the end of each session with 0 representing a missed appointment, 1 representing partial completion of session expectations, and 2 representing full completion. If there is a discrepancy, the tutor will explain her rating, and that rating will prevail. Missed appointments or practice exercises can be made up within a 2-week window with no point loss. Nia meets the conditions of the contract and gets her phone. She also makes good progress with writing and asks her parents if she can continue, to which they happily agree.

In Chapter 4 we noted that children's innate desire for competence, self-control, and relatedness are powerful intrinsic motivators; and intrinsic motivators are superior to extrinsic motivators in producing lasting behavior change. At the same time, we acknowledged that children, like adults, find some tasks tedious or unappealing and may need an extra boost, an extrinsic motivator, to overcome task avoidance. In this chapter we'll discuss how to decide whether a reward is needed and, if so, what type of reward suits the outcome you want.

Let's start with a brief review of the conditions that need to be in place prior to deciding a reward is needed.

1. *My child knows exactly what is expected.* That means that you've spelled out, in detail, the steps of the task, the time frame or deadline, and the expected outcome, and provided written and/or picture prompts.

2. *My child has the basic skills necessary to complete the task.* That means that the task is developmentally appropriate, and you have taught it using modeling and verbal scaffolding if there are multiple steps. The child has rehearsed the task and demonstrated, at least under supervision, that she understands and can independently complete the task.

3. *The task has been structured to accommodate my child's executive skill challenges.* If you followed Chapter 5 on environmental modifications, you likely have covered this. If your child struggles with organization, you've helped with an organizational structure for the task. If your child has difficulty with time management, together you've worked out time prompts, as Laila and her mom did in Chapter 6.

These conditions are important prerequisites so you know task avoidance is a motivation issue rather than a skill issue. The three scenarios above depict different ways you can use motivational strategies to help your child develop executive skills and complete tasks. Sometimes, as in the case of Mara, it can be as simple as remembering to say something positive about the child's effort. Or, as in the case of Grady, it can mean just ensuring that the child does the have-to before getting to the want-to. Sometimes, we admit, motivational strategies have to be a little more elaborate, as in the case of Nia, where a careful plan and monitoring are required, and the payoff is not already part of the child's preferred activities.

Motivation is important whether you're trying to encourage your child to follow the sequence of rules or steps in an intervention you've both designed or trying to encourage the child to use executive skills already within her behavioral repertoire. Our focus here is mainly on positive consequences, an outcome that the child looks forward to either during or after the task.

Reinforcing Executive Skills and Task Performance with Praise

For children, positive parental attention and appreciation for what they do is essential for healthy development. Knowing specifically what they are being recognized for leads to positive feelings, strengthens the parent–child relationship, and leads to a desire to engage in similar behaviors in the future. However, not all types of praise are equal in their effects on children. There is substantial research support for what is described as "process praise," which means specifically recognizing children for the effort they're making during a task or have made to achieve a result. As in the first scenario above, Mara's dad does this when he says, "I can see you're working hard to put each object on your placemat drawing." This may be as simple as providing praise and recognition.

Parents might say to their 5-year-old, for instance, "You remembered to brush your teeth after breakfast without my having to remind you. That's great!" If you're inclined to believe virtue should be its own reward, remember that we're dealing with kids here. They look forward to your approval, and getting it definitely encourages them to repeat the behavior, so you'll recognize the work they are doing or have done. (Besides, what adult do you know who doesn't appreciate praise for their effort, at least sometimes?)

We've found, in fact, that praise is one of the most underappreciated (and underused) tools for promoting behavior change that parents have at their disposal. Skilled behavior specialists generally recommend that for every corrective statement directed at a child, parents make three positive statements. In practice this is a difficult ratio to reach. Still, it's a goal worth working toward.

We should also point out that some kinds of praise are more effective than others. Global praise ("Good work!" "Nice job!") is less effective than more specific praise that is individualized to the child and to the behavior being reinforced. The box on page 108 outlines how praise can be delivered most effectively.

When Praise and Encouragement Alone Are Not Enough

Natural consequences and logical consequences can also work to motivate your child.

Natural Consequences

Natural consequences, by definition, are the natural or inevitable outcome of the child's decisions. Their advantage lies in the fact that they require no intervention on the part of the parent and are precursors of many of the reasons we follow rules as adults (paying bills on time, obeying speed limits, exercising, and the like). Some typical examples:

- If you wear your coat outside, you'll be warm.
- If you eat what we're having for dinner, you won't be hungry.
- If you do your homework, you won't have to stay after school to finish it.
- If you keep track of your baseball glove (or whatever belonging the child values), you won't have to buy a new one.

While natural consequences are an effective way to avoid power struggles around some issues, their use is not acceptable under certain conditions:

- When health or safety issues are involved (running into the street, touching hot objects, taking prescribed medication).
- Harm to others, property, animals (hitting others, abusing animals, breaking windows).
- Disrupting activity of others (acting up in, say, a restaurant or children's museum)

Effective Praise . . .

1. Is delivered during or immediately after the positive behavior occurs.

2. Specifies the particulars of the accomplishment ("Good job picking up your toys right away after I asked you") or the effort during the task ("You're working hard to pick up your toys").

3. Provides information to the child about the value of the accomplishment ("When you get ready for school quickly, it makes the morning go so smoothly!").

4. Lets the child know that they're working hard to accomplish the task ("I see that you really trying to control your temper with your brother!").

5. Orients the child to better appreciate their own task-related behavior and think about problem solving ("I like the way you thought about that and tried to figure out a good solution for the problem").

when the consequence involves multiple people, such as the whole family needing to leave the situation.

Additionally, you need to understand the characteristics of your child so you're not subjecting them to a consequence that is an unrealistic expectation. For example, if your child struggles with the executive skill(s) involved in the behavior, it is important that you've addressed the three prerequisites listed above to ensure that you're dealing with a motivational as opposed to a skill issue.

Logical Consequences

Logical consequences are the actions that a parent takes with a child in response to an unacceptable behavior in a situation. They differ from natural consequences in that they are not the inevitable outcome of a child's behavior (as is being cold after refusing to put on a coat). Instead they are implemented by a parent when a child chooses to continue a behavior rather than follow an expectation or a rule that has been set by the parent.

• Seven-year-old Tonya wants to go to a children's museum where a reservation is required. Her dad presents her with time options, and she chooses one. He explains that she will need to be ready on time, so they don't arrive too late for their reservation. The next day, 30 minutes before they need to leave, her dad tells her that if she wants to go, she needs to be dressed by then. He reminds her again in 15 minutes, and at 5 minutes he reminds her one more time and sets a visual timer for her. When the timer goes off, Tonya is still playing with her toys and hasn't dressed. Dad calmly explains that they won't be able to go today but they can try again tomorrow if she is ready on time.

- Eleven-year-old Dom has a new video game. His mother has an established rule that gaming equipment needs to be used in the way for which it was designed. If not, the equipment will be put away. Dom successfully gets through the first level of the game but is not able to get to level 2. Frustrated, he throws the game controller. His mom removes it and says that he can try again tomorrow.

Experts agree that to be effective and fair to the child, logical consequences should be based on the three Rs: relevant, realistic, respectful. *Relevant* means that the consequence has a logical relation to the behavior that the child can understand. In the two examples with Tonya and Dom, the consequences are directly related to the behaviors. *Realistic* means that the behavior and the consequence are in proportion to each other. Tonya and Dom can each try again the next time the opportunity presents itself. Unrealistic consequences would be no museum visits for 3 months or elimination of video games. *Respectful* means that the consequence is stated in a calm, matter-of-fact manner and tone, not as a threat, warning, or punishment. Comments that blame or shame the child ("How could you be so clumsy!" or "You're acting like a 2-year-old!") undermine the intent of the consequence and lead to resentment. Consequences speak for themselves and provide the child with the opportunity to make a different decision that better serves both your child and you.

You can establish rules and logical consequences for a variety of different situations and behaviors:

- Using toys/objects for their intended use and caring for them. If not, fixing or replacing them or removing them for a time.
- Cleaning up (after play, crafts, making food) before moving on to the next play activity.
- Coming home at designated time or coming home earlier the next time.
- Behaving in a socially acceptable manner (at a restaurant, sitting at the table, using inside voice, playing with chosen tabletop activities). If not, leaving the situation for a time and coming back to try again.
- Maintaining safe behavior while driving in a car (sitting in a booster seat, seat belt, inside voice, using chosen objects—books, music, soft toys). If unsafe behavior, driver stops if safely possible.
- Finishing a designated chore before play.

As we've noted for any consequence, positive or negative, before implementing them you need to be sure the task you expect the child to do is developmentally appropriate and within the child's skill repertoire, and explain specifically what behaviors are expected for that situation or task.

Something Fun at the Finish Line

Sometimes there are no obvious natural or logical consequences, or you prefer not to use them because there is an easier path to get to an outcome that satisfies both your child's and your needs. In the example about Grady practicing trumpet, missing or ending the trumpet lessons might be a logical consequence, but it seems somewhat drastic. Instead Grady and his parents agree on a "first—then" solution—first practice and then play video game—and this resolves the issue. This strategy is also known as the Premack principle or "Grandma's law" ("first dinner and then dessert") referred to in Chapter 4. The basic idea is doing something less appealing for the opportunity to do something more appealing. In more technical terms, it *kindles a positive drive state* that helps undermine any negative thoughts or feelings we might have about the task in front of us. In other words, it has an energizing effect.

For this strategy to be effective, there are a few principles to keep in mind. As with any consequence, the payoff needs to be proportional to the task demand. A 2-hour chore for 10 minutes of a video game is not proportional (nor is 1 hour of a video game proportional to a 5-minute chore if your child suggests this). The payoff needs to be some activity that your child values and that you can live with. The task needs to be completed in the way you both agree on, and the payoff needs to come immediately after the task is completed. See the box below for a more effective way to incentivize children to perform tasks.

Wording Incentives as Positives Rather Than Negatives

Children are often told, "If you don't pick up your toys, you can't go out-side to play" or "If you don't load the dishwasher, you can't play your video game." The focus of these statements is on punishment and the negative consequence of not doing something rather than the positive consequence of doing something. We strongly recommend you turn it around to emphasize the positive: "As soon as you pick up your toys, you can go outside to play" or "As soon as the dishwasher is loaded, you can play your video game." The difference may seem subtle, but it's impor-tant. When you stress access to a desired activity rather than lack of access to a desired activity, you're keeping your child's eyes on the prize. The behavioral data we've collected show that this shift really is effec-tive: we've seen increases in direction following and decreases in task refusal and power struggles when adults use positive statements with kids rather than negative ones.

Using More Formal Incentive Systems

While praise, natural and logical consequences, or having something to look forward to are our preferred motivational strategies, they may not always be enough to motivate children to use difficult skills or participate in challenging situations. In this case, you may find it helpful to use a more formal incentive system.

When to consider using formal reward systems:

- When you want your child to try something that you think they would find helpful or you think they could learn to like, such as the example of Nia going to tutoring. In this circumstance, it's important to be aware of your own expectations. The objective is not to pressure your child to engage in an activity because it satisfies your desire.
- When, because of executive skill challenges, your child struggles to consistently initiate tasks that are very effortful for him, such as chores, and "first—then" strategies have not been effective. This is often true for a child with ADHD.
- When your child needs to complete a nonpreferred task in a limited time period, such as a school project or an application for an activity she wants to attend.

Conditions:

- We recommend that formal reward systems be short-term or limited to the completion of a specific demand (as in Nia's case).
- They should be specific to the behavior and the situation they were designed for (such as completion of specific chores by a certain time after school). It is important for children to understand this, so they don't develop an expectation that any time they complete any task, they will receive a reward.
- The value of the reward for the specific task, once agreed upon by child and parents, is not open to negotiation unless the task demand changes. The objective here is to ensure that neither party decides on their own to insist on an incentive change.

If you have decided on a formal incentive system, follow these steps:

Step 1: Describe the Problem Behavior and Set a Goal

This may sound familiar because it's identical to the initial steps listed in the previous chapter on teaching executive skills. As you may remember, it's important to describe the problem and goal behaviors as specifically as possible. For example, if doing chores after school is the objective, the goal might be "Joe will complete daily chores without reminders before 4:30 in the afternoon." If you have specific expectations for what constitutes an acceptable job, be sure to include those.

Step 2: Decide on Possible Rewards and Contingencies

The first step in designing a system of rewards and contingencies is to talk with your child about what you want them to do and what rewards they would like to earn. Letting your child choose the type of reward increases the likelihood of success since you are assured they've chosen what they value. Your role is to establish the economy—that is, the type or rate of pay for task completion. There are a few options here. In Nia's case, as noted, she chose a one-time payoff (phone), which came with the agreed-upon completion of tutoring. For children with shorter time horizons or the need for more immediate reinforcement, "payment" per task (such as each day the chore is completed) is preferable.

The objective of the system is to incentivize the child to make the effort to start and to establish the habit. Discuss the time frame that it will be in place and the date that it will end. For habit building, 4–8 weeks should be sufficient. If the task has its own timeline or deadline (as in Nia's case), the incentive is delivered upon completion. Your job is to set the amount of pay for the task. Some children prefer incentive systems that have a "menu" of rewards to choose from. In this case, with your child you create a system in which points can be earned for the goal behaviors and traded in for the reward the child wants to earn. The bigger the reward, the more points the child will need to earn it. The menu, depending on what the child wants, can include larger rewards that may take a week or a month to earn and smaller rewards that can be earned daily. Rewards can include "material" reinforcers (such as favorite foods or small toys) as well as activity rewards (such as the chance to play a game or go to an event with a parent or friend). If maintaining the habit is still a problem, it will be necessary to build "first—then" contingencies into the system—access to a preferred activity after a task is done (such as the chance to watch a favorite TV show or the chance to play with a friend). An example of how this process might be applied to the problem of completing chores is shown on the facing page (top).

Step 3: Write a Behavior Contract

The contract should say exactly what the child agrees to do and exactly what the parents' role and responsibilities will be. Along with points and rewards, be sure to praise your child's successful efforts for following the contract. Also be sure the contract is one you can realistically oversee. For instance, if both parents work and are not at home, you won't be able to monitor whether your child is beginning his chores right after school, so an alternative contract may need to be written. An example of how this might be applied to the problem of completing chores is shown on the facing page (bottom).

Blank forms that you can use to design incentive systems and write behavior contracts are included at the end of this chapter.

Step 4: Evaluate the Process and Make Changes If Necessary

Once the contract is in place and your child has started, if he is consistently successful 75% or more of the time, then you are on the right track. If not, then you will need to

Sample Incentive Planning Sheet

PROBLEM BEHAVIOR

Forgetting to do chores after school

GOAL

Complete chores by 4:30 p.m. without reminders

POSSIBLE REWARDS
(Child earns 1 point for each day the goal is met)

Daily (1 point)	Weekly (5 points)	Long-term
Extra TV show	Mom will make favorite dessert	Buy video game (20 points)
Extra video game time	Have friend spend night on weekend	Eat out (15 points)
Play game with Dad	Chance to choose dinner menu	

POSSIBLE CONTINGENCIES/PENALTIES

Can play with friends after school as soon as chores are done

Access to TV/video games after chores are done

examine where the breakdown might be. Does the task demand need to be modified? Does the rate of pay need to be adjusted? Does the child need additional skill instruction? In general it's common to have to tinker with the rules of the contract, the points allotted, or the specific rewards chosen before the contract works the way you want it to.

Parents often ask how they can develop this kind of system for one child in the family and not for all children because it may seem to be "rewarding" children with

Sample Behavior Contract

Child agrees to: complete chores by 4:30 P.M. without verbal reminders.

To help child reach goal, parents will: place a chore list on kitchen table before child comes home from school.

Child will earn: 1 point for each day he completes chores without verbal reminders.
Points can be traded in for items on the reward menu.

If child fails to meet agreement, child will: not earn any points for that day.

problems while neglecting those without. We have found that most siblings are understanding of this process if it's explained to them carefully. If there are problems, however, you have several choices:

1. Set up a similar, time-limited system for other children with appropriate goals (*every* child has *something* he or she could be working to improve).
2. Make a more informal arrangement by promising to do something special from time to time with the other children in the family, so they don't feel left out.
3. Have the child earn rewards that benefit the whole family (such as eating out at a preferred restaurant).

Using Motivational Strategies to Reinforce Executive Skills in General

All the examples we've given you focus on a specific target behavior to be improved (remembering to do chores, finishing projects, picking up toys, and so on). You can use the same strategies to focus on helping your child develop executive skills more broadly rather than addressing single behaviors. If you decide you want to work on task initiation—for instance, every time your child starts a task without the need for reminders—you can reinforce the child for that. "Thanks for emptying the dishwasher right after you came home from school" and "I like the way you started your homework at 5:00, just as we agreed on" are examples of specific praise that focuses on task initiation. If you feel you need to use a more powerful reinforcer, then each time your child starts something right away, or at the time agreed on, or without the need for more than one reminder, you can put a token or coin in a jar. When the jar is full (or the child has earned the agreed-upon number of tokens/cash), the reward is earned. As above, use these systems for a specific, limited time.

If you've stuck with us to this point, you should now understand the three broad approaches to managing your child's executive skill weaknesses. In the next section we move from "big picture" to practical applications. So if you're not yet sure how to use what you've learned so far, keep reading. We will give you teaching routines and vignettes drawn from our experience as parents and clinicians that solve the array of problems that arise in daily living because children have less-than-perfect executive skills. We have provided an Incentive Planning Sheet and a Behavior Contract on pages 115–116 for you to use. You may find them helpful.

Incentive Planning Sheet

PROBLEM BEHAVIOR

_____
_____
_____
_____
_____

GOAL

_____
_____
_____
_____
_____

POSSIBLE REWARDS

Daily	Weekly	Long-term
_____	_____	_____
_____	_____	_____
_____	_____	_____
_____	_____	_____
_____	_____	_____
_____	_____	_____
_____	_____	_____

POSSIBLE CONTINGENCIES/PENALTIES

_____
_____
_____
_____

From _Smart but Scattered, Second Edition,_ by Peg Dawson, Richard Guare, and Colin Guare. Copyright © 2025 The Guilford Press. Permission to photocopy this material, or to download enlarged printable versions (_www.guilford.com/dawson4-forms_), is granted to purchasers of this book for personal use; see copyright page for details.

Behavior Contract

Child agrees to: _____

_____

_____

_____

To help child reach goal, parents will: _____

_____

_____

_____

Child will earn: _____

_____

_____

_____

If child fails to meet agreement, child will: _____

_____

_____

_____

From *Smart but Scattered, Second Edition*, by Peg Dawson, Richard Guare, and Colin Guare. Copyright © 2025 The Guilford Press. Permission to photocopy this material, or to download enlarged printable versions (*www.guilford.com/dawson4-forms*), is granted to purchasers of this book for personal use; see copyright page for details.

PART III

Putting It All Together

8

Advance Organizer

In Chapters 5–7 you learned the ABCs of designing interventions to improve your child's executive skills: change the *antecedent* (modify the environment), address the *behavior* directly (teach the skill), and change the *consequence* (provide incentives). Pretty straightforward, but where do you begin? How much are you really going to have to do to make a significant difference in your child's life?

At the risk of sounding like a broken record, before you embark on an intervention, ensure that these three conditions have been met:

1. My child knows exactly what is expected of her.
2. My child has all basic skills to complete the task.
3. I've structured the task and made the environmental changes necessary to accommodate my child's executive skill challenges.

As we've been promising since the beginning of this book, we're going to make the process of helping to improve your child's executive skills manageable by offering several approaches. How much you actively do will be your choice. You'll be able to have a measurable impact on your child within the bounds of your available time and energy.

We are, in fact, so thoroughly committed to this process that the first and most important rule of thumb we want to offer is this:

First, Do the Minimum Necessary to Put Your Child on a Path to Success

Sure, you can use everything we've explained in the last four chapters and combine all the possible approaches to intervention from Chapters 10–20 to devise a multicomponent plan. Eventually you may decide to do that. But you're reading this book to make your life easier at the same time as you're giving your child a boost toward the skills needed to be successful. So try the minimum intervention first:

• *If you can devise simple environmental modifications that your child will eventually internalize on her own, by all means do it.* A note on the kitchen table that says *Please walk the dog as soon as you get home from school* is an example of an environmental modification. If you leave the note for 3 weeks and then don't leave it, does your child still remember to walk the dog? If so, her own working memory is kicking in. If you ask your child to estimate how long it will take them to do their math homework and you compare those estimates to the actual time and see that your child is becoming more accurate, you know the child is refining time management skills. (See Chapter 5 for a detailed discussion of how to modify the environment to enhance executive skill development.)

• *Or if you think your child already has a particular skill but needs to be encouraged to use it, a motivational strategy alone may be sufficient.* Maybe you've worked with your daughter to set up a folder system to help her keep track of homework assignments, but she keeps stuffing the work into random books and notebooks. A motivational strategy might look like this: Have her show you the folders when she finishes her homework and say, "You're working really hard to organize your homework. Good job." Kids value positive recognition for their efforts. Having her show you her folders when she finishes her homework lets her know you're interested and you appreciate her work. If this isn't enough, the next step is a first—then option, such as "As soon as you finish your folders, you can . . . [do a preferred activity]." See Chapter 7 for further instructions on how to use strategies to motivate kids.

• *If you believe your child might benefit substantially just from some scaffolding and game playing, give that a shot first.* Learning how to win and lose gracefully (that is, develop emotional control) is particularly well suited to game playing. Chances are, though, that there are some skills your kids will need help to develop that require a multipronged approach. Take, for example, long-term school assignments. Breaking down an assignment into subtasks and timelines is something that many kids simply need help with. Being shown options and then being walked through one that fits for them a few times as practice may be all they need to acquire these skills. Or consider the skill of time management. If your child struggles to manage time because she doesn't know how long it takes to do certain tasks, you can work with on her time estimation skills and then build in some practice, and that may be all she'll need to become skilled at time management. Chapters 10–20 will show you how to teach each of the 11 executive skills when the problem is that the child isn't sure how.

But what if you help your child learn a skill and practice it and the child still doesn't use it? This is a sure sign that you need a multipronged approach. Sometimes just understanding how the process works isn't enough, and the child finds that particular skills demand so much effort that he avoids them. For those cases, Chapters 10–20 also illustrate how you can put together a program that incorporates motivational techniques and troubleshooting so that even the tasks that seem "impossible" to your child right now eventually become manageable.

Next, Learn the Principles That Underlie Effective Strategies

When your child is struggling with a skill that requires a more targeted approach, you can count on the guidelines provided in this chapter. These principles form the foundation for all the strategies you'll learn to use in this book. Read this chapter before you start using any intervention with your child. Come back to it when a strategy you're trying isn't working; it may be because you've forgotten an important guideline and need to tweak the strategy to integrate it.

Now Tackle Specific Daily Routines

In our work, parents bring up a certain predictable set of daily problems associated with executive skill challenges over and over. Parents of preschoolers and early-elementary-school-age children often complain about their child's inability to get through a morning routine, get ready for bed efficiently, clean up bedrooms or playrooms, or control their temper. Parents of children in upper elementary school and middle school often complain about their kids' failure to get their homework done, keep their notebooks organized, or carry out long-term projects. We know that battles over these regular routines can ruin your day and your child's—day after day and week after week. You can all get pretty quick relief by attacking these routines directly with the instructional schemes we've created for you. *That's why we strongly recommend that you try using the ready-made interventions in Chapter 9 as your next step after you've tried the minimal help listed above.* Chapter 9 gives you detailed plans, including any forms or checklists you need to implement the plan, for 15 different daily routines that often cause problems for kids with weak executive skills. We add a few more strategies for school-related issues in Chapter 23.

Choosing a Routine to Tackle First

You'll find it easy to dive in if you look through the list of routines at the beginning of the chapter and immediately zero in on one that feels like the bane of your existence. Maybe the battle over getting ready for school leaves your child too upset to concentrate during the first couple hours of school, and as a result his reading grades are taking a nosedive. Or trying to wrestle your child into bed at night leaves you so worked up that you rarely get a good night's sleep. In cases like these you know which routine to tackle first.

But what if you look through the list of daily routines and can point to a dozen of them that cause you and your child trouble every day? How do you know where to start? Here are a few ideas:

- *Start with the problem that, if cleared up, would make your child's life—and yours!—go so much more smoothly.* Because improved quality of life is one of our bottom lines, this is often the best place to start. Maggie wasn't sure it mattered that much to 6-year-old Bess's well-being that bedtime felt like a wrestling match (in fact, in her worst moments she thought, incorrectly as it turned out, that Bess thoroughly enjoyed this battle of wills). But it left Maggie exhausted, unable to fall asleep herself, and feeling like an incompetent parent who missed the cuddling during bedtime stories when her little girl was 4. So she chose bedtime as the routine to tackle first.

- *Start with a problem that is small and can be tackled easily.* The benefit of this approach is that you can achieve some quick success and build your and your child's confidence to try something a little more challenging. Brad chose helping his son Trey do the chore of feeding the dogs every night. It was a simple chore that took very little time, but Trey never seemed to remember to do it and then drove his father crazy responding with "Just a minute!" numerous times when reminded. You too can work with your child to break down a routine we've laid out to make it even simpler by targeting a very simple chore to address.

- *Give your child a choice of what to tackle first.* This appeals to us because it increases the child's ownership of the problem and the solution—and it taps the child's desire for mastery and control. Jessie decided she wanted help with practicing the piano. Her grandparents were coming to town for her recital, and her desire to perform well for them served as a built-in incentive.

- *Choose one where the implementation can be shared.* If you and your spouse agree on the target problem and you can share the burden for solving it, the effort required of you alone is lessened, which makes it more likely that the intervention will work. Read through the routine and decide who will do what when. Make sure you agree on the details since, as we all know, the devil is in the details. For the Gonzales family, homework was perfect. One parent would help their son with getting his math done while the other cooked dinner, then the cook would help him stick to his reading assignment while the other parent did the dishes.

- *Think about long-term goals.* This is especially important with older children, where adulthood is beginning to appear on the horizon. When I realized that my then 13-year-old son (this is Peg talking) had some significant executive skill problems in a number of domains, I wasn't sure what to focus on. I finally asked myself, *What skills will be absolutely critical for both success in college and success on the job?* With that in mind, I decided a clean bedroom was a low priority, while meeting deadlines and remembering everything he had to get done were high priorities. Once I'd made that decision, I began monitoring his homework by asking him two questions when he came home from school every day: *What do you have to do? When are you going to do it?*

Which Executive Skills Will You Be Building in Your Child?

Each routine covered in Chapter 9 lists up front the executive skills that the routine demands. You'll notice that all these routines, while designed to address one particular problem in daily life, actually aim at working on a number of executive skills simultaneously. Kids who have trouble getting through a morning routine, for instance, often struggle with task initiation (they're slow to get started), sustained attention (they have trouble persisting long enough to get it done), and working memory (they lose track of what they're supposed to be doing). By developing an intervention to deal with one problem, then, you're actually working to improve several executive skills simultaneously. You can probably guess that in time this means you may see improvements in other routines involving the same executive skills without directly intervening in those routines. (As we've noted, though, don't expect this to happen overnight or even this month. Sometimes, for some kids, you'll have to keep the aids in place for quite a while before the skills are internalized.)

Finally, Target Specific Executive Skill Weaknesses

If your child's problems are pretty pervasive, especially if Chapter 2 helped you identify just one or two executive skill weaknesses behind all the trouble, or the routines that cause the greatest problems aren't covered in Chapter 9, you'll want to go beyond following our instructions and design your own strategies. Some of you may want to use the ready-made routines in Chapter 9 *and* design your own plans. Each of Chapters 10–20 goes into depth on a particular skill, giving you additional information on it, helping you look more closely at your child's struggles in the skill, and then showing you how other parents and children have devised effective interventions. You can pick any problem where your child struggles and with them design a plan of attack that will either help develop the skill discussed in that chapter or help the child practice and enhance the skill when the child has it but doesn't use it well. Each of these chapters also gives some general tips for strengthening the skill outside of a fully drawn intervention scheme.

How Do You Decide Which Executive Skills to Target?

If you start by using the plans we've created for Chapter 9, you'll probably notice that the routines your child needs help with almost all entail the same executive skills. This is one way to determine which individual skills to work on further. You also have the questionnaires that you used to assess your child's executive skills in Chapter 2 to go on. Finally, you can confirm your initial assessment of your child by filling in the brief questionnaire at the beginning of each of the skills chapters that discusses the skill you believe your child lacks.

These questionnaires are similar to the one you completed in Chapter 2, but this time we ask you to rate how well or how often you feel your child exhibits each of the behaviors listed, so you'll know whether all you need is the general tips or whether you should design your own full-blown intervention strategies. If you decide to craft your own intervention, you can draw from all the ideas in Chapters 4–7. Because we're such strong believers in checklists, we've put one together to help you remember all the elements you need to at least consider when creating a plan to help your child cope with their particular problem or particular executive skill weakness. It is shown on the facing page. In case you need a refresher about the meaning of any of the items on the checklist, we've noted where in the book the item is discussed.

Tips for Success in Designing Your Own Program

Whether you use our interventions from Chapter 9 or design your own—or both—your plan is more likely to succeed if you keep these ideas in mind:

- *Help your child own the plan.* Involve your child as much as possible from the outset in designing the intervention. Listen to her input, incorporate her suggestions, and honor her requests whenever possible. Be willing to compromise to increase your child's ownership of the plan. Remember, one of the forces that shape children's behavior is a drive for mastery and control—use this to your advantage whenever you can.

- *Remember the importance of goodness of fit.* Keep in mind that what you think would work for you may not be a good fit for your child. We've found in particular that organizational schemes that work for one individual have no appeal to another. Ask your child what will work for him and offer options to choose from if he's not sure.

- *Take opportunities to brainstorm with your child.* Brainstorming itself builds executive skills. If your child can't think of anything that might work for them, turn it into a brainstorming session or offer choices and see which one feels right to your child.

- *Expect to have to tweak your strategies.* Assume that the first plan you design will need to be adjusted. For each of the routines we present in the next chapter, we list some modifications and adjustments you may want to consider. In the skills chapters (Chapters 10–20), many of the scenarios we present show how the initial attempts met with some success but also needed to be tinkered with to produce the maximum benefit.

- *Practice, role-play, or rehearse the procedure before putting it in place.* This ensures that your child understands the plan and has all the skills needed and that any tools or accommodations needed are in place (timers, picture strips, labels, storage containers, and others). This will be particularly important if the target executive skill is response inhibition or emotional control. Because things can happen quickly in real

Designing Interventions

Intervention steps	Reference page(s)

1. Establish behavioral goal.

Problem behavior: _____   94

Goal behavior: _____   94

2. What environmental supports will be provided? (Check all that apply.)

☐ Change physical or social environment (e.g., add physical barriers, reduce distractions, provide organizational structures, reduce social complexity).   76–78

☐ Change the nature of the task (e.g., shorten it, build in breaks, give something to look forward to, create a schedule, build in choice, make the task more fun).   78–80

☐ Change the way adults interact with the child (e.g., rehearsal, prompts, reminders, coaching, praise, debriefing, feedback).   80–85

3. What procedure will be followed to teach the skill? _____   86–103

Who will teach the skill/supervise the procedure? _____

What steps will the child follow? _____

1. _____

2. _____

3. _____

4. _____

5. _____

6. _____

4. What incentives will be used to encourage the child to learn, practice, or use the skill? (Check all that apply.)   104–116

☐ Specific praise   106–108

☐ Something to look forward to when the task (or a piece of the task) is done

☐ A menu of rewards and penalties   112–113

Daily reward possibilities: _____

_____

_____

Weekly reward possibilities: _____

_____

_____

Long-term reward possibilities: _____

_____

_____

From *Smart but Scattered, Second Edition,* by Peg Dawson, Richard Guare, and Colin Guare. Copyright © 2025 The Guilford Press. Permission to photocopy this material, or to download enlarged printable versions (*www.guilford.com/dawson4-forms*), is granted to purchasers of this book for personal use; see copyright page for details.

life and because the problem behavior often occurs in emotionally charged situations, the more practice the child can get when emotions are not at their peak, the more likely the child will be able to follow the script in the heat of the moment.

● *Always use lots of praise and positive feedback.* As we've noted, "process praise" is a powerful motivator on its own for children. Always begin with that. If something else is needed, "first—then" strategies are the next option, combined with continued praise.

● *Use visual reminders whenever possible.* All too often verbal reminders "go in one ear and out the other." When you do use verbal cues, use them to refer your child to visuals such as picture schedules, lists, checklists, written mottos, or slogans: "Check your list." "What comes next on your schedule?"

● *Start small(er)!* Begin with a behavior that's a minor annoyance and build in lots of success up front so that you and your child experience success right away. When you move on to bigger problems, still plan for success by making the initial goals attainable. Your long-term goal may be to get your son to do all his homework independently without needing your presence, but a reasonable first step might be to get him to work by himself for a few minutes. If you know you tend to overreach, take your first idea for a goal and cut it in half (half the time, half the work, half the challenge, half the improvement).

● *Whenever possible, measure progress by finding something to count, then graph the results.* If you're not sure whether the program is working, figure out a way to collect data to answer the question. Graphs, by the way, can be incredibly reinforcing to children (actually, to people of all ages). Some examples of behaviors that can be counted and graphed are completed homework assignments per week, number of "meltdowns" per day, number of school days per week that the child remembered everything they had to bring to and from school, number of times an unexpected change of plans was handled without crying, and number of evenings per week that homework was finished before the agreed-upon time.

What If Your Child Wants No Part of Your Plans?

If after reading through the teaching routines, scenarios, and behavior plans you're all gung-ho to try something but your child wants no part of it, here are some things to try:

● *Ask your child's opinion.* What does your child think would be a way to manage the problem?

● *Reduce the initial task demand.* Children balk at tasks that look very effortful to them. The objective is to start small, so the child sees the task demand as easily manageable, such as starting room cleaning with only putting dirty clothes in a hamper. We know that the effortfulness of a task decreases with repetition, so as the child masters one step, you can add another small step. The objective is that at the beginning of the task your child be able to see the end in sight.

• *Try negotiating.* Be willing to give up something to get something in return (but make sure both sides are satisfied). If you're skeptical that the child's plan will work, let them try it out for a limited time and then revisit the result and decide on changes if necessary.

• *If your child resists all your attempts to engage her in developing a behavior plan (this is most likely to occur in adolescence), you can still build in logical or natural consequences.* To get to the privileges your child wants, arrange it so that she has to go through you ("I'll be happy to take you to the mall, so you can hang out with your friends as soon as you clean your bedroom").

• *Consider more powerful reinforcers.* We've found that parents and teachers often err on the side of stinginess. Remember that what we're often asking children with executive skill deficits to do is tasks that require huge efforts from them. If the task looks bigger to them than the reward, they'll continue to resist the task. If you've reduced the task demand and it's still a no-go, make sure that what comes after the task is followed by something they value.

• *If nothing seems to work and the problems are severe enough, seek outside help such as a therapist, coach, or tutor.* Chapter 21 offers suggestions for how to do this.

The Game Plan at a Glance

1. First try modifying the environment (Chapter 5), using scaffolding and games (Chapter 6), or providing incentives (Chapter 7).

2. If that's not enough, learn the principles and guidelines behind effective strategies for building executive skills (Chapter 8).

3. Start intervening by using our ready-made plans to tackle especially problematic daily routines (Chapter 9).

4. If that's not enough, work on specific executive skills (Chapters 10–20).

   • Follow general tips for helping the child use weak skills more effectively and consistently.

   • If the child lacks the skill altogether, design your own interventions, following the "Designing Interventions" framework on page 125 of this chapter.

9

Ready-Made Plans
for Teaching Your Child
to Complete Daily Routines

The following 15 routines are the ones that children tend to struggle with most. We've grouped them starting with home routines, followed by tasks requiring emotional control, flexibility, and response inhibition. Glance through the list and you'll undoubtedly zero in on the areas where you and your child need help. Refer back to Chapter 8 if you identify several and don't know where to start. We've given the chapter number for each executive skill the routine addresses if you decide you want to do more targeted work on specific skills.

In Chapter 6 we described in some detail a process parents can use to teach children executive skills they struggle with. In this chapter we offer suggestions for how to teach skills by embedding them in specific daily routines or through adopting a consistent approach for handling problem situations (such as problems handling temper or anxiety).

A Reminder about the Child's Role

Although we have met with success using a "top-down" approach to teaching children routines that incorporate executive skills, our larger goal is to give children as much control over the whole process as we can for a number of reasons. First of all, this helps them exercise some important executive skills, in particular planning, goal-directed persistence, and metacognition, all skills involved in problem solving. Second, we want them eventually to be able to apply this problem-solving approach independently, and having them participate in designing an intervention is a great way to practice this skill. And finally, when children are consulted and viewed by their parents as collaborators in the process, not only do they have more ownership over the outcome, but they also may bring ideas to the table that their parents wouldn't have considered.

So we suggest that whatever intervention you would like to try should begin with a discussion with your child. Here are some steps you might consider building into that discussion:

- Describe the problem in a nonjudgmental way.
- Talk about why it's a problem and what positive effect you think might come from trying to change the behavior.
- Ask the child for help in coming up with a strategy to solve the problem that you're both comfortable with.
- Come up with a mutually agreed-upon game plan for implementing the intervention that includes walking through the steps from start to finish (mentally, verbally, or physically rehearse).
- Ask the child how they would like to be cued both to begin the routine and to complete each step in the routine. While verbal cues to begin a routine may

work best, you may combine visual and verbal cues once the child begins the routine ("Check your list for what to do next"). There are also apps available, such as Choiceworks, that can be used to list the steps in the routine, estimate how much time will be needed for each step, and to count down the time, signaling when the child should finish one step and go on to the next.

- Agree on a start time to begin the intervention.

Adapting the Interventions for Your Child's Age

In some cases the ages for which the interventions are appropriate will be dictated by the developmental task involved in the routine or by the school curriculum. We don't expect first graders to study for tests (except spelling tests), to do long-term projects, or to write papers, so these routines were not designed for that age group (these routines are included in Chapter 23, since they are school-related routines). Other routines may be applicable for a range of ages. Because many of the routines were written for children in the middle of the age range covered by this book (mid-elementary school), here are some suggestions for how to adjust the strategies for younger and older children where that seems appropriate.

General guidelines for developing instructional routines for young children:

- Keep them short.
- Reduce the number of steps involved.
- Use pictures as cues rather than written lists or written instructions. This might mean taking a picture of the child doing the routine steps, drawing pictures, or finding clip art online.
- Be prepared to provide cues and supervision, and in some cases you'll need to help the child follow the routine, working side by side.

General guidelines for developing instructional routines for older children:

- Make them full partners in the design of the routine and the troubleshooting that may be required to improve the routine.
- If there's a difference of opinion, negotiate rather than dictate.
- Whenever possible, use visual cues rather than verbal cues (because the latter sound a lot like nagging to children).

A note about checklists: In the routines that follow, we provide checklists. They are just samples; you can use them as is or just as a model, with your own tasks listed in the left column. You may also want to consider using pictures in place of words—even older children who can read often prefer pictures. We also like laminated checklists that have two columns, To Do and Done, with the list as well as each item backed with Velcro, so that the child can move the item from the To Do column to the Done column.

1. Getting Ready in the Morning

Executive skills addressed: Task initiation (Chapter 15), sustained attention (Chapter 14), working memory (Chapter 11).

Ages: Specifics we've included are for ages 7–10, but this routine is very easy to customize for younger and older children just by changing the sophistication of the tasks. (For younger kids, it's a bit more involved than that—see recommendation regarding pictures.)

1. Sit down with your child and together make a list of the things to be done before leaving for school in the morning (or just starting the day for younger kids).
2. Decide together the order in which the tasks should be done.
3. Turn the list into a checklist. (The checklists on pages 132–133 are samples; you can use them as is or as models, with your own tasks listed in the left column.)
4. Make multiple copies and attach them to a clipboard or post them where the child would like.
5. Talk through with your child how the process will work from the moment the child wakes up. Explain that in the beginning you will cue your child to do each item on the list and that the child will check off each item as it is completed. Ask the child how they would like to be cued.
6. Rehearse or role-play the process so that your child understands how it will work— that is, walk through each step, with the child pretending to do each step and check it off.
7. Determine what time the whole routine should be finished to get to school on time (or to have some time to play before going to school or to get to whatever the child needs to do).
8. Put the system to work. *Having agreed on a cueing system*, you should initially cue your child to begin the first step, watch as they do the step, prompt to check off the step on the checklist, praise the child for completing each step, and cue your child to do the next step. Continue the process with supervision until the entire routine is completed.
9. Once the child has internalized the process and is able to complete the routine independently within time constraints, the checklist can be faded.

Fading the Supervision

1. Using the child's preferred cueing system, cue your child to begin and supervise throughout the routine, providing frequent praise and encouragement as well as constructive feedback.

Morning Routine Checklist

Task	Number of reminders/ tally marks (////)	Done (✓)
Get up		
Get dressed		
Eat breakfast		
Put dishes in dishwasher		
Brush teeth		
Brush hair		
Get backpack ready for school		
Other:		
Other:		

From *Smart but Scattered, Second Edition*, by Peg Dawson, Richard Guare, and Colin Guare. Copyright © 2025 The Guilford Press. Permission to photocopy this material, or to download enlarged printable versions (*www.guilford.com/dawson4-forms*), is granted to purchasers of this book for personal use; see copyright page for details.

Getting Ready for School Checklist

Task	Done (✓)
All homework completed	
All homework in appropriate place (notebook, folder, and so on)	

Items to go to school	Placed in backpack (✓)
Homework	
Notebooks/folders	
Textbooks	
Silent reading book	
Permission slips	
Lunch money	
Sports/PE clothes/equipment	
Notes for teacher	
Assignment book	
Other:	
Other:	

From *Smart but Scattered, Second Edition,* by Peg Dawson, Richard Guare, and Colin Guare. Copyright © 2025 The Guilford Press. Permission to photocopy this material, or to download enlarged printable versions (*www.guilford.com/ dawson4-forms*), is granted to purchasers of this book for personal use; see copyright page for details.

2. Cue your child to begin, make sure they start each step, and then go away and come back for the next step.

3. Cue your child to begin and check on them intermittently (every two steps, then every three steps, and so on).

4. Cue your child to begin and have them check in with you at the end.

Modifications/Adjustments

1. Use explicit praise to let the child know what's going well: "You did a nice job going through the routine step by step" or "I liked the way you used the checklist to keep track of everything you had to do."

2. If more than praise is needed for the child to follow the routine, use a first—then strategy (such as "If you finish the routine with time to spare, you'll be able to work on your LEGO project").

3. Have the child set the timer (or model it for them first, then hand it off)—at the beginning of each step—and challenge the child to complete the step before the timer rings.

4. Adjust the time or the schedule as needed. If on-time completion is still an issue, discuss other options with the child (like waking earlier, prepping the night before, dropping something) and come to a mutual decision about what to try next.

5. Rather than making a checklist, write each task on a separate index card and have the child hand in the card and get a new one as each step is completed. (Involve the child in this whether it's written or in pictures. They need as much decision making and ownership as possible.)

6. For younger children, use pictures rather than words, keep the list short, and assume that you'll need to continue to cue the child (see the "Fading the Supervision" list above regarding cueing).

7. The same approach can be adapted for children who need help specifically with making sure they're taking everything to school that they need. A sample checklist for this is provided on page 133.

2. Bedroom Cleaning

Executive skills addressed: Task initiation (Chapter 15), sustained attention (Chapter 14), working memory (Chapter 11), organization (Chapter 17).

Ages: Specifics we've included are for ages 7–10, but this routine is very easy to customize for younger and older children just by changing the sophistication of the tasks. At all ages, the child should partner with you in making decisions for each step below.

1. Sit down with your child and together make a list of the steps involved in cleaning their bedroom. They might look like this:

  - Put dirty clothes in laundry
  - Put clean clothes in dresser/closet
  - Put toys away on toy shelves or in boxes/bins
  - Put books on bookshelves
  - Clean off desk surface
  - Throw away trash
  - Return things to other rooms (dirty dishes to kitchen, towels to bathroom, and so on)

2. Turn the list into a checklist (provided on page 136 or create your own). You may want to create a checklist that includes pictures showing what the bedroom looks like when it is clean (neatly made bed, floor clear of toys or clothes, desktop, dresser top clear of clutter).

3. With the child, decide when the chore will be done.

4. Decide with the child what kinds of cues and reminders will be given before and during the task.

5. With the child, decide how much help the child will get in the beginning (the long-term goal should be for the child to clean the room alone).

6. Decide how the quality of the task will be judged; having pictures for what the clean room should look like can help with this discussion.

7. Put the routine in place with the agreed-upon cues, reminders, and help.

Fading the Supervision

1. Cue your child to begin and supervise throughout the routine, providing frequent praise and encouragement as well as constructive feedback.

2. Cue your child to begin, make sure they start each step, and then go away and come back for the next step.

3. Cue your child to begin, then check on them intermittently (every two steps, then every three steps, and so on).

4. Cue your child to begin and have them check in with you at the end.

Modifications/Adjustments

1. Use explicit praise to let the child know what's going well (such as "You did a nice job going through the routine step by step" or "I liked the way you used the checklist to keep track of everything you had to do").

2. If more than praise is needed for the child to follow the routine, use a first—then strategy (such as "Once the bedroom is clean, you'll be able to play with your friend").

Bedroom-Cleaning Checklist

Task	Number of reminders/ tally marks (////)	Done (✓)
Put dirty clothes in laundry		
Put clean clothes in dresser/closet		
Put toys away (toy shelves, toy box)		
Put books on bookshelves		
Tidy desk		
Throw away trash		
Return things to other rooms (for example, dishes, cups, towels, sports stuff)		
Other:		
Other:		

From *Smart but Scattered, Second Edition*, by Peg Dawson, Richard Guare, and Colin Guare. Copyright © 2025 The Guilford Press. Permission to photocopy this material, or to download enlarged printable versions (*www.guilford.com/ dawson4-forms*), is granted to purchasers of this book for personal use; see copyright page for details.

3. If even with your constant presence, cueing, and praise, the child can't follow the routine, begin by working alongside your child, sharing each task.

4. If even that is too much, consider using a backward chaining approach—you clean the entire room except for one small piece and have the child do that piece with supervision and praise. Gradually add in more pieces for the child to do until the child is doing the entire job.

5. Make the room easier to clean—use storage bins that the child can "dump" toys into and label each bin.

6. Take a photograph of what a "clean room" looks like, so when your child completes the task, you can ask them to rate their performance by comparing their work to the photo.

7. For younger children use pictures of each step rather than words; reduce the number of steps; assume the child will need help rather than expecting them to work alone.

3. Putting Belongings Away

Executive skills addressed: Organization (Chapter 17), task initiation (Chapter 15), sustained attention (Chapter 14), working memory (Chapter 11).

Ages: Specifics we've included are for ages 7–10, but this routine is very easy to customize for younger and older children just by changing the list of belongings.

1. With your child, make a list of the items your child routinely leaves out of place around the house.

2. Identify the proper location for each item.

3. With your child, decide when the item will be put away (for example, as soon as I get home from school, after I finish my homework, just before bed, right after I finish using it, and the like).

4. Decide with your child on a "rule" for reminders—how many reminders are allowed before a penalty is imposed (for example, the belonging is placed off limits). A sample checklist is on page 138.

5. Decide where the checklist will be kept.

Fading the Supervision

1. Remind your child that you're working on learning to put things away where they belong.

2. Put the checklist in a prominent place and remind your child to use it each time they put something away.

Putting Belongings Away Checklist

Belonging	Where does it go?	When will I put it away?	Number of reminders/ tally marks (////)	Done! (✓)
Sports equipment				
Outerwear (jackets, gloves, and so on)				
Other clothing				
Shoes				
Homework				
Backpack				
Other:				
Other:				

From *Smart but Scattered, Second Edition*, by Peg Dawson, Richard Guare, and Colin Guare. Copyright © 2025 The Guilford Press. Permission to photocopy this material, or to download enlarged printable versions (*www.guilford.com/dawson4-forms*), is granted to purchasers of this book for personal use; see copyright page for details.

3. Praise or thank your child each time they put something away.

4. After your child has followed the system for a couple of weeks, with lots of praise and reminders from you, fade the reminders. Keep the checklist in a prominent place, but now you may want to impose a penalty for forgetting. For example, if a toy or a desired object or article of clothing is not put away, your child may lose access to it for a period of time. If it's an object that can't be taken away (as in a school backpack), then impose a fine or withdraw a privilege.

Modifications/Adjustments

1. Use explicit praise to let the child know what's going well ("You put all your belongings away!" or "I liked the way you used the checklist to remind you of the things you had to put away").

2. If more than praise is needed for the child to follow the routine, use a first—then strategy (such as "When everything is put away, we'll be able to read a story before bed").

3. If remembering to put items away right after use or at different times during the day is too difficult, arrange for a daily pickup time when all belongings need to be returned to their appropriate locations.

4. For younger children, use pictures, keep the list short, and assume the child will need cues and/or help for a longer period of time.

4. Completing Chores

Executive skills addressed: Task initiation (Chapter 15), sustained attention (Chapter 14), working memory (Chapter 11).

Ages: Any age; even preschoolers can be assigned simple, short chores.

1. Together with your child, make a list of chores that need to be done.

2. Talk with your child about how long it will take to do each chore. (Since estimating this can be challenging, it may be better to watch the child perform each step a couple of times and use that as baseline.)

3. Decide with your child when (day and/or time) the chore needs to be done.

4. With your child, create a schedule to keep track of the chore. A sample schedule is on page 140.

5. Decide where the checklist will be kept.

Completing Chores

	Chore	How long will it take?	When will you do it? Day Time
1.			
2.			
3.			
4.			

	Sunday	Monday	Tuesday	Wednesday	Thursday	Friday	Saturday
	Chore done (✓)	**Chore done** (✓)	**Chore done** (✓)	**Chore done** (✓)	**Chore done** (✓)	**Chore done** (✓)	**Chore done** (✓)
1							
2							
3							
4							

From *Smart but Scattered, Second Edition*, by Peg Dawson, Richard Guare, and Colin Guare. Copyright © 2025 The Guilford Press. Permission to photocopy this material, or to download enlarged printable versions (*www.guilford.com/dawson4-forms*), is granted to purchasers of this book for personal use; see copyright page for details.

Fading the Supervision

1. Using a cueing system the child selects, prompt your child to begin each chore and supervise throughout, providing frequent praise and encouragement as well as constructive feedback.

2. Cue your child to begin, make sure the child starts each step, and then go away and come back for the next step.

3. Cue your child to begin, then check on them intermittently (every two steps, then every three steps, and so on).

4. Cue your child to begin and have them check in with you at the end.

Modifications/Adjustments

1. Use explicit praise to let the child know what's going well (for example, "You remembered to do your chores at 4:00 as we agreed").

2. If more than praise is needed for the child to follow the routine, use a first—then strategy ("As soon as you finish your chores, you can play Roblox for half an hour," for example).

3. Set a kitchen timer—or have the child set the timer—at the beginning of each step and challenge the child to complete the step before the timer rings.

4. Adjust the time or the schedule as needed—for example, wake the child up earlier or see if any items on the list can be dropped or done the night before.

5. Rather than making a checklist, write each task on a separate index card and have the child hand in the card and get a new one as each step is completed.

6. For younger children, use pictures rather than words, keep the chores very brief, don't give too many chores, and assume the child will need cues and/or help to complete the chore.

5. Maintaining a Practice Schedule*

Executive skills addressed: Task initiation (Chapter 15), sustained attention (Chapter 14), planning/prioritizing (Chapter 16).

Ages: Mainly 8–14; for younger children, activities like dance, music, and sports should be designed more for fun than for skill acquisition, although younger kids do build skills during ballet lessons, soccer, tumbling classes, and the like.

1. Ideally this process should begin when your child first decides on a skill they want to develop that requires daily or consistent practice. Before you and the child decide

---

*For a musical instrument, sport, or other skill that requires consistent practice.

to go ahead with this, have a conversation about what will be required to master the skill (or to get good enough for it to be enjoyable!). Talk about how often your child will need to practice, how long practice sessions will last, what other responsibilities the child has, and whether there is enough time in the schedule to make consistent practice possible.

2. Create a weekly schedule for when the practice will take place. A sample is on the facing page.

3. Talk about what cues or reminders your child would like to receive to remember to start the practice.

4. Talk about how you and your child will decide whether the process is working. In other words, what are the criteria for success to signal that your child should continue?

5. Decide how long you will keep at it before deciding whether to continue. Many parents have strong feelings that when a child decides to take up something like a musical instrument or a sport (especially if money is involved, such as buying an expensive instrument), they should "sign on" for enough time to make the expense and commitment worth it. Given that many children tire of these kinds of activities within a relatively short period of time, it makes sense to come to some agreement in advance for the minimum amount of time you expect your child to stick with it before you can discuss giving it up.

Fading the Supervision

1. Cue your child to begin the practice at the agreed-upon time and to mark the checklist when they have finished. Place the checklist in a prominent place so that it alone can eventually act as the cue.

2. Use a written reminder and the checklist. If your child doesn't begin within 5 minutes of the agreed-upon time, provide a verbal reminder. If the child *does* begin on time, provide positive reinforcement for this.

Modifications/Adjustments

1. You and your child may want to pick a start time that's easy to remember—such as right after dinner or right after a favorite daily TV program. This way the previous activity actually serves as a cue to begin the next activity.

2. If your child is having trouble remembering to start the practice without reminders, have the child set a kitchen timer, alarm clock, or watch alarm as a reminder, or use a voice assistant like Alexa or Siri to do so if these are available.

3. If your child resists practicing as much as you originally agreed on, consider changing the schedule rather than giving up. Make the practice sessions shorter, schedule them for fewer days, break them in two with a brief break between them, or

Learning a New Skill/Maintaining a Practice Schedule

Before you begin, answer the following questions:

1. What do I want to learn?

2. Why do I want to learn this?

3. What will be involved in learning the skill (lessons, practice, and so on), and how much time will be involved?

What needs to be done	When will this happen?	How much time will it take?
Lessons		
Practice		
Other (for example, games, exhibitions, recitals)		

4. Will I have to give up anything I'm doing now to fit this into my schedule?

If you decide you want to go ahead, plan your schedule by filling in the boxes that follow. Write what time each activity will take place and how long it will last. You can use this to keep track of your practices as well by crossing off each practice after you've finished it.

	Monday	Tuesday	Wednesday	Thursday	Friday	Saturday	Sunday
Lessons							
Practice							
Games, exhibitions, recitals							

From *Smart but Scattered, Second Edition*, by Peg Dawson, Richard Guare, and Colin Guare. Copyright © 2025 The Guilford Press. Permission to photocopy this material, or to download enlarged printable versions (*www.guilford.com/dawson4-forms*), is granted to purchasers of this book for personal use; see copyright page for details.

give them something to look forward to when the practice is finished (for example, schedule the practices *just before* a preferred activity).

4. If you find yourself thinking you need to add a reinforcer to make the practices more attractive to your child, it may be time to rethink the whole process. If your child is reluctant to practice as much as is needed to acquire the skill, this is a signal that your child may not care so much about learning the skill after all. Many times it is parents who want children to learn something (particularly a musical instrument) and the process is not being driven by the child at all. If this is the case, be up front about it with your child—and then add the reinforcer to persuade your child to work on the skill.

6. Bedtime

Executive skills addressed: Task initiation (Chapter 15), sustained attention (Chapter 14), working memory (Chapter 11).

Ages: Specifics we've included are for ages 7–10, but this routine is very easy to customize for younger and older children just by changing the sophistication of the tasks.

1. Talk with your child about what time bedtime is. Make a list of all the things that need to be done before bedtime. This might include picking up toys, getting out clothes for the next day, making sure the child's backpack is ready for school (see Homework on page 148), putting on pajamas, brushing teeth, and washing face or bathing.
2. Turn the list into a checklist or picture schedule. A sample is on the facing page.
3. Talk about how long each task on the list will take. If you want, time each task with a stopwatch so you know exactly how long each task takes.
4. Add up the total amount of time and subtract that from the bedtime hour, so you know when your child should begin the bedtime routine (for example, if bedtime is 8:00 P.M. and it will take a half hour to complete the routine, your child should start the routine at 7:30).
5. Prompt your child to begin the routine at the agreed-upon time.
6. Supervise your child at each step, encouraging them to "check your list to see what's next" and providing praise for completion of each task.

Fading the Supervision

1. Cue your child to begin and supervise throughout the routine, providing frequent praise and encouragement as well as constructive feedback.
2. Cue your child to begin, make sure they start each step, and then go away and come back for the next step.

Bedtime Routine Checklist

Task	Number of reminders/ tally marks (////)	Done (✓)
Pick up toys		
Make sure backpack is ready for school		
Make a list of anything you have to remember to do tomorrow		
Get clothes ready for next day		
Put on pajamas		
Wash face or bathe		
Brush teeth		
Other:		
Other:		

From *Smart but Scattered, Second Edition*, by Peg Dawson, Richard Guare, and Colin Guare. Copyright © 2025 The Guilford Press. Permission to photocopy this material, or to download enlarged printable versions (*www.guilford.com/dawson4-forms*), is granted to purchasers of this book for personal use; see copyright page for details.

3. Cue your child to begin, check on them intermittently (every two steps, then every three steps, and so on).

4. Cue your child to begin and have them check in with you at the end.

Modifications/Adjustments

1. Use explicit praise to let the child know what's going well (such as "You were able to begin your bedtime routine right on schedule").

2. Build in rewards or penalties. For instance, if your child completes the routine at or before the specified bedtime, they earn a little extra time before the lights have to go off. If they do not complete the routine by bedtime, the next night they have to begin the routine 15 minutes earlier.

3. Set the kitchen timer or give your child a stopwatch to use to help the child keep track of how long each step is taking.

4. Rather than making a checklist, write each task on a separate index card and have the child hand in the card and get a new one as each step is completed.

5. For younger children, use pictures rather than words and assume the child will need cueing and/or supervision.

7. Desk Cleaning

Executive skills addressed: Task initiation (Chapter 15), sustained attention (Chapter 14), organization (Chapter 17), planning/prioritizing (Chapter 16).

Ages: Specifics we've included are for ages 7–10, but of course most 7-year-olds don't spend a lot of time at a desk, so if you need to customize for other ages, it will likely be for older children—just make the tasks more sophisticated.

First Steps: Cleaning the Desk

1. Take everything out of the desk.

2. Decide what items will go in which drawer. Make labels to put on the drawers.

3. Put appropriate items in the correct drawers.

4. Have a bin near the desk to hold paper that can be recycled.

5. Decide what items should go on top of the desk (a pencil holder, stapler, wire baskets for papers in current use and for things that need to be filed, and the like). Consider putting a bulletin board next to the desk to hold reminders as well as mementos.

6. Place items where your child wants them.

7. Take a picture of what the desk looks like to use as a model. Put the photo on the wall or bulletin board near the desk.

Steps for Maintaining a Clean Desk

1. Before beginning homework or any other desk project, make sure the desk looks like the photo. If not, put things away so the desk does look like the photo.

2. After finishing homework, put everything away so that the desk again looks like the photograph. This step could also be built into a bedtime routine.

3. Once a week, go through the baskets and decide what needs to stay in the basket, what can be filed, and what should be thrown away/recycled.

4. Create a checklist that lists the tasks involved in maintaining a clean desk. A sample is below.

Fading the Supervision

1. Using your child's chosen cueing system, cue your child for each step in the maintenance procedure and supervise throughout the routine, providing frequent praise and encouragement as well as constructive feedback.

2. Cue your child to begin, make sure they start step 1 of the procedure, and come back at the end to make sure they finished. Do the same with step 2. At step 3, stay with your child to assist in basket cleaning.

3. Cue your child for all three steps of the maintenance procedure but leave and check in at the end.

4. Remind your child to begin the procedure. At a later point (such as just before bed), check in to make sure the desk is clean. Provide praise and constructive feedback.

Clean Desk Checklist

	Monday	Tuesday	Wednesday	Thursday	Friday	Saturday	Sunday
Desk surface picked up							
Baskets cleared							
Desk matches photograph							

From *Smart but Scattered, Second Edition*, by Peg Dawson, Richard Guare, and Colin Guare. Copyright © 2025 The Guilford Press. Permission to photocopy this material, or to download enlarged printable versions (*www.guilford.com/dawson4-forms*), is granted to purchasers of this book for personal use; see copyright page for details.

Modifications/Adjustments

1. Use explicit praise to let the child know what's going well (for example, "I know this isn't easy for you, but you've done such a nice job cleaning off your desk!").

2. As your child follows the process, continue to refine it. For instance, there may be better ways of organizing things on top of the desk or in the drawers, and these changes should be incorporated into the process.

3. Visit an office supply store to see what kind of materials might help your child establish and maintain a system for keeping the desk uncluttered and materials readily available for use.

8. Homework

Executive skills addressed: Task initiation (Chapter 15), sustained attention (Chapter 14), planning/prioritizing (Chapter 16), time management (Chapter 18), metacognition (Chapter 20).

Ages: 7–14.

1. Explain to your child that making a plan for homework is a good way to learn how to make plans and schedules. Explain that when the child gets home from school, before doing anything else, they will make a homework plan using the form that you will provide (the form appears on the facing page).

2. Homework planning steps:
   a. Write down all assignments (this can be shorthand because more detailed directions should be in your child's agenda book or on worksheets).
   b. Make sure your child has all the materials needed for each assignment.
   c. Determine whether the child will need any help to complete the assignment and who will provide the help.
   d. Estimate how long each assignment will take.
   e. Write down when he or she will start each assignment.
   f. Show the plan to you so you can help make adjustments if needed (for example, with time estimations).

3. Using your child's preferred cueing system, cue your child to start homework at the time listed in the plan.

4. Monitor your child's performance throughout. Depending on the child, this may mean staying with the child from start to finish or checking up periodically.

Fading the Supervision

1. Cue your child to make the plan and to begin the routine, providing frequent praise and encouragement as well as constructive feedback. If necessary, sit with your child as they do the homework.

Daily Homework Planner

Date:

Subject/ assignment	Do I have all the materials?	Do I need help?	Who will help me?	How long will it take?	When will I start?	Done (✓)
	Yes ☐ No ☐	Yes ☐ No ☐				
	Yes ☐ No ☐	Yes ☐ No ☐				
	Yes ☐ No ☐	Yes ☐ No ☐				
	Yes ☐ No ☐	Yes ☐ No ☐				
	Yes ☐ No ☐	Yes ☐ No ☐				
	Yes ☐ No ☐	Yes ☐ No ☐				

From *Smart but Scattered, Second Edition*, by Peg Dawson, Richard Guare, and Colin Guare. Copyright © 2025 The Guilford Press. Permission to photocopy this material, or to download enlarged printable versions (*www.guilford.com/dawson4-forms*), is granted to purchasers of this book for personal use; see copyright page for details.

2. Cue your child to make the plan and to start homework on schedule. Check in frequently, providing praise and encouragement.

3. Cue your child to make the plan and start homework on schedule. Ask your child to check in with you when the homework is done.

Modifications/Adjustments

1. If your child resists writing the plan, you do the writing, but have your child tell you what to write.

2. If your child tends to forget assignments that may not be written down, modify the planner to list every possible subject and talk about each subject with your child to jog their memory about assignments.

3. Build in breaks if the child runs out of steam before the homework is done. The breaks should be time-limited (you and your child should agree on how long they should last). Building in physical activity for breaks can make it easier to focus when your child gets back to work.

4. Create a separate calendar for long-term projects so that your child can keep track of the work that needs to be done on them (see Long-Term Projects from page 302 on).

5. Use explicit praise to let the child know what's going well (for example, "I like the way you've been able to get your homework done before dinner—you get to do fun stuff after dinner!").

6. For younger children, simply establishing a set time and place to do homework may be sufficient because they tend to have only one or two assignments per night. Asking them to estimate how long it will take to do each assignment may be useful because this helps train time management skills.

9. Organizing Notebooks/Homework

Executive skills addressed: Organization (Chapter 17), task initiation (Chapter 15).

Ages: 6–14.

1. With your child, decide on what needs to be included in the organizational system: A place to keep unfinished homework? A separate place to keep completed homework? A place to keep papers that need to be filed? Notebooks or binders to keep notes, completed assignments, handouts, worksheets, and so on? A sample list is in the worksheet on the facing page.

2. Once you've listed all these elements, decide how best to handle them, one at a time. For example, you and your child might decide on a colored folder system, with a different color for completed assignments, unfinished work, and other papers. Or you might decide to have a separate small three-ring binder for each subject or one large

Setting Up a Notebook/Homework Management System

System element	What will you use?	Got it (✓)
Place for unfinished homework		
Place for completed assignments		
Place to keep materials for later filing		
Notebooks or binder(s) for each subject		
Other things you might need: 1. 2. 3. 4.		

From *Smart but Scattered, Second Edition,* by Peg Dawson, Richard Guare, and Colin Guare. Copyright © 2025 The Guilford Press. Permission to photocopy this material, or to download enlarged printable versions (*www.guilford.com/dawson4-forms*), is granted to purchasers of this book for personal use; see copyright page for details.

binder to handle all subjects. You may want to visit an office supply store to gather ideas.

3. Gather the materials you need—from the house if you have them on hand or from the office supply store if you don't. Materials should include a three-hole punch, lined and unlined paper, subject dividers, and small Post-it packages your child might want to use to flag important papers.

4. Set up the notebooks and folders, labeling everything clearly.

5. At the beginning of each homework session, have your child take out the folders for completed assignments, unfinished work, and material to be filed. Have your child make a decision about each piece of material and where it should go. Complete this process before beginning homework.

6. When homework is completed, have your child place homework in the appropriate folder and file anything else that needs to be saved.

Fading the Supervision

1. Using your child's preferred cueing system, cue your child to begin homework by following the "organizing" process. Supervise each step of the process to make sure all steps are followed and checked off on a checklist. A sample is provided below.

2. Cue your child to begin homework with the organizing process and remind the child to check off each step when done. Check back periodically and check in at the end of homework to make sure the checklist is done and that materials have been stored appropriately.

3. Cue at the beginning, check in at the end, and do occasional spot checks of notebooks, folders, and other files.

Modifications/Adjustments

1. As much as possible, involve your child in the design of the organizing system. We've discovered that what works well for one person is a disaster for another because it's not a good fit.

2. Redesign the elements that aren't working right. Again, involve your child in the troubleshooting. "How could this work better for you?" is the way to approach this.

Maintaining a Notebook/Homework Management System

Task	Monday	Tuesday	Wednesday	Thursday	Weekend
Clean out "to be filed" folder					
Go through notebooks and books for other loose papers and file them					
Do homework					
Place all assignments (both finished and unfinished) in appropriate places					

From *Smart but Scattered, Second Edition*, by Peg Dawson, Richard Guare, and Colin Guare. Copyright © 2025 The Guilford Press. Permission to photocopy this material, or to download enlarged printable versions (*www.guilford.com/dawson4-forms*), is granted to purchasers of this book for personal use; see copyright page for details.

3. Streamline or simplify the system as much as possible. For instance, keeping all incomplete homework in one folder might work better than separating homework by subject.

4. For people who are not naturally organized, it can take a long time for this process to become a habit. Keep in mind that supervision over the long haul may be necessary.

10. Learning to Control Temper

Executive skills addressed: Emotional control (Chapter 12), response inhibition (Chapter 10), flexibility (Chapter 13).

Ages: Any age.

1. Together with your child, make a list of the things that happen that cause your child to lose his or her temper (these are called *triggers*). You may want to make a long list of all the different things that make your child angry and then see if they can be grouped into larger categories (when told "no," when the child loses a game, when something promised doesn't happen, and so on).

2. Talk with your child about what "losing your temper looks or sounds like" (for example, yells, swears, throws things, kicks things or people, and the like). Decide which ones of these should go on a "can't do" list. Keep this list short and work on only one or two behaviors at a time.

3. Now make a list of things your child can do instead (called *replacement behaviors*). These should be three or four different things your child can do instead of the "can't do" behaviors you've selected.

4. Put these on a "Hard Times Board" (see the example on the next page).

5. Practice. Say to your child, "Let's pretend you're upset because Carlos said he would come over to play and then he had to do something else instead. Which strategy do you want to use?" (See the more detailed practice guidelines that follow.)

6. After practicing for a couple of weeks, start using the process "for real," but initially use it for only minor irritants.

7. After using it successfully with minor irritants, move on to the more challenging triggers.

8. Connect the process to a reward. For best results, use two levels of rewards: a "big reward" for never getting to the point where the Hard Times Board needs to be used, and a "small reward" for successfully using a strategy on the Hard Times Board to deal with the trigger situation.

Sample Hard Times Board

TRIGGERS: WHAT MAKES ME MAD

1. When I have to stop doing something fun
2. When it's time to do a chore
3. When my plans don't work out

CAN'T DOS

1. Hit somebody
2. Break anything

WHEN I'M HAVING A HARD TIME, I CAN:

1. Draw a picture
2. Read a book
3. Listen to music
4. Play with the dog

From *Smart but Scattered, Second Edition*, by Peg Dawson, Richard Guare, and Colin Guare. Copyright © 2025 The Guilford Press. Permission to photocopy this material, or to download enlarged printable versions (*www.guilford.com/dawson4-forms*), is granted to purchasers of this book for personal use; see copyright page for details.

My Hard Times Board

TRIGGERS: WHAT MAKES ME MAD

1.
2.
3.

CAN'T DOS

1.
2.

WHEN I'M HAVING A HARD TIME, I CAN:

1.
2.
3.
4.

From *Smart but Scattered, Second Edition*, by Peg Dawson, Richard Guare, and Colin Guare. Copyright © 2025 The Guilford Press. Permission to photocopy this material, or to download enlarged printable versions (*www.guilford.com/dawson4-forms*), is granted to purchasers of this book for personal use; see copyright page for details.

Practicing the Procedure

1. Use real-life examples. These should include a variety representing the different categories of triggers.

2. Make the practice sessions "quick and dirty." For example, if a coping strategy is to read a book, have your child open a book and start reading, but don't spend more than 20–30 seconds on this.

3. Have your child practice each of the strategies listed on the Hard Times Board.

4. Have brief practice sessions daily or several times a week for a couple of weeks before putting it into effect.

Modifications/Adjustments

1. At first you may need to model the use of the strategy. This means talking aloud to show what your child might be saying or thinking as the child implements the strategy.

2. There may be times when, despite having a procedure in place, your child still loses control and can't calm down or use any of the strategies on the Hard Times Board. In this case, remove the child from the situation (physically if necessary). Tell the child in advance that you will do this, so that your child knows what to expect. Say, "If you hit or kick or scream, we're always going to leave."

3. If your child is fairly consistently unable to use the strategies effectively, it may be time to consider seeking professional help; see Chapter 21.

11. Learning to Control Impulsive Behavior

Executive skills addressed: Response inhibition (Chapter 10), emotional control (Chapter 12).

Ages: Any age.

1. Together with your child, identify the triggers for the impulsive behavior (watching TV with siblings, open-ended play with friends, or whatever). You can use the worksheet on the next page if you like.

2. Agree on a rule for the trigger situation. The rule should focus on what your child can do to control impulses. Build in choice if you can—in other words, you and your child should come up with a couple of different things the child can do in place of the unwanted impulsive response.

3. Talk about what you might do to signal to your child that you think they are on the verge of "losing control" so that they can back off or use one of the coping strategies agreed on. This works best when the signal is a relatively discrete visual signal (for example, a hand motion) that can alert your child to the problem situation.

The things I do without thinking include:

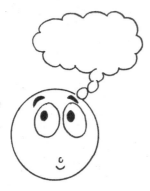

Common situations where I act without thinking are:

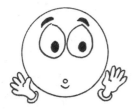

What I will do to stay controlled:

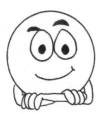

From *Smart but Scattered, Second Edition*, by Peg Dawson, Richard Guare, and Colin Guare. Copyright © 2025 The Guilford Press. Permission to photocopy this material, or to download enlarged printable versions (*www.guilford.com/dawson4-forms*), is granted to purchasers of this book for personal use; see copyright page for details.

4. Practice the procedure. Make this a "Let's pretend" role play. "Let's pretend you're outside playing with your friends and one of them says something that makes you mad. I'll be your friend and you be you." If this is hard for your child, you may want to play your child in this role play to model how the child will handle the situation.

5. As with the other skills involving behavior regulation, practice the procedure daily or several times a week for a couple of weeks.

6. When you and your child are ready to put the procedure in effect in "real life," remind the child about it just before the trigger situation is likely to occur (for example, "Remember the plan," "Remember what we talked about").

7. Review how the process worked afterward. You may want to create a scale that you and your child can use to assess how well it went (5—Went without a hitch! to 1— *That* didn't go real well!).

Modifications/Adjustments

1. If you think it will make the process work more effectively or more quickly, tie the successful use of a replacement behavior to a reinforcer. This may best be done using a "response cost" approach. For example, give your child 70 points to begin the day. Each time your child acts impulsively, subtract 10 points. You can also give bonus points if your child gets through a specified period of time without losing any points.

2. If impulsivity is a significant problem for your child, begin by choosing one time of day or one impulsive behavior to target to make success more likely.

3. Be sure to praise your child for showing self-control. Even if you're using tangible rewards, social praise should always accompany any other kind of reinforcer.

12. Learning to Manage Anxiety

Executive skills addressed: Emotional control (Chapter 12), flexibility (Chapter 13).

Ages: All ages.

1. Together with your child, make a list of the things that happen that cause your child to feel anxious. See if there's a pattern and whether different situations can be grouped into one larger category (for example, a child who gets nervous on the soccer field, when giving an oral report in school, and playing in a piano recital may have *performance* anxiety—that is, the child gets nervous when they have to perform in front of others).

2. Talk with your child about what anxiety feels like, so the child can recognize it in the early stages. This is often a physical feeling—"butterflies" in the stomach, sweaty hands, faster heartbeat.

3. Now make a list of things your child can do instead of thinking about the worry

(called *replacement behaviors*). These should be three or four different things your child can do that either are calming or divert attention from the worries.

4. Put these on a "Worry Board" (an example appears on the facing page).

5. Practice. Say to your child, "Let's pretend you're getting nervous because you have a baseball tryout and you're worried you won't make the team. Which strategy do you want to use?" (See the more detailed practice guidelines that follow.)

6. After practicing for a couple of weeks, start using the process "for real" but initially use it for only minor worries.

7. After using it successfully with minor worries, move on to bigger anxieties.

8. Connect the process to a reward. For best results, use two levels of rewards: a "big reward" for never getting to the point where the Worry Board needs to be used and a "small reward" for successfully using a strategy on the Worry Board to deal with the trigger situation.

Practicing the Procedure

1. Use real-life examples. These should include a variety representing the different categories of triggers.

2. Make the practice sessions "quick and dirty." For example, if a coping strategy is to practice "thought stopping," have the child practice the following self-talk strategy: Tell her to say, loudly and forcefully (but to herself), "*Stop!*" This momentarily interrupts any thought. As soon the child has done this, have her think of a pleasant image or scene. Practice this a few times daily. When the problem or anxiety-provoking thought occurs, use this strategy, and continue repeating it until the thought stops.

3. Have your child practice each of the strategies listed on the Worry Board.

4. Have brief practice sessions daily or several times a week for a couple of weeks before putting it into effect.

Modifications/Adjustments

1. Possible coping strategies for managing anxiety might include deep or slow breathing, counting to 20, using other relaxation strategies, thought stopping or talking back to your worries, drawing a picture of the worry, folding it up, and putting it in a box with a lid, listening to music (and maybe dancing to it), challenging the logic of the worry. For further explanation for these, type "relaxation for kids" into a search engine and check out the websites that come up. Another helpful resource is a book written for children and parents to read together: *What to Do When You Worry Too Much* by Dawn Huebner, PhD.

2. Helping children manage anxiety generally involves a procedure sometimes called *desensitization*, in which the degree of anxiety to which the child is exposed is low

Sample Worry Board

I GET WORRIED WHEN . . .

1. *I have a test at school*
2. *I have to kick a soccer ball in a game*
3. *I have to talk in front of a group*

WHEN I GET NERVOUS . . .

1. *My heart beats too fast*
2. *My stomach feels queasy*
3. *I have trouble thinking clearly*

WHEN I'M FEELING WORRIED OR NERVOUS, I CAN . . .

1. *Draw a picture of my worry and then tear it up*
2. *Use a relaxation technique*
3. *Talk back to my worries*
4. *Listen to music*

From *Smart but Scattered, Second Edition*, by Peg Dawson, Richard Guare, and Colin Guare. Copyright © 2025 The Guilford Press. Permission to photocopy this material, or to download enlarged printable versions (*www.guilford.com/ dawson4-forms*), is granted to purchasers of this book for personal use; see copyright page for details.

My Worry Board

I GET WORRIED WHEN . . .

1.
2.
3.

WHEN I GET NERVOUS . . .

1.
2.
3.

WHEN I'M FEELING WORRIED OR NERVOUS, I CAN . . .

1.
2.
3.
4.

From *Smart but Scattered, Second Edition*, by Peg Dawson, Richard Guare, and Colin Guare. Copyright © 2025 The Guilford Press. Permission to photocopy this material, or to download enlarged printable versions (*www.guilford.com/ dawson4-forms*), is granted to purchasers of this book for personal use; see copyright page for details.

enough so that with some support he can get through it successfully. For example, if a child is afraid of dogs, you might begin by asking him to look at a picture of a dog and model what he might say to himself ("I'm looking at this picture, and it's a little scary when I think of there being a real dog, but I'm managing OK, I'm not getting too scared. I can look at the picture OK"). The next step might be to have the child be inside a house with a dog outside and talk about what that's like. Very gradually bring the dog closer to the child. A similar approach can be used with other fears and phobias. The exposure has to be very gradual; you don't move to the next step until the child feels comfortable with the current step. The critical elements in guided mastery are physical distance and time—in the beginning, the child is far removed from the anxiety-provoking object and the exposure is for a very short time. The distance is then reduced and the time increased gradually. It's also helpful to have a script (something the child is to say in the situation) and a tactic he can use (such as thought stopping or something he can do to divert his attention).

3. The kinds of worries or anxieties that this approach will work with are (1) separation anxiety (being unhappy or worried when separated from a loved one, usually a parent); (2) handling novel or unfamiliar situations; and (3) obsessive or catastrophic thinking (worrying about something bad happening). This approach should work with all three, although the coping strategies for each may vary.

13. Learning to Handle Changes in Plans

Executive skills addressed: Emotional control (Chapter 12), flexibility (Chapter 13).

Ages: Any age.

Helping your child accept changes in plans without anger or distress involves some advance work and lots of practice. Whenever possible, present your agenda for your child ahead of time, before the child has formulated their own plan for that time period. Meanwhile, you start introducing the child to small changes on a regular basis, gradually increasing the child's tolerance for surprises over time.

1. Sit down with your child and establish a schedule of activities and tasks. This might mean creating some organization and routine for the day, or it might mean simply making a list of events that are already part of a routine. Include any activity that is a "have to" as far as you're concerned (mealtimes, bedtime, and so on) and any regular activity (such as lessons and sports). You can use the form on the facing page or make one of your own.

2. Try not to attach precise times to the activities unless necessary (as with sports events and lessons), using time ranges instead. For example, dinner might be around 5:00 P.M., which could be between 4:30 and 5:30.

Managing Changes in Plans or Schedules

DAILY SCHEDULE

Date: _____

Time	Activity

Surprise:

From *Smart but Scattered, Second Edition*, by Peg Dawson, Richard Guare, and Colin Guare. Copyright © 2025 The Guilford Press. Permission to photocopy this material, or to download enlarged printable versions (*www.guilford.com/dawson4-forms*), is granted to purchasers of this book for personal use; see copyright page for details.

3. Talk with your child about the fact that changes or "surprises" can always come up despite plans and schedules established in advance. Give examples: instead of fish, we have pizza for dinner; you get to play outside for an extra 20 minutes; we have to go to the dentist today.

4. Create a visual for the schedule, such as activities written on a card or a series of pictures, and post it in at least two places, such as the kitchen and your child's room. Make a card that says "Surprise!" on it and explain that when a change is coming, you will show him the card, say what the change is, and write it in the "Surprise" section on the schedule. (Even when a change comes up that's a surprise to everyone, you can pull out the card and follow the same process.)

5. Review the schedule with your child either the night before and/or the morning of the day.

6. Start to introduce changes. For each one, show the Surprise! card and then note the change in the Surprise section of the form. Initially these should be pleasant, such as extra playtime, going out for ice cream, playing a game with a parent. Gradually introduce more "neutral" changes (apple juice for orange juice, one cereal for another, and the like). Eventually include less pleasant changes (can't do a planned activity because of weather).

Modifications/Adjustments

If the Surprise! card and the gradual introduction of changes are not sufficient, there are a few other approaches to consider. When possible, introduce the change well before the event. This gives your child time to adjust gradually rather than quickly. Depending on her reaction to less pleasant change (crying, resisting, complaining), talk about other behaviors the child could use that would allow for protest in an acceptable way (such as filling out a Complaint Form, see below). You also can provide a reward for success-fully managing the change. Keep in mind that reactivity to change decreases with the amount of exposure that the child has and the success she has in negotiating it. As long as the exposure is gradual and does not initially involve situations that are frustrating or threatening, your child can become more flexible.

14. Learning Not to Cry over Little Things

Executive skills addressed: Emotional control (Chapter 12), flexibility (Chapter 13).

Ages: Any age.

When children cry over little things, they're generally trying to communicate that they want sympathy, and they're using this method of getting it because they've found it effective in the past. So the goal of this intervention is not to teach kids to be tough

Complaint Form

Date: _____

Nature of complaint:

Why you think the situation was unfair:

What you wish had happened:

From *Smart but Scattered, Second Edition,* by Peg Dawson, Richard Guare, and Colin Guare. Copyright © 2025 The Guilford Press. Permission to photocopy this material, or to download enlarged printable versions (*www.guilford.com/dawson4-forms*), is granted to purchasers of this book for personal use; see copyright page for details.

little soldiers or anything of the sort, but to help them find ways other than crying to get what they want. The goal is to get them to use words instead of tears in those situations where crying does not appear to be an appropriate response.

1. Let your child know that crying too much makes people disinclined to spend time with him or her and that you want to help the child find other ways of handling feelings when upset so that this doesn't happen.

2. Explain that your child needs to use words instead of tears when upset. This can be done by having your child label their feelings ("I'm upset," "I'm sad," "I'm angry," and the like).

3. Let your child know that it may be helpful to explain what caused these feelings (for example, "I'm upset because I was hoping to go to DeDe's house, but when I called, no one was home," or "I'm mad because I lost the game").

4. When your child is able to use words, respond by validating the child's feelings (for example, "I can see you're upset. Not being able to play with a friend must be a big disappointment to you"). Statements like this will communicate to the child that you understand and sympathize.

5. Let your child know in advance what will happen when an upsetting situation arrives. This should include giving the child a script for handling the situation. You might say, "When you feel like crying, you can use words like 'I'm angry,' 'I'm sad,' 'I need help,' or 'I need a break.' When you use words, I'll listen and try to understand your feelings. If you start to cry, though, you're on your own. I'll either leave the room or ask you to go to your bedroom to finish crying." At first you may periodically need to remind your child of the procedure to prepare the child to follow the script when an upsetting situation occurs.

6. As soon as your child starts to cry, make sure they get no attention from anyone for crying. This means no attention from *anyone* (siblings, parents, grandparents, and others), so you should make sure everybody likely to be involved understands the procedure. Without the attention for crying, it will gradually diminish (although it may get worse initially before it gets better).

7. The goal here is not to extinguish *all crying* (because there are legitimate reasons for children to cry). A rule of thumb for judging when it may be appropriate to cry is to think about the average child of your child's age. Would crying be a natural response in the situation at hand? Crying is appropriate, for instance, when dealing with physical pain or when a serious misfortune befalls your child or someone your child is close to.

Modifications/Adjustments

If crying is firmly entrenched, you may want to build in a reinforcer to help your child learn to use words instead of tears. Depending on the age of your child, you could give the child stickers or points for using words instead of tears or for going a certain amount of time without crying. To determine how long that time should be, it would be helpful to take a baseline, so you know how frequently your child cries now. A log to help you track how often the crying occurs, how long it lasts, and the precipitating event is included on the facing page. At the bottom of the log is a "contract" you can make with your child to handle crying. Depending on the age of the child, the contract can be completed with words, pictures, or both.

15. Learning to Solve Problems

Executive skills addressed: Metacognition (Chapter 20), flexibility (Chapter 13).

Ages: 7–14; even though metacognition in its most advanced form is one of the latest skills to develop, you can do problem solving with younger kids too (see, for example, the widely respected program called *I Can Problem Solve*, by Myrna B. Shure, PhD, for preschoolers).

1. Talk with your child about what the problem is. This generally involves three steps: (a) empathizing with the child or letting the child know you understand how they feel ("I can see that makes you really mad" or "That must be really upsetting for you"); (b) getting a *general* sense of what the problem is ("Let me get this straight—you're upset because the friend you were hoping to play with can't come over"); and (c) defining the problem more narrowly so that you can begin to brainstorm solutions ("You have a whole afternoon free, and you can't figure out what to do").

2. Brainstorm solutions. Together with your child, think of as many different things as you can that might solve the problem. You may want to set a time limit (like 2 minutes) because this sometimes speeds up the process or makes it feel less like an open-ended task. Write down all the possible solutions. Don't criticize the solutions at this point because this tends to squelch the creative thinking process.

3. Ask your child to look at all the solutions and pick the one the child likes best. You may want to start by having your child circle the top three to five choices and then narrow them down by talking about the pluses and minuses associated with each choice.

4. Ask your child if they need help carrying out the choice.

5. Talk about what will happen if the first solution doesn't work. This may involve choosing a different solution or analyzing where the first solution went wrong and fixing it.

6. Praise the child for coming up with a good solution (and then praise again after the solution is implemented).

Upset Log

Date	Time	Duration of upset	Precipitating event

Here's what I can do instead of crying:

Here's what will happen if I can keep from crying when I'm upset:

Here's what will happen when I cry over little things:

From *Smart but Scattered, Second Edition,* by Peg Dawson, Richard Guare, and Colin Guare. Copyright © 2025 The Guilford Press. Permission to photocopy this material, or to download enlarged printable versions (*www.guilford.com/dawson4-forms*), is granted to purchasers of this book for personal use; see copyright page for details.

Modifications/Adjustments

This is a standard problem-solving approach that can be used for all kinds of problems, including interpersonal problems as well as obstacles that prevent a child from getting what they want or need. Sometimes the best solution will involve figuring out ways to overcome the obstacles, while at other times it may involve helping your child come to terms with the fact that they cannot have what they want.

Sometimes the problem-solving process may lead to a "negotiation," where you and your child agree on what will be done to reach a solution that's satisfactory. In this case you should explain to your child that whatever solution you come up with, you both have to be able to live with it. You may want to talk about how labor contracts are negotiated so that both workers and bosses get something they want out of the bargain.

After you've used the process (and the Solving Problems Worksheet on the facing page) with your child for a number of different kinds of problems, your child may be able to use the worksheet independently. Because your goal should be to foster independent problem solving, you may want to ask your child to fill out the worksheet alone before coming to you for your help (if needed). Eventually your child will internalize the whole process and be able to solve problems "on the fly."

Solving Problems Worksheet

What is my problem?

What are some possible things I could do to solve my problem?

What will I try first?

If this doesn't work, what can I do?

How did it go? Did my solution work?

What might I do differently the next time?

From *Smart but Scattered, Second Edition*, by Peg Dawson, Richard Guare, and Colin Guare. Copyright © 2025 The Guilford Press. Permission to photocopy this material, or to download enlarged printable versions (*www.guilford.com/dawson4-forms*), is granted to purchasers of this book for personal use; see copyright page for details.

10

Building Response Inhibition

Response inhibition is the capacity to think before you act—to resist the urge to say or do something before you've had a chance to evaluate the situation. In adults, the *absence* of this skill is more apparent to the casual observer than the presence of the skill because most of us maintain a level of self-control that enables us to function well at home and at work. Most of us have learned on the long road to adulthood, often through painful experience, how to think before acting. When we spot someone who does stand out due to a lack of response inhibition, we have a multitude of metaphors and other expressions to describe the resulting behavior: we say the person "shoots from the hip" or "flies off the handle," or we just comment "Open mouth, insert foot."

Some of us exercise this executive skill quite well until we find ourselves in an emotionally charged situation. In this day of instant communication, angry texts or emails that the sender instantly regrets—or regrets after receiving an equally angry response—are a common product of weak response inhibition. Our ability to think before acting also suffers when we're physically impaired by too much alcohol, too little sleep, or too much stress. If you tend to jump to conclusions, or you act before you have all the necessary facts, or you blurt out whatever pops into your mind without thinking, you may be challenged in response inhibition yourself. To help your child overcome response inhibition challenges when you share the weakness, see the suggestions in Chapter 3.

How Response Inhibition Develops

As we said early in this book, response inhibition emerges first in infancy. In its most rudimentary form, response inhibition allows an infant to "choose" to respond or not respond to whatever is before the baby. Prior to its emergence, babies pretty much respond to their immediate environment. If something enters their visual field, they fixate on it, at least long enough to make sense out of it. With response inhibition comes the capacity to ignore or not be deterred by interruptions if there's something else they are working toward. Once language develops, the capacity to inhibit responding becomes more developed because they can internalize rules given to them by others (for example, "Don't touch the hot stove").

Just as goal-directed persistence, in its most advanced and complex form, may be the culminating executive skill that defines a mature adult, response inhibition is the fundamental executive skill that enables all other executive skills to develop. Children at the mercy of their impulses struggle to initiate, sustain attention, plan, organize, or problem solve effectively. One who develops a strong ability to inhibit impulses has a significant advantage in school, making friends, and ultimately setting and achieving goals.

Developing response inhibition in young children often begins with teaching "wait" and "stop." And there are some natural ways that parents of young children teach this concept. As a young child (this is Peg talking), I remember being made to take a nap at an age when I didn't think I needed to nap anymore. I complained about it, but I remember lying down on my bed and watching my mother set a kitchen timer. "You can get up when the bell rings," she instructed me. What was she doing? Teaching me to wait.

By the way, there are childhood games that have been around for generations if not centuries that teach the same skill. Think about "Simon Says" or "Red Light Green Light." Those games require the children playing them to listen to the instructions and make a decision: Are they going to act or stop or wait? Perhaps you can think of other childhood games that teach the same lesson.

A famous study conducted many years ago by a Stanford University psychologist named Walter Mischel, known as "the marshmallow test," showed that kids vary in their ability to inhibit responses when very young and that those variations predict different levels of performance later in development. Three- to 5-year-olds were left alone in a room with one marshmallow and given the choice of eating it or waiting until the researcher returned and getting two marshmallows. Through a one-way mirror, the researchers watched some of the children control their impulse to eat the single marshmallow by talking to themselves, avoiding looking at the marshmallow, or finding other ways to divert their attention from the candy. When the researchers followed up many years later, they found that those children who had good response inhibition as preschoolers were earning better grades on their report cards, were less likely to be in trouble with the law, and were more successful in other ways.

Sesame Street at one point hired the marshmallow test researcher as a consultant to help them create content to teach young children to wait. They produced some engaging parodies that are as entertaining for parents as for children. Check them out by going to YouTube and typing *Sesame Street executive functioning* into the search engine.

While children become more adept at using most executive skills over time and with age, the development of response inhibition may not follow so steady a trajectory. Response inhibition, it seems, may be more susceptible to disruption in adolescence. Neuroscientists studying how the brain changes during the teen years have found that there is something of a "disconnect" between the lower centers of the brain, where emotions and impulses are processed, and the prefrontal cortex, where rational decisions are made. Only slowly, over the course of adolescence, and even into adulthood, do these connections become stronger and faster (through pruning and myelination, as described in Chapter 1), enabling young people to temper their emotions with reason. Until those connections are firmly in place, youngsters are more likely to make decisions rashly and based on "gut feelings" without the anchoring influence of sound judgment that the frontal lobes provide.

Meanwhile, teenagers are undergoing other developmental changes that challenge impulse control. Gaining autonomy is a critical developmental task that's facilitated when teens become more strongly influenced by their peers and at the same time begin to challenge parental authority. Unfortunately, while this shift is helping teens become independent, it's also potentially leading the teens to be more impulsive. And to make matters even more complicated, society as a whole starts to loosen the controls, allowing teenagers a lot more freedom in how they spend their time and who they spend it with. Inevitably, this loosening of control, as essential as it is, can lead to bad decisions. If we're lucky, bad decisions will result in good lessons learned and no permanent damage to our children or anybody else. But we can increase our luck in this area if we actively help our children learn to control their impulses.

How does your child's ability to control her impulses stack up against what's developmentally appropriate? The rating scale in the questionnaire on the facing page can help you answer this question, confirming or denying your preliminary assessment from Chapter 2 by giving you the chance to look a little more closely at how often your child is able to use this skill.

If you gave your child mostly 2s or higher for each ability for her age, you can probably say your child is not seriously deficient in response inhibition but would benefit from some tweaking. If you gave the child all 0s or 1s, you probably need to teach the skill directly. To help you design your own intervention strategy, we provide a fairly detailed scenario depicting situations that parents frequently seek our help with. Following the description of an intervention we've used, we give you a template, or outline, that breaks the intervention down by the kinds of elements we discussed in the first half of the book. In each case we describe environmental modifications, a skill instruction sequence, and an incentive to help reinforce the child for using the skills. Don't forget to use our suggestions in Chapter 3 for boosting your success with such interventions when you and your child have a weakness in response inhibition.

A Good Place to Start

The essence of response inhibition, especially in young children, is being able to wait or stop. So we recommend that parents begin by teaching "wait/stop." This can be easily incorporated in situations that arise naturally. Here are a couple of examples from personal experience (this is Peg talking):

How Well Can Your Child Inhibit Impulses?

Use the following scale to rate how well your child performs each of the tasks listed. At each level, children can be expected to perform all the tasks listed fairly well to very well.

Never or rarely	Does but not well (about 25% of the time)	Does fairly well (about 75% of the time)	Does very well (always or almost always)
0	1	2	3

PRESCHOOL/KINDERGARTEN

☐ Acts appropriately in situations where danger is obvious (e.g., not running into the road to retrieve a ball, looking both ways before crossing street)

☐ Can share toys without grabbing

☐ Can wait for a short period of time when instructed by an adult

LOWER ELEMENTARY (GRADES 1–3)

☐ Can follow simple classroom rules (e.g., raising hand before speaking)

☐ Can be in close proximity to another child without need for physical contact

☐ Can wait until a parent gets off the phone before telling the parent something (may need reminders)

UPPER ELEMENTARY (GRADES 4–5)

☐ Handles conflict with peers without getting into physical fights (may lose temper)

☐ Follows home or school rules without an adult's immediate presence

☐ Can calm down or de-escalate from emotionally charged situation when prompted by an adult

MIDDLE SCHOOL (GRADES 6–8)

☐ Able to walk away from confrontation or provocation by a peer

☐ Can say no to a fun activity if other plans have already been made

☐ Resists saying hurtful things when with a group of friends

From *Smart but Scattered, Second Edition,* by Peg Dawson, Richard Guare, and Colin Guare. Copyright © 2025 The Guilford Press. Permission to photocopy this material, or to download enlarged printable versions (*www.guilford.com/dawson4-forms*), is granted to purchasers of this book for personal use; see copyright page for details.

- A mom in an airport telling her young daughter that she will be able to eat the special treat just purchased at a food court "as soon as we get to the gate." (I kept an eye on the pair—the daughter waited until they got to the gate, which took about 2 minutes.)
- A mom arriving at a beach and halting her toddler son before he dashed off into the water. "Wait just a minute," she said, and this command stopped her son in his tracks. She set down the blanket, towels, and lunch cooler, which took about a minute, and then told her son, "OK—we can go in the water now."

Even with older children, waiting is a skill worth practicing. The wait time can be stretched for longer periods. When I was 14 (Peg talking again), I desperately wanted to get my ears pierced. My father told me that if I waited until my birthday and still wanted to get my ears pierced, he would consider it. That conversation took place in January—my birthday wasn't until September. When my birthday came, I got my ears pierced.

Building Response Inhibition in Everyday Situations

- *Always assume that the youngest children have very limited impulse control.* This may seem like stating the obvious, but when you have a kid who's smart but scattered, emphasis on *smart*, it's remarkably easy to forget that native intelligence doesn't translate to response inhibition when the child in question is only 4, 5, or 6. Even though response inhibition starts to develop in infancy, preschool and primary-grade children have a lot of competing drives to contend with, whether it's the desire to have a four-scoop ice cream cone instead of a single scoop, to stay up late because they don't feel even a little bit tired, or to dart across the school parking lot to see their best friend when the lot is teeming with cars trying to get back on the road. Whether it's removing temptations by controlling snacks, establishing routines such as consistent bedtimes, making rules about behavior (such as displaying good table manners and sharing toys with a playmate), or providing close supervision in situations where impulses might get a child in trouble (such as in that busy parking lot), setting limits for our kids introduces the youngest kids to impulse control and thus encourages response inhibition.

- *Help your child learn to delay gratification by using formal waiting periods for things she wants to do or have.* Learning to wait for something is the foundation for the more sophisticated executive skills we want children to develop over time. If your child has trouble waiting, set a timer and let her know when the bell rings she can have or do what she's asked for. Make the time lag small initially and gradually increase the time delay. First—then schedules accomplish the same goal ("First do your spelling homework, then you get to play a video game").

● *Offering children the opportunity to earn some things they want is another way to teach them to delay gratification and inhibit impulses.* If this is hard for them, give them a visible means to mark their progress, such as a graph or sticker chart.

● *Help children understand that there are consequences for weak impulse control.* In some cases the consequences will be naturally occurring events (if your son keeps hitting his playmates, they will soon not want to play with him anymore), while in other cases you will need to impose consequences ("If you can share the Xbox with your brother, you can continue to play with it").

● *Prepare your child for situations that require impulse control by reviewing them in advance.* Ask, "What are the rules for playing video games?" or "What might you do if there's a long line of kids waiting to go down the biggest slide at the water park?"

● *Practice response inhibition in role-playing situations.* Kids, just like adults, may have more trouble controlling impulses than usual when the situation is emotionally charged or they're overtired or overstimulated (such as during holidays). In those cases in particular, pose a predictably dicey dilemma and play the role of someone who might challenge your child's ability to think before acting or speaking.

● *Cue your child before he enters a situation that calls for a specific behavior you're targeting and then recognize him for exhibiting self-control.* Let's say you're working hard at helping your child avoid getting into fights when he goes outdoors to play with neighbors. Before your son goes outside, ask, "What behavior are we working on?" If he's not sure, review the expectations (keep them simple) and have him repeat them. Then watch how things go so you can offer specific praise quickly after your child shows that he's practicing self-control. It's important for you to be right there (or at least able to watch from a short distance, such as through a window), so you can observe the behavior directly rather than relying on your child's report. Being present is also important because you need to be able to reinforce your child's positive behavior as it occurs.

● *Remember to praise your child for waiting.* We are pretty quick to correct children when they do something wrong, but we often forget to acknowledge good behavior. Here are some examples of things you could say: "Nice job waiting," or "You really had something you wanted to say, but you were able to wait until Dad finished talking before you said anything," or "I appreciate your waiting until I got off my Zoom call before you started playing a video game."

● *Use storybooks or other media to teach children about response inhibition.* The *Sesame Street* videos referenced above can be a great conversation starter. Although they are obviously geared toward preschoolers, we know middle school teachers who've used them successfully to teach this skill in the classroom (such as by introducing them in a way that acknowledges they may seem "babyish" but challenging students to apply the lessons to age-appropriate issues). The Resources at the end of the book include a list of picture books that have response inhibition as a theme. *See routine 11 in Chapter 9 for a general teaching sequence to help children learn to control impulsive behavior.*

A Parent's Fondest Dream:
Reducing Interruptions during Phone Calls

Mekhi, an active 6-year-old, is the younger of two children in his family. He can play for short periods of time alone but likes it better if he has a friend to play with or one of his parents is available. His 9-year-old sister has little patience for the games he wants to play. His parents, particularly Mom, are especially frustrated by Mekhi's interrupting when they're on the phone or when someone comes to the door. For example, Mekhi might be looking at a book when the phone rings. As soon as his mother picks it up, Mekhi is there. Sometimes it might be a repeated question: "Mom, can you play a game with me?" Or he might be complaining about his sister's being mean to him. Often he tugs on her arm, sits in her lap, or touches her face. Mekhi's father gets similar interruptions but is less bothered by them because he's not around as often and Mom gets the brunt of this behavior.

Mekhi's parents have tried a number of techniques to get around these disruptions. If the phone call is short, they alternate between ignoring Mekhi and telling him to be quiet. Once in a while, if the call is important, they will try to "buy" quiet behavior with the promise of a new toy. Sometimes they will put the call off until later. When Mekhi is particularly noisy, they threaten a consequence when they get off the phone. They haven't had much success with any approach and would like to see Mekhi begin to manage this behavior on his own.

Mekhi's parents ask Mekhi if he could help them solve a problem. They describe their problem and explain that it's important for them to be able to talk and listen to other people on the phone. They give a few examples, and Mekhi also gives an example of when he talks on the phone. His parents ask if Mekhi could think of something he could do instead of talking to them during phone calls. He suggests playing with trucks or watching TV. TV time is already limited to a certain part of the day, so the parents ask for another idea, and Mekhi chooses LEGOs. Mekhi makes a card with drawings of trucks and LEGOs and with help writes the words underneath each picture. They will keep the card by the phone, and when the phone rings or when Mom or Dad need to make a call, they will show it to Mekhi, and he will choose one or the other activity. For the first few weeks his parents make "practice" phone calls or ask family or friends to call occasionally so Mekhi can practice his plan. They realize that in the early stages the calls need to be short. They also realize that they need to reinforce Mekhi's desirable behavior frequently (at least twice a minute) by telling him that he's doing a good job playing. Whenever they failed to do this in the first few days, Mekhi stopped playing and came to them. From this they recognized that they had to praise him before he interrupted them. They make a deal with him that if he does a good job, he can pick out some new LEGOs or trucks to add to his collection.

Intervention Steps

Step 1: Establish a Behavioral Goal

Target executive skill(s): Response inhibition

Specific behavioral objective: Engage in independent play and do not interrupt when parents are on the phone.

Step 2: Design Interventions

What environmental supports will be provided to help reach the target goal?

- Availability of preferred toys
- Picture card of play choices
- Parent cue to choose when phone rings

• • •

What specific skill will be taught, who will teach the skill, and what procedure will be used to teach it?

Skill: Response inhibition (learning to play independently instead of seeking out parents when they are on the phone)

Who will teach the skill? Parents

Procedure:

- Mekhi chooses two preferred play activities.
- Parents make up picture cards for these activities.
- When parents are going to make or answer a phone call, they present card and Mekhi chooses one activity.
- Parents, during call, praise him for continuing to play.

• • •

What incentives will be used to help motivate the child to use/practice the skill?

- Parents praise Mekhi for playing.
- Parents add to Mekhi's toy collection for these activities if he does well.

Keys to Success

- *Don't wait to reinforce the behavior you're looking for.* Parents sometimes feel silly praising a child for sticking with the chosen activity when the child has been involved with it for only a minute. But as Mekhi's parents quickly discovered, if you wait, you're leaving a window wide open for your child to abandon the activity and come looking for attention, in which case the whole exercise has already gotten off on the wrong foot.

- *Don't assume that quick success means the problem has been solved.* In most cases, if you follow the plan and pay attention to your child at short intervals, you will see success quickly. It's then far too easy to get overconfident—or simply to forget to praise your child because you're not being interrupted. But if you abandon this exercise prematurely, the old behavior pattern is bound to return—and then you're likely to decide the plan simply failed. Attention must be faded gradually (for example, from every 30 seconds to every 45 or 60 and so on) until your child can engage in the activity for 5–10 minutes or more without interrupting. How long the child can stay with the activity is somewhat dependent on age, so with younger children (kindergarten to early elementary grades), you should continue to check in at least every few minutes.

11

Enhancing Working Memory

Working memory is the capacity to hold information in mind while performing complex tasks. We rely on working memory all the time. It's the ability to run out to the store to buy a few things and remember what they are without having to write them down. When you remember to stop by the dry cleaner on your way home from work, you're using working memory. When you look up a phone number and remember it long enough to make the call, you're using working memory. When your spouse asks you to do something and you say, "I'll do it as soon as I finish loading the dishwasher," and then you actually remember to do it, chances are your working memory is pretty good. Odds are it's not so good, however, if you can't remember anyone's birthday, you tend to return home with only half your errands done unless you have a written itinerary, and you'll do anything to avoid having to introduce people at a cocktail party because you can't remember anyone's name. In that case, be sure to use the tips in Chapter 3 to help you enhance your child's working memory when you have the same weakness.

How Working Memory Develops

Working memory begins to develop fairly early in infancy. When you're playing with a baby and you hide a favorite toy under a blanket, you know the baby is using working memory if he lifts the blanket to retrieve the toy. This is because the baby is able to hold an image of the toy in mind as well as the memory of what you did to hide it.

Children develop *nonverbal* working memory before they develop *verbal* working memory because this skill begins to emerge before language does. When children develop language, however, their working memory skills expand because now they can draw on both visual imagery and language to retrieve information.

We tend naturally to limit our expectations for working memory in very young children. Before the age of 3, we generally expect children to remember only things that are in close proximity—either in time or in space. If we want them to do something, we don't say, "Would you mind putting your toys away after you finish watching *Barney*?" (unless we also expect to cue them once *Barney* is over). And while we might ask them to put all their blocks in the toy box while we're standing in the playroom with them, we generally don't instruct them to go to their bedroom and do a similar task all by themselves.

Gradually we're able to stretch both time and distance in terms of what we expect our children to be able to remember. One caution: In the work we've done with schools for children with complex learning disabilities or dyslexia, those teachers tell us that working memory is particularly challenging for this group of students—and there is a lot of research to support that observation. This suggests that these children may need cues, prompts, and reminders for longer than we think we should have to provide them. There are some children whose working memory skills may never "work" as well as we'd like. In this case, the long-term goal should be for these children to identify those situations where working memory challenges get them in trouble and to develop a compensating strategy (an environmental modification) that works for them.

In the questionnaire on the facing page, you can evaluate where your child might fall on the developmental ladder based on the kinds of tasks children are capable of carrying out independently at various childhood stages. Using this scale will give you a closer look than the scales in Chapter 2 did at how well your child uses the skill of working memory.

A Good Place to Start

Probably the most important thing to understand about working memory is that it allows for the temporary storage of information but is restricted in two important ways: (1) by the length of time information can be held in memory and (2) by the amount of information it can manage at any one time. The research consensus is that working memory develops over the course of childhood, and adult capacity is 4–5 items. The amount of information retained can be increased to some extent by "chunking"—by combining pieces of information into groups. Think of telephone numbers: 10 numbers are a lot to hold on to, so we chunk them into sets of three, each of which has no more than four numbers in it (for example, 708-555-1555).

What this tells us is that working memory is limited in general, so the working memory of a child who struggles with this executive skill is even more limited. A good place to start then is to understand that if we are relying on our children to recall verbal instructions of any appreciable length, more often than not we're going to be disappointed if not frustrated. Below we provide lots of suggestions for how to work around weaknesses in working memory, but our first piece of advice is this: whenever possible, pair the verbal with a visual.

How Good Is Your Child's Working Memory?

Use the following scale to rate how well your child performs each of the tasks listed. At each level, children can be expected to perform all the tasks listed fairly well to very well.

Never or rarely	Does but not well (about 25% of the time)	Does fairly well (about 75% of the time)	Does very well (always or almost always)
0	1	2	3

PRESCHOOL/KINDERGARTEN

☐ Runs simple errands (e.g., gets shoes from bedroom when asked)

☐ Remembers instructions that were just given

☐ Follows a routine with only one prompt per step (e.g., brushing teeth after breakfast)

LOWER ELEMENTARY (GRADES 1–3)

☐ Able to run an errand with two to three steps

☐ Remembers instructions that were given a couple of minutes earlier

☐ Follows two steps of a routine with one prompt

UPPER ELEMENTARY (GRADES 4–5)

☐ Remembers to perform a routine chore after school without reminder

☐ Takes books, papers, assignments to and from school

☐ Keeps track of changing daily schedule (e.g., different activities after school)

MIDDLE SCHOOL (GRADES 6–8)

☐ Able to keep track of assignments and classroom expectations of multiple teachers

☐ Remembers events or responsibilities that deviate from the norm (e.g., permission slips for field trips, special instructions regarding extracurricular activities)

☐ Remembers multistep directions, given sufficient time or practice

From *Smart but Scattered, Second Edition*, by Peg Dawson, Richard Guare, and Colin Guare. Copyright © 2025 The Guilford Press. Permission to photocopy this material, or to download enlarged printable versions (*www.guilford.com/dawson4-forms*), is granted to purchasers of this book for personal use; see copyright page for details.

Here's an example: We did some work at the American School in London a while back. At the secondary level, the school uses a co-teaching model, with a support teacher as well as a general education teacher in every classroom. A support teacher for an English teacher reported that whenever the teacher he was supporting began giving verbal instructions for a class activity, the support teacher immediately went to the whiteboard and wrote the instructions in a brief bulleted list. This approach certainly helped the students with learning disabilities he was there to support—but it probably helped many other students in the class as well.

Building Working Memory in Everyday Situations

- *Make eye contact with your child before telling him something you want him to remember.*

- *Keep external distractions to a minimum if you want your child's full attention* (for example, turn off the television or turn down the volume).

- *Have the child repeat back to you what you just said, so you know she has heard you.*

- *Use visual or written reminders*—picture schedules, lists, and schedules, depending on the age of the child. Prompt the child at each step to "check your schedule" or "look at your list." Consider keeping packs of sticky notes available so that you can quickly add a visual reminder to verbal instructions. We met a mother who got tired of nagging her son about taking out the trash. He kept putting her off by saying, "As soon as I get to a stopping point in the game I'm playing," but then he'd forget to follow through. She finally took a sticky note and wrote TRASH on it, walked by where he was sitting, and slapped the note on his shirt without saying a word. Not only was this a successful strategy, but the mom reported that he actually told her that the reminder helped.

- *Use silicone bands that children can slip on their wrist to help them remember.* We met a teacher who had students select a different-colored band for each subject, then slip a band on their wrist if they had homework in that subject. Her rationale: the students may forget to open their assignment books, but at some point in the evening they'll see those bands on their wrist and be reminded of the work they have to do.

- *Post a large whiteboard calendar in a prominent place in your house.* The calendar *can* be used to remind the family of regularly scheduled activities (like dance classes every Thursday) or for special activities (a field trip this Friday). Parents may prompt children to "check the calendar," but if they're worried that a child will glance at it and say they complied with the request, they can ask to child to read aloud what's on today's schedule.

• *Rehearse with the child what you expect him to remember just before the situation* (for example, "What do you need to say to Aunt Mary after she gives you your birthday present?").

• *Help the child think about ways to help her remember something important that she thinks will work for her.* Children in middle school can use cell phones for text messages or any of a number of reminder apps to remember things they have to do. We've known students who text themselves as a way of remembering something important. It's also possible to arrange for the text to be sent at a specific time (such as just before they have to do what they're trying to remember to do).

• *With older students, teach them the concept of "offloading."* This refers to the idea that the brain doesn't have to work as hard when you can find a way to "offload" some of the tasks you're asking it to do. Examples: The brain doesn't have to allot space to remembering homework assignments when we write them down. It doesn't have to work at remembering something we have to do after school if we build an alarm into our smart phone to remind us. This may be a hard sell with some teenagers, especially those with ADHD, who see any extra step as not worth the time or energy. These kids also may have an inflated sense of their own capabilities. In the research this is referred to as *positive illusory bias.* The youngster may think, "I don't have to write down my homework because I'll remember it." They put a positive spin on their working memory skills—but, sadly, it's an illusion.

• *Beware of computer training programs that promise that children can enhance their working memory by spending a few weeks playing computer games.* While it's tempting to think there is an all-purpose exercise program that will strengthen working memory, the research on the impact of computer gaming programs yields mixed results at best. The summaries of research that we've seen indicate that while playing video games to enhance working memory may yield positive results, primarily the research shows that kids who play these games get better at playing the games but the evidence that it generalizes to other situations (consistently remembering gym clothes on PE days, for example) is scanty.

Having said this, there's certainly no harm in playing memory games with children. Card games such as Concentration, Lotto, or Memory games (Amazon offers an array of these) are fun to play and may increase children's ability to focus in the moment and remember important information. And you can enhance their benefit by talking with children about what strategies they used to help them remember. I remember (this is Peg talking) my mother playing a game with my brothers and me when we were quite young in which she would place several disparate objects on a tray (spoon, block, toy soldier, and so on), show us the tray for a short period of time, then block our view of the tray and remove a single object. She then asked us to identify what object she'd removed. Again, it was fun to play and may have helped increase our powers of observation and working memory.

- **Consider using a reward for remembering key information or a natural or logical consequence for forgetting.** For example, a child might be allowed to earn time on a video game for each day he brings home all his homework materials. Rewards and consequences are useful when your child's working memory is only mildly underdeveloped. If a child has more significant working memory weaknesses, then compensatory strategies and rewards may be necessary. Our rule of thumb is that an intervention (including one that employs rewards) should yield the desired result 75–80 percent of the time to be considered successful.

- **Remember to praise your child for remembering something or for using a strategy to remember something.** Here are some examples: "I like the way you remembered to put everything in your backpack as soon as you finished." "You remembered to get your teacher to sign off on your assignment book every day this week—what strategy did you use to help you to remember?" "You remembered to check your work before putting your math homework in your homework folder. I see that you were able to fix a couple of mistakes."

Ending the Waiting Game: Teaching Your Child to Get Dressed without Dawdling

Annie is a bright 8-year-old second grader who can be absent-minded at times but is one of the more advanced students in her class. She has a variety of interests and is a good friend to her peers. Her mother would like to see her develop more independence, particularly around recurring tasks such as picking out clothes and getting dressed for school. Because Annie's best friend, Sarah, has been managing the dressing process for the better part of a year, Mrs. Smith doesn't think this is an unrealistic expectation for Annie. She and Annie have talked about it, and Annie has said she'd like to do it, particularly because she'd like to choose her own clothes.

However, each morning a familiar pattern unfolds: "Annie, it's time to start getting dressed." "OK, Mom," Annie says as she heads upstairs. Mom busies herself getting ready for work and after about 10 minutes calls to Annie. "Annie, how's it coming?" "OK, Mom," comes the reply. After another 5 minutes, Mom calls out, "Annie, you need to move it along." "OK" comes the reply again. Shortly after that Mom goes upstairs to find Annie sitting on the floor drawing, still in her pajamas. "Annie!" says Mom with great frustration while grabbing some clothes. Annie begins to protest the choices, but her mom silences her and stays long enough to see that Annie is well into getting dressed before telling her to be downstairs "in 1 minute!"

In a calmer moment, Annie and her mother talk it over and decide that Mom will watch Annie go through this task to decide what might help. Although a bit slow, Annie is able to pick out her clothes and get dressed without major problems. However, in spite of her good intentions, when Annie tries to manage the task on her own, her mother still ends up frustrated at having to give Annie repeated reminders.

They decide to try another approach. If Annie agrees to work with her on a plan, Mom agrees to let Annie pick out some new clothes she has wanted. First they make a list of the steps in the dressing process and Annie writes these down. Annie says that sometimes it's hard for her to choose what to wear, so they decide to put out a choice of two outfits the night before and Annie picks out a place where they will be kept. They then do a pretend walk-through, and Mom takes a digital photo of each step. Annie matches the steps she wrote to the pictures and hangs the "picture board" next to her closet. (If you think your child would struggle with a two-choice option, let her pick one set of clothes.)

In the beginning, Annie thinks that besides cueing her that it's time to get dressed, it would help if Mom came upstairs with her to watch her get started and then left. Mom reluctantly agrees, provided that it's temporary. The final issue is time. Morning is usually rushed, and when Annie is slow, her mother gets upset. They buy an inexpensive digital timer, and Annie feels like 12–15 minutes is plenty of time to finish. Mom agrees. Because Annie sometimes gets lost in the process, she sets the timer for 5-minute intervals; that way, even if she gets involved with something else, the timer can be a cue. As an added check, when her mother hears the timer, she yells to Annie, "What step?" and Annie says where she is in the sequence.

Over the first few weeks, Annie has one or two mornings where Mom has to prod her, but overall they're both pleased. Annie feels comfortable with Mom not going upstairs with her, but she still likes the verbal check-ins and the praise from Mom when she does a good job. They also plan a shopping trip together.

Intervention Steps

Step 1: Establish a Behavioral Goal

Target executive skill(s): Working memory

Specific behavioral objective: Annie will complete her morning dressing routine within 15 minutes with no more than one adult prompt.

Step 2: Design Interventions

What environmental supports will be provided to help reach the target goal?
- Advance selection of clothes
- Timer
- Parent observation and prompts in early stages of the plan

• • •

What specific skill will be taught, who will teach the skill, and what procedure will be used to teach it?

Skill: Working memory (follow a daily morning routine)

Who will teach skill? Mother

Procedure:

- Mother and Annie meet to discuss the problem and desired outcome.
- They make a list of steps, and Annie writes them down.
- Two outfits are selected the night before.
- Annie does a walk-through, and Mom takes a picture of each step.
- Annie matches the written steps to the pictures and posts the sequence next to her closet.
- Annie decides on the time needed, and they get a timer.
- Mom agrees to cue her and watches her start for a week or so.
- Mom checks in when the timer beeps at each 5-minute interval.
- Mom keeps track of the number of reminders needed each day.

• • •

What incentives will be used to help motivate the child to use/practice the skill?

- Praise from mother
- Purchasing new clothes

Keys to Success

- *Be enthusiastic and thorough in the early stages.* This system is usually successful when first implemented because it's novel and provides systematic cueing as well as an incentive. When it breaks down, it's often because parents haven't monitored the system closely enough in the initial stages.

- *Err on the side of cueing for too long.* In our experience, many kids need ongoing cueing, and when parents are reluctant to provide it, initial gains often disappear. If your child "relapses" when you start to pull back on cueing, step it up and fade out of this role very gradually, in baby steps.

The Absent-Minded Athlete: Teaching Your Child to Keep Track of Sports Equipment

It's 7:30 Monday morning, and Jake, a 14-year-old eighth grader, is on his phone texting his friends. Because he is dressed, has eaten, and says his stuff (school backpack and soccer bag) is ready, his dad is OK with him doing this until the bus comes at 7:45. He has a soccer game today, and to be on the safe side Dad says, "Jake, check your soccer bag to make sure you have everything." "No problem" comes the reply as he continues to text his friends. A couple of minutes before the bus comes his father cues Jake and his sister to get ready. When Jake comes into the hall, his father asks if he has checked his soccer stuff, and he quickly opens the bag and rummages through it. "What did you do with my shin guards?" he accuses his father in a panic. Irritated and unable to resist the urge, Dad replies that he wore them to work. Jake, frustrated, says, "My coach will kill me, and I won't be able to play." The bus arrives, and Dad tells him they'll try to work something out, although he's not sure what. At the game his coach is upset with him and tells him that he can't play. Just before the game starts, his father meets a parent who has an extra pair of shin guards. He debates whether to let Jake suffer the consequences of not playing, but because this has happened before and it hasn't solved the problem, he doesn't want to see him in more trouble with his coach. He gives the guards to his son, but they agree that this will not happen again.

That night they talk about a system to help Jake organize and remember equipment. Because he is a three-sport athlete, this is basically a year-round problem. Dad suggests a list that he can use to check off equipment as he packs his bag. While this might help him know if he has what he needs in his bag, it doesn't solve the problem of organizing his equipment so that it is readily available when he needs it. His father jokes that maybe he should just sleep with his equipment on the night before a game so he can just pack it in the morning and know he has everything. Jake says that maybe they should make a cutout of Jake that wears the sports gear. That's a lot of work, so they settle on using a coat rack, with a designated spot for each item. This gives him a place to store his equipment and easily see what's missing. They agree to put labels on the rack for each piece of equipment needed, and Dad agrees to cue Jake the night before to check the rack and pack. For his part, Jake agrees that when Dad cues him to do this the night before, he will do it and not wait until the morning. They also agree that if he doesn't follow through and forgets something, Dad won't rescue him.

Intervention Steps

Step 1: Establish a Behavioral Goal

Target executive skill(s): Working memory

Specific behavioral objective: Jake will organize his sports equipment before each game and have the equipment he needs for each game with no more than one adult prompt.

Step 2: Design Interventions

What environmental supports will be provided to help reach the target goal?

- A coatrack that will be labeled with equipment needed for practice and games
- Reminder from his dad the night before a game to check and pack his equipment

• • •

What specific skill will be taught, who will teach the skill, and what procedure will be used to teach it?

Skill: Working memory (remember all required sports equipment for practice and games)

Who will teach the skill? Father

Procedure:

- Jake and Dad meet and agree on a plan for organizing the equipment.
- Dad supplies Jake with a coatrack.
- Jake makes labels and hooks for all equipment and puts them on the coatrack.
- He tries one practice run with his father watching.
- Dad agrees to cue him to get equipment ready the night before.
- For 2 weeks, Dad checks with him after he has given the cue to ensure that he has followed through.

• • •

What incentives will be used to help motivate the child to use/practice the skill?

- Jake will be able to participate in sports without experiencing consequences from coaches for not having equipment.

Keys to Success

- *Don't rely on your child's statement that they have acted on your cue. In this example the coatrack served as a reminder and an organizing* tool for Jake. While this may be enough in most cases, children with working memory weaknesses, when asked about or cued to remember something, will often indicate that they have done what they need to do or will take care of it and then proceed to forget. Therefore you'll need to follow up the cue with a check to see if your child has in fact acted on the cue. Acting at the time that the cue is given is key, which may involve your checking on a more frequent basis until the desired behavior is established.

12

Improving Emotional Control

Emotional control is the ability to manage emotions to achieve goals, complete tasks, or control and direct your behavior. If this is a strength for you, you're not only able to handle the daily ups and downs of life easily but can maintain your cool in more emotionally charged situations as well—whether it's a confrontation with a hot-tempered boss or with a teenage son challenging parental authority. Having the skill to control your emotions means not only being able to control your temper, but also being able to manage unpleasant feelings such as anxiety, frustration, and disappointment. Being able to control your emotions also means being able to tap into positive emotions to help you overcome obstacles or to keep you going during difficult times. It's not hard to see how important this skill can be to success during childhood and beyond.

Some of us demonstrate the skill in some settings but not in others. Most of us, kids and adults alike, have a "public self" and a "private self," and different rules seem to govern each of these personas. Does your child hold it together at school but then fall apart at home? Do you keep your cool at work but let your guard down with your family? This shift isn't uncommon, and it's not always a problem. But it can be. If either you or your child finds controlling your emotions such a strain that you can't make the effort once you're within the confines of home and family, feelings are likely to get hurt or chronic tension may be chipping away at your family. In that case explosions over the kinds of tasks that your child struggles with due to executive skill deficits may be a major problem for you. That's an indication that boosting emotional control is a priority for you and/or your child. If taking an objective look at the situation tells you that a lack of emotional control on your part is contributing to your child's problem, you might consider consulting a therapist for help.

How Emotional Control Develops

In early infancy, babies need parents to respond to their physical needs (food, bottle, diaper change) as they arise, and when these needs are met consistently and predictably, babies' reactions are regulated and predictable. Of course there are always times when adults can't supply immediate relief, so babies gradually learn to soothe themselves. There are some exceptions to this typical developmental progression. Colicky babies, for example, show increased signs of distress—excessive crying, arched back, clenched fists, and so on—thought to be associated with physical discomfort or overstimulation. Most infants seem to outgrow this phase and learn self-soothing techniques just like other babies.

In toddlerhood and the preschool years, however, you can begin to see individual variations in emotional regulation abilities. Some little kids go through the "terrible twos" with only mild tantrums, while others have emotional meltdowns whose frequency or intensity challenges even the most unflappable parents. At around age 3, most children learn and expect rituals, such as a precise sequence of steps they want to happen every night at bedtime. Despite these expectations, you'll notice that some children can roll with changes in the routine while others get very agitated if the sequence is disrupted in any way. Kids with low emotional control can therefore appear to be very rigid. If your child fits this description, you might benefit from reading Chapter 13 too; there's a lot of overlap between the emotional control and flexibility skills.

In elementary school, children whose ability to manage their emotions is challenged frequently encounter social problems; they may have trouble sharing toys, losing at games or sports, or not getting their way during make-believe games with friends. Kids who have good emotional control are the ones you'll notice can make compromises, accept winning and losing at games with equanimity, and may act as peacemakers in altercations between peers.

Adolescence brings new challenges for emotional control as it does for many other executive skills. This age group as a whole is more susceptible to breakdowns in the ability to handle stress. Teenagers rely on the prefrontal cortex to tell the rest of the brain how to behave. In times of stress, in the words of one brain researcher, "they are using up prefrontal cortex like crazy." This means the part of the brain responsible for managing executive skills becomes overloaded as teenagers try to inhibit responses (see Chapter 10), tap into working memory (Chapter 11), and control their emotions all at the same time. No wonder teenagers often make slow or bad decisions or, worse, bad *fast* decisions. Teens who lag behind in developing emotional control will be at an even bigger disadvantage, experiencing more than their share of emotional turmoil during a phase of development that's marked by emotional ups and downs. You can help him boost his emotional control using the strategies in this chapter.

It's well worth the effort: teenagers who can manage their emotions are less likely to argue with teachers or coaches, can handle performance situations (games, exams) without excessive anxiety, and can bounce back quickly from disappointment.

How does your child's ability to manage her emotions match what might be considered developmentally appropriate? The rating scale in the questionnaire on the facing page can help you answer this question, confirming or denying your preliminary assessment from Chapter 2 by giving you the chance to look a little more closely at how often your child is able to use this skill.

A Good Place to Start

As parents, when we're confronted with a child who's upset, our first instinct is often to reassure them. If our child says, "I'll never be able to figure out this math problem—I'm so stupid," we may rush to say respond, "No, you're a smart kid. I know you'll be able to get it with a little more thought." Or when our child says, "Nobody likes me; I never get invited for play dates," we want to remind them that they have lots of friends, and we may even name them. When we do that, though, we miss the opportunity to let our children know that we understand what they're feeling. If we start by acknowledging their feelings, not only are we letting our kids know that we "get them," we're also helping our children label their feelings accurately. And, it turns out, simply labeling feelings can have a powerful effect.

When external events trigger a strong emotion, this activates a part of the brain known as the *amygdala*. This is the "fight, flight, or freeze" part of the brain. It's the part of the brain that alerts us to danger so that we can act to protect ourselves. Back when humans were hunters and gatherers, we lived in a world where physical dangers occurred frequently and could be life-threatening. When the amygdala is notified of danger, it mobilizes all our physical and psychic resources to take action to protect ourselves from that danger.

In the 21st century most of the events that trigger strong emotions are not life-threatening. Luckily, we can respond by accurately assessing what is happening. And a key way to do this is to label the emotion we're feeling. When we do that, it turns out that labeling the feeling diminishes its power over us. Brain imaging studies show that simply identifying the feeling decreases the activity in the amygdala, which makes the feeling less intense—and therefore more manageable. Dan Siegel, a clinical professor of psychiatry at UCLA and the author of many books on neurobiology and the impact of mindfulness on the brain, uses the expression "Name it to tame it" to capture the value of connecting feelings with words.

So instead of jumping in to reassure our children when they are clearly unhappy or upset, start by helping them identify the feelings they're experiencing. We might say things like "You sound frustrated" or "I'm sensing you're feeling pretty discouraged" or "Are you feeling lonely?" Don't worry if we guess the wrong feeling—our kids will correct us, and this will give them the chance to talk further about what's going on. But if we think the child might be able to label the feeling without help from us, we might ask, "How does that make you feel?" and give them the chance to put the feeling into words.

How Well Does Your Child Regulate Emotions?

Use the following scale to rate how well your child performs each of the tasks listed. At each level, children can be expected to perform all the tasks listed fairly well to very well.

Never or rarely	Does but not well (about 25% of the time)	Does fairly well (about 75% of the time)	Does very well (always or almost always)
0	1	2	3

PRESCHOOL/KINDERGARTEN

☐ Can recover fairly quickly from a disappointment or a change in plans

☐ Can use nonphysical solutions when another child takes a toy they were playing with

☐ Can play in a group without becoming overly excited

LOWER ELEMENTARY (GRADES 1–3)

☐ Can tolerate criticism from an adult (e.g., a teacher reprimand)

☐ Can deal with perceived "unfairness" without becoming overly upset

☐ Can adjust behavior quickly depending on the situation (e.g., calming down after recess)

UPPER ELEMENTARY (GRADES 4–5)

☐ Doesn't overreact to losing a game or not being selected for an award

☐ Can accept not getting what they want when working or playing in a group

☐ Acts with restraint in response to teasing

MIDDLE SCHOOL (GRADES 6–8)

☐ Can "read" reactions from friends and adjust behavior accordingly

☐ Can anticipate outcomes and prepare for possible disappointment

☐ Can be appropriately assertive (e.g., asking teacher for help, inviting someone to dance at a school dance)

From *Smart but Scattered, Second Edition*, by Peg Dawson, Richard Guare, and Colin Guare. Copyright © 2025 The Guilford Press. Permission to photocopy this material, or to download enlarged printable versions (*www.guilford.com/dawson4-forms*), is granted to purchasers of this book for personal use; see copyright page for details.

Once we've helped them label their feelings accurately, we should still avoid jumping in with either assurance or a quick solution. Open-ended questions can keep the conversation going and may eventually lead the child to decide how they want to handle the situation. So we might ask, "Do you want to talk more about this?" or "Where do you want to go with this?" And if our children rebuff our questions, we let it be. The conversation might end with us telling them, "I'm around if you want to talk about this."

Improving Emotional Control in Everyday Situations

• *With younger children, regulate the environment.* You can reduce the likelihood that the child's emotions will get out of control by building in routines, particularly around mealtimes, naptimes, and bedtimes. Avoid placing the child in situations where she is likely to become overstimulated or find ways to remove her quickly from those situations when you sense she's beginning to lose control.

• *Prepare your child by talking with him about what to expect and what he can do if he starts to feel overwhelmed.* Some problem situations are simply unavoidable but can be defused with a little advance work.

• *Help your child develop coping strategies.* What options for escape can you and they come up with? Younger kids may be able to come to an agreement with the teacher or other supervising adult about a signal that means the child needs a break. At home, you and your child might agree that when things get too hot to handle, the child can say something like "I need to go to my bedroom for a few minutes to be alone" to tell you a break is needed. Simple self-soothing strategies can include picking up and holding a favorite stuffed animal (for a younger child) or listening to soothing music.

• *Consider mindfulness meditation techniques.* Relaxation techniques, such as deep breathing and progressive relaxation, which involves alternately tensing and relaxing the major muscle groups in the body, can be helpful. A favorite book of ours that introduces mindfulness meditation to children is *Sitting Still Like a Frog*, by Eline Snel. It comes with an audio CD of brief guided meditations, which can make a relaxing addition to a bedtime routine. There are also YouTube resources, which can be found by typing "guided meditation for kids" into your search engine.

• *Help your child develop a script to follow for problem situations.* This doesn't have to be complicated, just something short she can say to herself to help her manage her emotions. It's helpful to model these kinds of self-statements. For instance, if your child gives up without trying when a homework assignment appears difficult, you might say, "Here's what you might say to yourself before starting this: *I know this will be hard for me, but I'm going to keep trying. If I get stuck after trying hard, I will ask for help. Or: I'll do the parts I understand first, then ask for help.*" Children who struggle with emotional control are more prone than peers to dissolve in tears or throw a tantrum when confronted with tasks they find frustrating or difficult.

● **Work with your child to "talk back" to their negative feelings.** This is a favorite technique of Lynn Lyons, coauthor of *Anxious Kids, Anxious Parents.*

● **Read stories in which characters exhibit the behaviors you want your child to learn.** *The Little Engine That Could* is a good example of one that models the positive emotions (in this case the determination represented by "I think I can, I think I can") that kids with emotional control challenges often have trouble accessing. Children's librarians may be a good resource to consult. In the Resources at the end of the book are a number of children's books with the theme of emotional regulation. (Amazon lists a bunch of similar books.)

If these efforts don't alleviate the problem, you may want to work with a counselor or therapist trained in cognitive behavioral therapy. We also recommend two books that explain this approach within the context of specific emotional control problems: *What to Do When You Worry Too Much* and *What to Do When You Grumble Too Much*, both written by Dawn Huebner. They are written for children and parents to read together and include exercises children can do to help them understand the problem and develop coping strategies. (There are both YouTube and Facebook resources from Dawn also.)

Smart and Showing It: Beating Test Anxiety

Kayla is a 14-year-old eighth grader. She has always been a very responsible girl, the oldest of three children in her family, and her parents expect her to do well. Kayla plays basketball and has a small group of close friends she has known since elementary school. She is a B student and has to put in a fair amount of effort for the grades she gets. Math in particular can be a struggle, especially this year with prealgebra.

Kayla has a major test coming up in math and is a wreck just thinking about it. She has really studied the material and has gone over the problems she didn't understand with one of her friends. She feels like she understands the material now, but this hasn't decreased her worry about not doing well on the test. Her mother sees that Kayla is on edge, but Kayla says she is "just tired." She feels like if she tells her parents she's worried, they will just focus on how important it is to do well, and this will only make her more anxious. Kayla doesn't sleep well the night before the test, and her stomach is churning when she gets to class. She is able to answer the first few questions but then "blanks" on two major problems. Kayla does what she can, and while relieved that the test is over, she knows she didn't do well. Her fears are confirmed when she gets her test grade, a D, and she is frustrated because she realizes that she knew how to do the problems but just panicked. She tells her parents, and they blow up. Her father says, "If this happens in high school, you can forget about college if you get grades like that." Kayla breaks down, telling her parents how hard she worked and how she "froze" when it came to the test. Seeing her reaction, her parents realize that demanding she do better will only make the situation more stressful for her.

Together, Kayla and her parents work out a plan. Because not all demands lead to major worry, they discuss how to tell when her worries reach a point that they hurt her performance. Kayla suggests she use a scale of 1 to 10, then she decides it will be a problem if her anxious feelings get above 4. In that case, Kayla says, it would help her if she could tell her parents something is bothering her. But it won't help if they stress about it or offer their standard solution, "You need to study more!" Her parents agree to listen, ask if there is some way they can help, and try not to stress. If they act otherwise, they suggest that Kayla remind them of their role, and she agrees to this.

From past experience, her parents know that Kayla's worry about performance demands decreases if she has a plan beforehand, so they discuss this with her. Kayla agrees and proposes the following plan to handle her anxiety about tests:

- For any subject she is worried about, she will meet with the teacher prior to any tests, explain that she sometimes gets anxious about tests, and ask if the teacher recommends any specific study techniques to help her master the material.
- If, as with math, she has ongoing difficulty, she will try to set up a schedule to review material with the teacher regularly.
- She will meet with her counselor to see if she has any strategies to manage stress and worrying.

Her parents think this is a very good plan, and they are impressed with Kayla's thoughtfulness and problem solving. For the next math test Kayla follows the plan. Her parents are more relaxed, which in turn helps Kayla. She is more comfortable taking the test, although a little disappointed with her grade, a C+. But her teacher, seeing her effort, offers the option of extra credit.

Intervention Steps

Step 1: Establish a Behavioral Goal

Target executive skill(s): Emotional control

Specific behavioral objective: Kayla will improve her performance on tests to Cs or higher.

Step 2: Design Interventions

What environmental supports will be provided to help reach the target goal?
- Scale to measure anxiety
- Nonjudgmental support from parents

- Teacher assistance with studying
- Guidance support with test anxiety strategies

• • •

What specific skill will be taught, who will teach the skill, and what procedure will be used to teach it?

Skill: Emotional control (reduction of anxiety)

Who will teach the skill? Teachers, guidance counselor, Kayla

Procedure:

- Kayla will meet with teachers to learn specific study strategies.
- For her most difficult subjects, she will meet on a regular basis with teachers.
- She will meet with her guidance counselor for stress management strategies.

• • •

What incentives will be used to help motivate the child to use/practice the skill?

- Improved grades
- Reduced anxiety

Keys to Success

- *Be supportive, but otherwise refrain from offering your opinions unless you have some expertise in test anxiety.* Stick to listening and providing whatever help your child asks for. Going beyond that and giving advice about what she should do will likely only add to the pressure an anxious child already feels and be counterproductive.

- *Get whatever concrete help is available from teachers, the school psychologist, and any other professionals you may need to consult.* Kayla found it helpful when her teachers were available and could provide encouragement and offer concrete study tips. A school counselor/ psychologist should also have some helpful strategies and be able to work through them with a child suffering from test anxiety. If your child reports that the school counselor has not been able to help, ask your pediatrician to refer you to someone your child can work with on a short-term basis to learn such strategies.

Staying in the Game:
How to Discourage Poor Sportsmanship

Aiden is an active 7-year-old in second grade, the youngest in a family with three kids. Since he was a toddler, Aiden has liked physical activities, especially sports, and he is clearly talented for a boy his age. He's excited about being able to play on "real" teams now and looks forward to games. At home when he has free time, Aiden wants his parents or siblings to play and practice with him. However, with his family and with his teams, Aiden expects to do well. When he or his team doesn't perform the way he expects, he can explode, complaining loudly, crying, and sometimes throwing equipment. When this happens, his coach sits him out or his parents remove him. After some time he settles down, but this action hasn't eliminated the behavior altogether; it still happens often enough to be a major concern to his parents. They've discussed stopping all sports participation but are reluctant to take this step because playing is so important to Aiden. At the same time they realize they won't have any choice if Aiden can't learn to tolerate errors and losing as part of sports.

After talking the situation over with one of the coaches and with friends who have two young sons involved in sports, they decide on a plan. They first sit down with Aiden and explain that if he is to continue to play sports, they need to work out a way to help him change his behavior. Although he doesn't want to admit there's a problem, he agrees to a plan because he doesn't want to give up sports. The plan includes the following:

● *When he's upset about his own performance, Aiden can express his frustration using agreed-upon behaviors.* These include clenching his fists, crossing his arms and squeezing, and repeating a phrase of his choosing over and over quietly. If the frustration involves his team or a teammate, any public comment must be encouraging (for example, "Good try," "It's OK," and the like).

● *Together Aiden and his parents write out scenarios for a few different situations that have happened,* substituting the use of his new strategies for his old behaviors.

● *Aiden and his parents role-play what will happen by actually having him make a "mistake,"* such as missing a basket or dropping a ball and then use one of his new strategies. They coach him through this and praise him for using the strategy.

● *Before each game or practice, one of his parents reviews the rules and strategies with Aiden and has him say how he will handle a frustrating situation if it comes up.* At the end of the game/practice Aiden and his parents go over how he has done. If he's had no outbursts, he earns points toward eventually going to see one of his favorite professional teams play.

● *Aiden agrees to try not to tantrum, scream, use disrespectful language, or throw things if he gets frustrated.* Any of these behaviors will result in his immediately leaving the game/practice and then missing the next one scheduled.

Aiden is not completely successful in his first few weeks of games and practice, but his coach and parents note a major reduction in his outbursts and are confident that they're on the right track.

Intervention Steps

Step 1: Establish a Behavioral Goal

Target executive skill(s): Emotional control

Specific behavioral objective: Aiden will not engage in tantrums after he makes errors or loses in a sport.

Step 2: Design Interventions

What environmental supports will be provided to help reach the target goal?

- Scenarios/social stories with acceptable behavior endings
- Clearly stated, written rules/expectations for Aiden's behavior
- Parent cueing prior to entering the situation

• • •

What specific skill will be taught, who will teach the skill, and what procedure will be used to teach it?

Skill: Emotional control (acceptable expression of anger/frustration)

Who will teach the skill? Parents

Procedure:

- Aiden, together with his parents, will read scenarios of successful outcomes for typical problem situations.
- Aiden and his parents will role-play the situation and use of a new strategy.
- Aiden and his parents will review behavioral expectations/rules prior to the game.
- Aiden and his parents will do a postgame review of his performance.
- Aiden loses a practice or game for engaging in problem behavior.

• • •

What incentives will be used to help motivate the child to use/practice the skill?

- Aiden is allowed to continue playing sports.

Keys to Success

Stick scrupulously to the game plan. This strategy's success depends on consistently following these steps:

1. Give the child an acceptable way to express his frustration.

2. Identify, with him, the situations where the behavior is most likely to occur.

3. Rehearse (role-play) the situation and cue the child on the appropriate behavior.

4. Cue him about your expectations just prior to entering the situation.

5. Remove him from the situation if necessary.

Skipping any one of these steps leaves the child vulnerable to losing control again since it's so hard for young children to "think on their feet" in frustrating situations.

13

Encouraging Flexibility

The executive skill of *flexibility* refers to the ability to revise plans in the face of obstacles, setbacks, new information, or mistakes. It relates to an adaptability to changing conditions. Adults who are flexible are able to "go with the flow." When plans have to change at the last minute due to variables beyond their control, they quickly adjust to problem solve the new situation and to make the emotional adjustment necessary (such as overcoming feelings of disappointment or frustration). Adults who struggle with flexibility are often described as being "thrown for a loop" when circumstances change unexpectedly. Those who live with these individuals, whether adults or children, often find it takes extra energy and planning on their part to reduce the impact of unexpected change on the family member who has flexibility challenges. If you're no more flexible (or only a little bit more) than your child, you'll find suggestions in Chapter 3 that will help you compensate for the shared weakness so you can help your child optimally.

How Flexibility Develops

We don't expect babies to be flexible, so we accommodate their schedules, feeding them when they're hungry and letting them sleep when they're tired. Fairly early on, however, parents begin to introduce more order and predictability so that they no longer have to ignore the schedules of the outside world to satisfy their baby's needs. By 6 months of age, for instance, most infants are following the sleep schedule of the family (that is, sleeping through the night as much as possible). Eventually, especially as solid food is introduced, we shape mealtimes as well, so they align more closely with family mealtimes.

As children progress from infancy to toddlerhood to the preschool years, we expect them to be flexible in a variety of situations—and most are. These include adjusting to new babysitters, starting preschool, and spending the night at a grandparent's house. We also expect them to adjust to unexpected changes in routines, deal with disappointments, and manage frustrations with a minimum of fuss. All these situations require flexibility, and some children handle them better than others. For the majority of children who struggle, parents find that it takes them a while to adjust to new situations, but they eventually do, and the next time a similar situation arises, it takes them a little less time to adjust. Somewhere between the ages of 3 and 5, most children have learned to manage new situations and unexpected events and either take them in stride or recover quickly if upset.

To assess how your child compares to other children of similar age, complete the questionnaire on the facing page.

A Good Place to Start

For children who struggle with flexibility, strong feelings often accompany situations when things don't go as planned. As with emotional control, your first step as a parent should be to acknowledge your child's feelings. "You were really counting on the store having the toy you saved up money for. It's really disappointing when you worked so hard for it and now the store doesn't have it!" That acknowledgment won't change the reality of the situation, but reflecting back the child's feelings is better than saying something like "It's no big deal. I'm sure the store will get more within the next few days." You may then be able to move on to "Let's make a plan for what to do instead. I know it won't be as good as what you were hoping for, but it will give us something to do while we wait."

Children who struggle with flexibility tend to be linear thinkers: there's only one solution to a problem, one right answer, one possible outcome when plans are made. Without even thinking about it, these children tend to lock in on that one solution or that one outcome. When you can anticipate that something may go awry, you can help children prepare for that in advance by painting an alternate picture and encouraging the child to come up with a plan for handling their disappointment. You might say to your daughter, "I know you're counting on your best friend coming for a sleepover on Friday night, but you haven't asked her yet, and her family might have other plans. Let's come up with a backup plan for what you can do instead." With inflexible children, if you talk about "Plan B" enough, they may eventually start thinking about backup plans on their own.

Finally, be sure to notice when your child makes a smooth adjustment. It could be as simple as "Hey, thanks for being flexible!" Or you might say, "I know that was hard for you, but you recovered quickly from something that must have really disappointed you."

Encouraging Flexibility in Everyday Situations

Especially when you're first working on this skill, you'll need to emphasize environmental modifications if your child has significant problems with flexibility. Youngsters who struggle with flexibility have difficulty handling new situations, transitions from one

How Flexible Is Your Child?

Use the following scale to rate how well your child performs each of the tasks listed. At each level, children can be expected to perform all the tasks listed fairly well to very well.

Never or rarely	Does but not well (about 25% of the time)	Does fairly well (about 75% of the time)	Does very well (always or almost always)
0	1	2	3

PRESCHOOL/KINDERGARTEN

☐ Can adjust to a change in plans or routines (may need warning)

☐ Recovers quickly from minor disappointments

☐ Is willing to share toys with others

LOWER ELEMENTARY (GRADES 1–3)

☐ Plays well with others (doesn't need to be in charge, can share, etc.)

☐ Tolerates redirection by teacher when not following instructions

☐ Adjusts easily to unplanned situations (e.g., a substitute teacher)

UPPER ELEMENTARY (GRADES 4–5)

☐ Doesn't "get stuck" on things (e.g., disappointments, slights, etc.)

☐ Can "shift gears" when plans have to change due to unforeseen circumstances

☐ Can do "open-ended" homework assignments (may need assistance)

MIDDLE SCHOOL (GRADES 6–8)

☐ Can adjust to different teachers, classroom rules, and routines

☐ Is willing to adjust in a group situation when a peer is behaving inflexibly

☐ Is willing to adjust to or accept a younger sibling's agenda (e.g., allowing them to select a family movie)

From *Smart but Scattered, Second Edition*, by Peg Dawson, Richard Guare, and Colin Guare. Copyright © 2025 The Guilford Press. Permission to photocopy this material, or to download enlarged printable versions (*www.guilford.com/dawson4-forms*), is granted to purchasers of this book for personal use; see copyright page for details.

situation to another, and unexpected changes in plans or schedules. Therefore helpful environmental modifications include the following:

- Reducing the novelty of the situation by not introducing a lot of change all at once.
- Keeping to schedules and routines whenever possible.
- Providing advance warning for what's coming next.
- Giving the child a script for handling the situation—rehearsing the situation in advance and walking the child through what's likely to happen and how she can use her script.
- Reducing the complexity of the task. Children who struggle with flexibility often panic when they think they won't remember everything they have to or when they think they won't succeed at what they're expected to do. Breaking tasks down so that they have to do only one step at a time will reduce the panic.
- Giving children choices. For some children, flexibility challenges arise when they feel someone is trying to control them. Offering choices for how to handle situations returns some of the control to them. Obviously you'll have to be able to live with whatever choice the child makes, so you need to carefully consider the options you present. A note of caution: many children who are inflexible struggle to make choices, especially when they are given too many at once. For them, limiting the choices to two may make sense. Or introduce the idea of choice by asking if having a couple of options would make the situation easier for them to manage.

As your child matures, you can use the following strategies to encourage greater flexibility:

- **Walk your child through the anxiety-producing situation,** offering maximum support initially so he never feels he is "on his own" in tackling the task. As he achieves success, confidence grows naturally, and the support is faded gradually. This approach is actually one that parents use all the time to help children adjust to new or anxiety-provoking situations. If your child has never gone to a birthday party and is apprehensive about it, you don't just drop him off and pick him up 2 hours later. You go in with him and stay for a while, until he's comfortable, and then you gradually pull yourself back and eventually leave the party. If your child is afraid of going into the water at the beach, you go in with her at first, holding her hand and letting her know you won't let go until she's ready. In other words, you provide physical support or your presence initially and then melt into the background as your child develops a comfort level and the confidence that he or she can manage the situation alone. The key is (and this should sound familiar) *offering the minimum support necessary for the child to be on a path toward success.*

- **Model flexible thinking.** When situations arise that don't go according to plan, comment on it and "think aloud," so your child hears how you handle it. "Oh! I was hoping to make pancakes for breakfast, but I see we don't have any eggs. Luckily I bought bagels yesterday and we can have those instead." Modeling flexible thinking is also a good strategy for helping children who struggle with flexibility handle homework challenges. Open-ended tasks (ones where there are multiple possible correct answers) are often difficult for these children. Many a parent has told us that a traditional spelling assignment—compose a sentence for each of your spelling words—can lead to meltdowns. One mother we know told us, "So I compose the sentence myself and my son writes it down." She felt terrible about doing that because she knew she was doing her child's homework for her. We suggested a different approach: "Try something like this. Think aloud, so your son hears your thought process. It might sound like this: I have to come up with a sentence for 'beautiful.' How can I do that? Well, let me start by thinking about what the word means. OK, it means 'pretty.' So what are some things that are beautiful? I think roses are beautiful. Roses are beautiful. There's my sentence!" Each repetition helps the child build a strategy to manage the task.

- *Use social stories to address situations where the child is predictably inflexible.* Social stories, developed by Carol Gray as a way to help children with autism understand social information so they can handle social interactions more successfully, can be used to help children with executive skill weaknesses as well. Social stories are brief vignettes that include three kinds of sentences: (1) descriptive sentences that relate the key elements of the social situation; (2) perspective sentences that describe the reactions and feelings of others in the situation; and (3) directive sentences that identify strategies the child can use to negotiate the situation successfully. For more information about social stories, visit Carol Gray's website (*https://carolgraysocialstories.com*).

- *Help your child come up with a default strategy for handling situations where her flexibility challenge causes the most problems.* These include simple measures like counting to 10, walking away from the situation to cool off and then returning, and asking a specific person to intervene.

The Lone Ranger: When a Teen Tries to Take Control of All of Her Own Plans

Hema is a 14-year-old eighth grader. She has always done better when she knows well in advance what is expected of her and what events or activities are scheduled. It's not unusual for her to have a meltdown when faced with unexpected changes in plans. Because Hema is older now, she has more opportunity to make her own plans and decisions, which she likes. Her parents see the upside and downside to this. The upside is that there are somewhat fewer conflicts because they are directly involved in fewer decisions. The downside is that Hema often makes decisions and plans without checking with her parents, even though the plans require parental involvement or consent. For example, in the most recent 2 months, she has invited friends for a sleepover, made plans to go to a party, and agreed to hang out with a friend at a video game arcade. In each case she did not check with her parents, and she exploded when told either that her plan could not happen or that they needed more details before giving permission. Hema's parents also get this reaction if they forget to give her advance warning (usually a day or two) about things like doctor or dentist appointments. As she has entered adolescence, the explosions have become more intense, with Hema screaming, throwing things, and telling her parents that she "hates" them. Depending on her behavior, her parents may end up grounding her, but this has not resolved the problem. The issue seems to involve Hema's setting a plan or agenda for how she will spend her time without realizing or considering that other people may have different plans. Once she sets her plan, anyone else's plan is an unexpected change, and she reacts negatively as she always has.

In a calm moment Hema and her parents talk and agree that they don't like the way things are going now. Hema says she would like more freedom in making choices. Her parents would like Hema to consider their plans and schedules as well as some basic rules they expect her to follow when she makes plans. Knowing that Hema does best with predictable routines and expectations, they propose the following:

• On days after school when she does not have a scheduled activity (such as play practice or an appointment) she can choose one of her "regular" activities—library, friend's house, or school game. She needs to call her mother to say where she is going, with whom, and how she will get there. When she arrives at the place, she will call her mother to let her know. If it's a friend's house, Mom will speak with the friend's parent. Once at a place, she cannot leave without permission, and her mother will pick her up or she will tell her mother who is going to drive her home. If she does not abide by these rules, she will forfeit her privilege (that is, the chance to do one of her regular activities) for 2 days.

• For special activities like dances, trips to the mall, sleepovers, and parties, Hema agrees to first tell them what she would like to do, including where she wants to go, with whom, for how long, and what transportation she'll need. She also needs to say who will supervise, and her parents will talk to this person to check. Her parents will let her know if this works and if not, why not, and suggest an alternative.

• Because communication is a key element of this plan, her parents agree to get Hema a cell phone, and she agrees not to use it during school hours.

• For appointments or activities they schedule for Hema, her parents will let her know at the time they schedule these and also remind her 2 days before the appointment.

• At least twice a week Hema and her parents will review the plan and decide whether any changes need to be made.

Along with this plan Hema's parents explain why having this information is important to them. She feels they are more careful than they need to be, but she's willing to give the plan a try.

Intervention Steps

Step 1: Establish a Behavioral Goal

Target executive skill(s): Flexibility

Specific behavioral objective: Hema will inform her parents if she chooses an agreed-upon activity or will ask permission before committing to activities that have not yet been agreed upon.

Step 2: Design Interventions

What environmental supports will be provided to help reach the target goal?

- Hema will have a list of "preapproved" activities.
- Her parents will provide Hema with a cell phone.
- Her parents will give Hema advance notice of appointments.

• • •

What specific skill will be taught, who will teach the skill, and what procedure will be used to teach it?

Skill: Hema will learn to take other people's agendas into consideration when making her own plans and will accept limits on her own plans.

Who will teach the skill? Parents

Procedure:

- Hema can choose from a list of activities that do not require advance permission and will let her parents know her choice.
- Activities outside this list always require that Hema get advance permission.
- Hema will communicate with her parents using a cell phone they provide.
- Her parents will give Hema advance notice of appointments/ obligations they schedule for her.
- Hema and her parents will meet twice a week to evaluate the plan.

• • •

What incentives will be used to help motivate the child to use/practice the skill?

- Hema will have increased control/choice over some activities.
- Hema will have advance notice of appointments.
- Hema will get a cell phone.

Keys to Success

- *Do your best to stick to the original agreement and follow through with consequences.* It would not be unusual for a 14-year-old to test/push the limits of this plan by not calling, calling late, or making a tentative plan and then running it by her parents. This could be accidental (forgetting to call) or intentional. It can be difficult to hold the line when this happens because it's natural to want to give your child more chances or to want to avoid a major tantrum. But unless you're consistent, this intervention won't get you and your child anywhere.

Handling Changes in Routines

Manuel is 5. He attends the afternoon kindergarten session, and his mother picks him up at 2:30 each day. Manuel has always been a creature of habit. His parents, who are not naturally organized, have learned that regular routines and organized spaces are important for Manuel. Getting him to try new activities requires a lot of coaxing, and he won't give something new a second chance if his first experience ends up at all negative. When he started to tip over while riding a bike without training wheels, he refused to try riding again, even though his dad caught him. In school it took a while, but he plays with peers and seems to enjoy himself. However, in other social situations with peers or adults, unless they're very familiar, Manuel tends to hide behind his mother or father. The afternoon pickup schedule can sometimes be a major problem for Manuel and his mother. They've established a regular routine for most days. After Mom picks him up, they stop for a snack at a nearby store. She puts a CD in that he likes to listen to, and they ride home the long way, so he can finish his snack. If the weather is good, he plays in the yard, and if not, he builds with blocks in the basement. Any change in this afternoon—stopping at the bank, picking up his sister at school, or taking her to an activity—makes Manuel cry and throw things, and he stays upset for a few hours. Although Manuel's mother understands his need for routine, she's tired of these outbursts. She understands that as he grows older, neither the family nor the rest of the world will be able to accommodate his routines, and they need to come up with strategies to increase his tolerance for change.

    The issue seems to be that Manuel is fixed on one plan or outcome when he's picked up. His mother decides to try getting him used to a few different pickup plans on a regular basis. She knows that surprises don't work for him, so first she introduces the idea: "Manuel, sometimes after I pick you up, we get your snack and come home. Sometimes I have to do something before we come home, like stop at the bank or pick up Maria. Most of the time I know the night before. How would you like me to let you know? I can just tell you or we could make up a plan using pictures." Manuel would rather nothing change, but his mom is determined, and he chooses pictures. They decide that they may eventually take photos. But to start, with his sister's help, he draws pictures of the car, home, the bank, Maria's school, and Maria playing soccer because these are the most likely stops. They put clear contact paper over each picture and Velcro the backs. Manuel's mother starts with changing the routine two days each week and then moves to three. Each night she and Manuel talk about what the plan for the next day is and he arranges the pictures into a "schedule." Before he goes to school the next day, they go over the schedule and she takes it with her in the car for after school. At first Manuel protests when it's a different day, but the protests are mild in comparison to before. Over time, Mom adds other errands and Manuel seems to have less and less difficulty with these after-school changes as long as he gets some advance warning. Mom is able to move the warning time to the morning before he leaves for school that day. Her goal eventually is to give Manuel the plan or schedule when she picks him up because this would allow her to be flexible in planning her day.

Intervention Steps

Step 1: Establish a Behavioral Goal

Target executive skill(s): Flexibility

Specific behavioral objective: Manuel will participate in schedule changes for his after-school pickup without tantrums.

Step 2: Design Interventions

What environmental supports will be provided to help reach the target goal?

- Manuel has pictures of possible after-school activities.
- Mother tells Manuel about the plan the night before.
- Mother reviews the schedule in the morning and takes it with her for pickup.

● ● ●

What specific skill will be taught, who will teach the skill, and what procedure will be used to teach it?

Skill: Flexibility around schedule changes

Who will teach the skill? Mother

Procedure:

- Mother tells Manuel that there will be schedule changes and asks him how he would like to be informed about these.

- Pictures of different activities are made.
- For each day, depending on the plan, the pictures are arranged into a schedule.
- The schedule is reviewed the night before, the day of, and in the afternoon when Manuel gets in the car.
- New activities/changes are added over time.

● ● ●

What incentives will be used to help motivate the child to use/practice the skill?

- No specific incentives are included in the plan.

Keys to Success

- *Don't expect your child to be flexible about changes in the intervention!* Remember, you're dealing with a child who has great difficulty with changes in daily routines. Once this new system is in place, it too can become a fixed expectation for the child. This means that if you don't use it, you might have to deal with a tantrum about changes in the intervention itself. Any significant change in the plan should be reviewed with the child so he knows what's coming.

- *Be prepared to add unheralded changes to the intervention.* Sometimes you just can't anticipate a change far enough ahead to prepare your child, yet she needs to learn to roll with these changes too. Once your child is demonstrating some ability to handle changes in schedule with equanimity, tell her well beforehand that on-the-spot changes can happen once in a while. Then start introducing some last-minute changes in the schedule, but stick to ones your child will like, such as going to get ice cream, at first. Then gradually introduce other types of changes.

14

Strengthening Sustained Attention

Sustained attention is the capacity to keep paying attention to a situation or task in spite of distractions, fatigue, or boredom. For us adults this means sticking with tasks at work or chores at home by screening out distractions whenever possible and getting back to work as soon as feasible when interruptions are unavoidable. If your ability to sustain attention is weak, you'll find yourself jumping from task to task, often failing to finish the first before beginning the second. You might look for excuses to stop working, such as checking your email every 5 minutes or suddenly remembering a phone call you need to make. If you think you lack this skill, your efforts to help your child develop it will benefit from the tips in Chapter 3.

How the Skill of Sustaining Attention Develops

Picture a very young child at the beach. Isn't it amazing that the simple act of dropping a pebble into the water or building a canal can be a source of endless fun? Hands-on activities that would quickly bore us (or their babysitters, older siblings, or grandparents) to death may enthrall your young child for a long time. In fact children's ability to sustain attention when very young depends completely on how much interest they have in the activity. Very young children can stick with tasks for a long time if the activity appeals to them.

From the perspective of executive skills, however, sustaining attention is a challenge when the activity is something the child considers uninteresting or difficult, like chores, schoolwork, or homework, or sitting through lengthy adult-oriented events such as weddings or religious services. That we don't expect young children to sustain attention long in these kinds of situations is why many houses of worship will have children attend only the first 10 minutes or so of a service before sending them off to a religion-related activity outside the worship area. It's also why teachers' organizations, such as the American

Federation of Teachers, recommend that children spend on homework no more than 10 minutes per grade level (10 minutes a night for first graders, 20 minutes a night for second graders, and so on). Good classroom teachers don't expect children to sit for long periods of time at their desks doing seatwork either, and skilled parents assign chores to younger children that can either be done quickly or be broken down into segments.

By the time children reach high school, they are expected to pay attention for longer periods of time in school and complete anywhere from 1 to 3 hours of homework a night. When schools made the switch to block scheduling a few years ago (longer classes that meet either for half the year or fewer times per week), it took teachers a while to modify their teaching style so that lectures were no longer the primary instructional method. Even teenagers have a hard time focusing on a 90-minute lecture.

To gauge how your child's attention compares to others of the same age, complete the questionnaire on the facing page.

A Good Place to Start

For children with short attention spans, our advice to parents is that *you have to start where the child is*. If your child's attention span is 10 minutes and you give her a 30-minute task to do, it's not going to go well. The child will work for 10 minutes and then likely drift off; you'll corral her back in, and maybe she'll work for another 10 minutes. Eventually the 30-minute task gets done, but neither you nor your daughter will be happy about it. Adjust what you're asking your child to do to fit her attention span: shorten the task or build in breaks, using either time or quantity as a measure. "How about you finish five math problems and then you can take a break?" or "Why don't we set a timer for 10 minutes and then we'll take a break from cleaning your bedroom?"

Then you and your child can gradually lengthen the amount of time. "The last few days, you've been doing five math problems followed by a break. Do you think you could try six problems today?" Or "We've been working for 10 minutes at this chore for a while now. Do you think you could work for 12 minutes this time?"

And then you can ask your child to set the parameters. "How many math problems can you do before you need a break?" or "How long do you think you can work before you need a break?"

Strengthening Sustained
Attention in Everyday Situations

• *Provide supervision.* Children can work longer when someone is with them, either offering encouragement or reminding them to stay on task. Maybe you can do some reading or paperwork of your own while your child is doing homework so that you're available to help your child stay on task while still spending the time productively.

• *Use a device that provides a visual depiction of elapsed time.* These devices can

How Well Can Your Child Sustain Attention?

Use the following scale to rate how well your child performs each of the tasks listed. At each level, children can be expected to perform all the tasks listed fairly well to very well.

Never or rarely	Does but not well (about 25% of the time)	Does fairly well (about 75% of the time)	Does very well (always or almost always)
0	1	2	3

PRESCHOOL/KINDERGARTEN

☐ Can complete a 5-minute chore (may need supervision)

☐ Can sit through a preschool "circle time" (15–20 minutes)

☐ Can listen to one to two picture books at a sitting

LOWER ELEMENTARY (GRADES 1–3)

☐ Can spend 10–30 minutes on homework assignments

☐ Can complete a chore that takes 10–20 minutes

☐ Can sit through a meal of normal duration

UPPER ELEMENTARY (GRADES 4–5)

☐ Can spend 30–60 minutes on homework assignments

☐ Can complete chores that take 30–60 minutes (may need a break)

☐ Can attend to sports practice, worship service, and the like for 60–90 minutes

MIDDLE SCHOOL (GRADES 6–8)

☐ Can spend 60–90 minutes on homework (may need one or more breaks)

☐ Can tolerate family commitments without complaining of boredom or getting into trouble

☐ Can complete chores that take up to 2 hours (may need breaks)

From *Smart but Scattered, Second Edition*, by Peg Dawson, Richard Guare, and Colin Guare. Copyright © 2025 The Guilford Press. Permission to photocopy this material, or to download enlarged printable versions (*www.guilford.com/dawson4-forms*), is granted to purchasers of this book for personal use; see copyright page for details.

be bought from Time Timer (*www.timetimer.com*) in clock or wristwatch form as well as a software version. Sand timers also work well—either physical sand timers or a sand timer app where the time can be set electronically.

- *Use a self-monitoring strategy.* Ample research has demonstrated that if you teach kids to monitor whether they're paying attention, their ability to attend improves. The most common way to do this is to sound tones at random intervals (the original study that demonstrated this had the tones sound anywhere from 15 to 90 seconds apart). When the child hears the tone, he is instructed to ask himself, "Was I paying attention?" He then answers the question by checking the appropriate column on a Yes/No checklist. There is an app available for the iPhone called the Original Beeper App that you can program for how long the work session will be, how frequently you want the tone to sound, and how quickly the child needs to respond to show that they were paying attention when the tone sounded. The app presents a variety of tones to choose from, and when the work session is over, the percentage of intervals on task is computed. Another option that works very similarly is iConnect (*https://iconnect.ku.edu*). Teachers often use this version to train self-monitoring in a school setting, but it can also be used in other settings and for other tasks besides schoolwork (for example, chore completion).

- *Make the task interesting.* Turn it into a challenge, a game, or a contest. Or ask your child if they can turn the task into a game. Many parents report to us that just adding a "beat the clock" element to any nonpreferred task can be motivating to children.

- *Offer praise for staying on task.* Instead of focusing on your child when she is off task (by nagging or reminding her to get back to work), provide attention and praise when your child is on task.

- *Give your child something to look forward to doing as soon as the task is finished.* Alternate between preferred and nonpreferred activities. This approach may need to be adjusted if you find your child rushing through the task and doing it poorly to get to the preferred task. This can be done by adding a quality standard that the child has to achieve to engage in the preferred task. We find this "first—then" option effective in most situations.

- *If the above are not effective, consider using incentive systems.* Rewards should be powerful, frequent, and varied. For instance, you might award points for completed work or for work completed within specific time parameters. It is best to use these systems sparingly, preferably for particularly challenging tasks like completion of a school project so that the child doesn't come to expect a reward for any task that demands attention. Alternatively, have a plan to fade the reward over time.

Delicate Negotiations:
Reducing Distractions during Homework

Andy is a seventh grader with a busy life. He plays soccer on his school team and a travel team. In addition, he has started to play bass guitar with some friends and eventually would like to have a band.

Andy would like to get good grades, but compared to his other activities, most of his homework assignments seem very boring. He's pretty much set aside time right after dinner to start his homework, and while he might start on time, he is easily sidetracked. Eventually he'll get back to work, but then he might get a snack or hear the TV on and watch Comedy Central. He usually gets through most of his homework eventually, but the quality varies. His bedtime keeps getting later and later because he works so inefficiently, and his dad invariably yells at him about not getting to bed at a reasonable hour. Andy finds studying for tests is the worst. The night before a test he'll start studying, but after no more than 10 or 15 minutes he'll decide he knows the material "as well as I'm ever going to" and will play video games, watch TikTok videos, or channel surf until he finds something to watch. His parents are very frustrated. They've considered depriving him of video game time or making him drop guitar, but they know both will trigger a huge fight. They dread that, and they're not sure it won't make things worse anyway.

After progress reports, his parents meet with his teachers and counselor, expressing their concerns. The parents and counselor discuss meeting with Andy to formulate a plan. At the meeting, his counselor tells Andy that she and his teachers feel he can do better, and he agrees. Reviewing what they see as distractions, Andy's laptop is number one, with video games a close second. The counselor reminds Andy and his parents that for middle school students the school recommends that computers be available when homework is complete. Andy uses his computer for some of his schoolwork, however. He proposes leaving an "away" message on his computer until 7:30 P.M. as a starting point, and his parents agree. Because he already sets aside time for homework, he agrees to set up a "schedule" so that he completes an assignment or part of an assignment before he takes a break. He thinks breaks of 10 minutes will work, and he will use a visible timer on his computer to keep track. To help him study for tests, he will meet with each of his teachers, and together they will develop a rubric outlining how to study in each subject along with estimated study time and a checklist to go with this. He also sets "reasonable" grade objectives for the next progress report, so he, his teachers, and parents can evaluate his strategies. His parents will email his teachers weekly to check on late or missing assignments. Andy agrees to let parents "cue" him twice a night if he is off track, and they agree to use a cue phrase that he suggests.

Intervention Steps

Step 1: Establish a Behavioral Goal

Target executive skill(s): Sustained attention

Specific behavioral objective: Andy will complete his assignments and study for tests to achieve his grade objectives for the quarter.

Step 2: Design Interventions

What environmental supports will be provided to help reach the target goal?

- Time-limited access to computer outside of using it for homework
- Visible time clock on computer
- Schedule for completion of assignments
- Rubrics from teachers for studying
- Two cues from parents
- Weekly feedback from teachers

• • •

What specific skill will be taught, who will teach the skill, and what procedure will be used to teach it?

Skill: Sustained attention to homework

Who will teach the skill? Parents and teachers

Procedure:

- Andy will use his computer for socializing and games after 7:30 P.M.
- Andy will set up an assignment schedule.
- He will allow himself timed 10-minute breaks.
- He will meet with teachers to establish study rubrics.
- Parents can cue him twice a night.
- Teachers will provide weekly performance feedback.

• • •

What incentives will be used to help motivate the child to use/practice the skill?

- Positive performance feedback from teachers
- Decreased conflicts with parents
- Improved grades

Keys to Success

- *Don't make any significant changes in the plan until your child has maintained improvements over one and preferably two marking terms (3–4 months). It's not unusual for this plan to work initially, making parents and teachers overconfident that the problem has been solved permanently. But if you drop the plan altogether or become a lot less vigilant,* your child's performance is likely to return, even if only gradually, to preplan levels. Then everyone involved usually concludes that the intervention didn't work.

- *Keep a reduced but still present level of monitoring in place for the whole year.* It may be hard to stick with it when things seem to be going so well, but it's only with this duration of reinforcement that many kids maintain long-term improvements in sustained attention.

Parent–Teacher Cooperation: Cutting Down on Distractions in School

Bella never seems to get her second-grade work done. The problem began last year in first grade once students were expected to complete seatwork independently. Her teacher made some accommodations, such as reducing the workload, because Bella was clearly a bright student who seemed to be able to master the lessons, even though she couldn't always get her work done. This year's teacher is not so inclined, though, and work completion is becoming a bigger issue. Mrs. Barker, her teacher, first raised the issue at the parent–teacher conference that accompanied the end of the first marking period. "Bella is such a social child," she said. "She seems to be able to keep track of everything else going on in the class and wants to help other students when they get stuck, but somehow can't find her way to getting through her own work."

Shortly afterward, Mrs. Barker started sending home with Bella the work that she hadn't finished in school with the instructions to get it done for homework. Her mother finds herself spending long homework sessions with Bella trying to get her through the work. This makes for a long day for both of them. Her mother feels that the daily homework assignments, which usually amount to about 10 minutes of math and 10 minutes of spelling, are reasonable, but when two or three unfinished worksheets are added on top of that, Bella balks, and this often leads to frustration and tears. Bella says she tries to get her work done in class, but she gets busy with other things. Her mother decides something needs to be done to address the fact that Bella is not getting her work done in school.

Bella and her mother meet with her teacher. They talk the problem over, and Mom says that at home Bella seems to do better when she breaks jobs into smaller chunks, and she sets a timer for Bella. Her teacher says that 5–10 minutes is about the maximum amount of time that Bella works before she gets distracted. She feels she can divide up Bella's work into shorter blocks, but she's still concerned that Bella will get distracted. They agree that when her teacher gives her independent work to do, she will cue Bella to set her timer. Her mother suggests that they make a checklist showing reading, math, and language arts work blocks. As soon as she finishes one part of the work Bella will give it to her teacher. Her teacher will praise her for the work completion, and Bella can check off one block. Her teacher will give her the next part and cue her to set her timer. If she finishes before the other children and her teacher says her work is acceptable, she can engage in a preferred activity from a list she has made. Because socialization can be a distraction, during work time Bella agrees she will move to a different area if cued by her teacher. If her work is not completed, she will use free time during the day or stay to complete it during homework club. Homework will continue to be completed at home. Mother and Bella set up a system that gives her a sticker for each day her work is finished during class time. Bella can then choose from a list of "special" activities once she earns a certain number of stickers.

Intervention Steps

Step 1: Establish a Behavioral Goal

Target executive skill(s): Sustained attention

Specific behavioral objective: Bella will complete assigned work in class within a specific time frame.

Step 2: Design Interventions

What environmental supports will be provided to help reach the target goal?
- Work will be divided into smaller blocks
- Timer and cues to set it
- Checklist for work
- Teacher cues

• • •

What specific skill will be taught, who will teach the skill, and what procedure will be used to teach it?

Skill: Sustained attention to work in class to increase work completion

Who will teach the skill? Teacher and mother

Procedure:
- Teacher agrees to break the work into smaller blocks of 5 minutes.
- Mother and Bella buy a small timer for school.
- Teacher cues Bella to set the timer at the beginning of work.
- Teacher and Bella create a checklist for each subject work block.
- Bella takes work to the teacher as soon as it's finished, the teacher praises her, and Bella checks it off.

- Teacher gives Bella the next work and cues her to set the timer.
- If Bella finishes early, she can choose from a list of preferred activities.
- If socializing is a distraction, the teacher cues Bella to move to a different area.
- Work not completed during class time will be done during free time or homework club.
- Bella earns stickers at home for on-time work completion and can choose from a list of special activities when she earns a certain number of stickers.

· · ·

What incentives will be used to help motivate the child to use/practice the skill?

- Praise from teacher
- Graph showing progress of on-time work completion
- Preferred activities in class for early work completion
- Stickers and special activities at home

Keys to Success

- *Make sure your child has the same assigned location in the classroom every day, so the teacher knows that if she is not there, she's probably off task.* We've used this system in public school classrooms for a number of years and found that success depends in good part on the teacher (or paraprofessional if there is one in class) maintaining the cueing and check-in system. The only way for this to be practical is for the student to be in a consistent location in the room.

- *Be sure to use an incentive system because it's the child who has to manage elements like setting the timer.*

- Make sure free time doesn't need to be used to complete work on a regular basis. This can be an effective strategy, but if it's needed all the time, you should meet with the teacher to determine where the plan has broken down.

15

Teaching Task Initiation

Task initiation is the ability to begin projects or activities without undue procrastination, in an efficient or timely manner. Adults have so many obligations that it might seem like all of us are good at initiating tasks—we have to be. Yet we know from our work with adults that this is not an easy skill for some people to develop, and even adults tend to put off until last the tasks they like least when a long to-do list is before them. This is not all that different from a child delaying homework until after playing one more video game—or leaving the least favorite homework assignment until the end of the evening. If procrastination and last-minute scrambling are particular problems for you, be sure to use the suggestions in Chapter 3 to increase your success when the two of you share this weakness.

How Task Initiation Develops

In the context of executive skills, task initiation does not apply to tasks we *want* to do but only to those we find unpleasant, aversive, or tedious—the ones we have to *make ourselves* do. When children are preschool age, we don't expect them to start this kind of work on their own. Instead we prompt them to do the task and then supervise them while they do it (or at least watch them get started).

Our first attempts as parents to get our children to begin tasks more independently comes through putting in place routines, such as morning or bedtime routines. Teaching your child that certain things have to be done at a set time each day in a set sequence is step one. Then, after a period of prompting and cueing (how long you need to do this will vary from child to child), your child internalizes the routine and is more likely to initiate it on his own or following a single reminder to "get started now."

Although it takes a long time to develop, task initiation is an important skill children need in school and beyond. Giving children developmentally appropriate chores to do is one of the best ways to begin teaching task initiation. Starting in preschool or kindergarten, this helps teach children that there are times when they have to set aside what they want to do in favor of something that needs to get done even though it may not be fun. This helps prepare them for school and for participation in extracurricular activities that sometimes necessitate setting aside preferred activities for something else.

In the questionnaire on page 220, you can evaluate where your child might fall on the developmental ladder, based on the kinds of tasks children are capable of carrying out independently at various childhood stages. This scale helps you take a closer look at the assessment you did in Chapter 2, focusing on how well your child uses this skill.

A Good Place to Start

One of our favorite ways to teach task initiation is to ask kids to make a plan with a *start time*—and then make sure they start the plan at the time they said they were going to start. One of the reasons this works is that *the brain learns by association*. When you connect two activities over and over again, then event A (stated start time) will trigger event B (actual start time). It's a variation on Pavlov's dog, which may be the most famous psychology experiment of all time. The Russian psychologist rang a bell and presented meat to the dog and the dog salivated (a predictable physiological response to the stimulus). After a while, Pavlov found that the sound of the bell alone led to the dog salivating—because the dog anticipated that the meat was coming.

If you use this approach with your child, you can't just ask the child what time they plan to start the task. Initially you will also need to prompt the child to begin the task at the agreed-upon time. If you institute this practice, especially when children are young, you may find, as many parents have reported to us, that it eliminates a lot of the fighting that used to take place when you were the one to establish the start time.

Once you've made the plan with the start time, you may also want to ask your child what cue or reminder to start the task at the agreed-upon time would work best for them. A parent recounted using this approach with her child around homework, and when the child stated what time he would begin, his mom suggested that he "tell Alexa to remind you." You may also want to ask your child if they want a reminder a few minutes before the stated start time, so they can finish what they're doing first.

Teaching Task Initiation in Everyday Situations

Before we make suggestions for strengthening task initiation in everyday situations, we want to stress the importance of giving children an array of options for being cued or reminded to start the task. We recommend that verbal prompts be kept to a minimum. This is because it's easy to become dependent on verbal prompts, and eventually it becomes difficult to distinguish between prompts and nags. Using picture schedules, timers, alarms, apps such as Choiceworks, or even having the child prompt Alexa or Siri

How Good Is Your Child at Task Initiation?

Use the following scale to rate how well your child performs each of the tasks listed. At each level, children can be expected to perform all the tasks listed fairly well to very well.

Never or rarely	Does but not well (about 25% of the time)	Does fairly well (about 75% of the time)	Does very well (always or almost always)
0	1	2	3

PRESCHOOL/KINDERGARTEN

☐ Will follow an adult directive right after it is given

☐ Will stop playing to follow an adult instruction when directed

☐ Can start getting ready for bed at set time with one reminder

LOWER ELEMENTARY (GRADES 1–3)

☐ Can remember and follow simple one- or two-step routines (such as brushing teeth and combing hair after breakfast)

☐ Can get right to work on a classroom assignment following teacher instruction to begin

☐ Can start homework at an agreed-upon time with a single prompt

UPPER ELEMENTARY (GRADES 4–5)

☐ Can follow a three- to four-step routine that has been practiced

☐ Can complete three to four classroom assignments in a row

☐ Can follow an established homework schedule (may need a reminder to get started)

MIDDLE SCHOOL (GRADES 6–8)

☐ Can make and follow a nightly homework schedule with minimal procrastination

☐ Can start chores at the agreed-upon time (e.g., right after school)—may need a written reminder

☐ Can set aside a fun activity when they remember a promised obligation

From *Smart but Scattered, Second Edition*, by Peg Dawson, Richard Guare, and Colin Guare. Copyright © 2025 The Guilford Press. Permission to photocopy this material, or to download enlarged printable versions (*www.guilford.com/dawson4-forms*), is granted to purchasers of this book for personal use; see copyright page for details.

(when families have this technology available to them) is preferable to having them rely on parents for verbal prompts to initiate.

With this in mind, here are some suggestions:

- *Reinforce prompt task initiation throughout the day.* When your child begins a task at an agreed-upon time, praise her for starting right away.

- *Provide visual cues to remind your child to begin the task.* This could be a written reminder on the kitchen table, so the child sees it when he gets home from school, or it could be one of the suggestions just given.

- *Break overwhelming tasks into smaller, more manageable pieces.* If the task seems too long or too hard, ask your child to select one piece to start with and gradually increase the number of steps she agrees to work on.

- *Create a routine for getting started.* A school psychologist we know was working with an elementary-school-age child on task initiation, and his favorite strategy was something they called 1-2-3 Start! He listed the first three things he planned to do, and then he started. If the task was particularly challenging or aversive, the first three steps might be tiny ("1. Put my name on my paper. 2. Turn to the right page in my math book. 3. Do the first problem.").

- *For children who* really *struggle with task initiation, practice this skill in isolation.* In other words, just practice getting started without the assumption that the task will get done. You might say to your child, "I can see that getting started on bedroom cleaning is really hard for you. Maybe it's because it seems like it will take forever. So how about we set an alarm, and when the alarm goes off we do one small piece of room cleaning just to practice getting started. You get to choose what that piece is." Let the child know that all you're doing is practicing getting started at an agreed-upon time. Obviously whatever the chosen task is, it should not be a preferred task. Agreeing to start playing video games at 5:00 will likely not get your child any closer to learning to begin tasks that are not preferred tasks. But this approach can be used with tasks such as chores or homework. A parent might object that "just getting started doesn't get the task done," but if you start with something the child is not doing now, then getting started is progress. If you build in a reward for getting started, you can gradually ask the child to work a little longer before they earn the reward.

Doing It Now Instead of Later:
How to End Procrastination on Chores

Seven-year-old Jack is the middle of three children in his family. He has a 10-year-old sister and a 3-year-old brother. Both parents work full-time, and Jack's stepfather has to travel often for his job. With three children at home and Mom often the only caretaker, Jack's parents expect the children to help out around the house with tasks appropriate for their age. Because his brother is only 3, chores are primarily the respon-sibility of Jack and his sister. Once she understands what is expected, Emily doesn't need frequent prompts or reminders to get chores done. Jack is a different story. More often than not he requires frequent cues to begin the task. For example, it's his job to clear the dinner table and pick up toys in the living room before bed. At the very least, his mother has to nag him repeatedly, and sometimes he responds only when she gets angry and threatens loss of computer time. Once he does get started, as long as he understands what the task involves, Jack is pretty good about completing it. But getting him started is like pulling teeth. And at a recent school conference it became clear that Jack has the same difficulty at school, particularly with tasks that require a lot of effort, even though he's not struggling academically. His teacher has taken to giving Jack "start times" to begin work, which has helped him.

Jack's parents, knowing that work demands are only going to increase as he gets older, decide that now is the time to address the issue. Taking a cue from his teacher, his parents talk with Jack about having start times for two of his chores, clearing the table and picking up toys. As an incentive they tell him that he can decide, within limits, how long before he starts a chore, and he can pick out a time he likes from a few choices. Jack chooses a Time Timer, which uses a decreasing red clock face to show time remaining. They agree on a 5-minute delay for the table and a 10-minute delay for toys. Initially his parents will cue Jack by giving him the timer. He wants to manage keeping track of the elapsed time and beginning the task, and his parents agree. As an added incentive, for every 5 days that Jack begins his chore on time, he can have a "free pass," meaning he can skip one task for that day. If he doesn't start his chore within 2 minutes after the timer has gone off, he'll stop any other activity he is doing until the chore is complete.

At first Jack's parents sometimes have to cue him to start once the timer goes off, but in general they see a definite improvement in his beginning tasks. After about a month, Jack no longer uses or needs the timer for clearing the table. They continue to use it for toy pickup, although his parents notice that when Jack is told he has 15 min-utes until bedtime, he often begins picking up at that point.

Intervention Steps

Step 1: Establish a Behavioral Goal

Target executive skill(s): Task initiation

Specific behavioral objective: Jack will begin two chores after an agreed-upon elapsed time with one cue.

Step 2: Design Interventions

What environmental supports will be provided to help reach the target goal?

- Jack will have a timer available to signal when to begin.
- Parents will provide a cue to set timer.

• • •

What specific skill will be taught, who will teach the skill, and what procedure will be used to teach it?

Skill: Task initiation on chores

Who will teach the skill? Parents

Procedure:

- Parents and Jack select the chores to practice the skill.
- Jack selects the start times for the chores.
- Jack chooses, and his parents buy, a timer to signal the start time.
- Before each chore, his parents present the timer as a cue to set the time.
- Jack monitors the time, and when the timer signal occurs, he begins the task.
- If the chore is not started within 2 minutes of the timer signal, Jack stops any other activity until the chore is complete.

• • • .

What incentives will be used to help motivate the child to use/practice the skill?

- Parent nagging is eliminated.
- Jack can earn a "free pass" for every 5 days of on-time task initiation.

Keys to Success

- *Be diligent about consistency during the initial "habit-building" period.* When this intervention breaks down, it's usually because the system wasn't followed consistently in the first few weeks.

- *Don't hesitate to reinstitute use of the cues and the timer for a few weeks* if your child stops initiating assigned chores or other tasks over a period of a month or more. Sometimes kids need a refresher course.

- *If you find constant cueing or nagging necessary, impose loss of smart phone or computer time or another valued privilege as a consequence.*

Laying the Groundwork for Success in High School and College: No More Procrastinating on Homework

It's about 4:30 on Tuesday afternoon, and Colby, an eighth grader, has just arrived home after lacrosse practice. He lugs his heavy backpack into his bedroom and throws it down on his bed. He knows he should check his assignment sheets to remind himself what homework he has but hears a bell on his cell phone that signals an incoming text, which he assumes is from one of his gaming friends. He tells himself he'll just check in, reminding himself he forgot to get the math assignment. Maybe his friend knows what it is.

His friend's text asks if he's interested in a few rounds of an online game with a group that he sometimes plays with. He decides he'll play for a half hour and then get started on his homework. Around 5:30 his mother checks in with him to ask about his homework and to let him know they will eat at around 6:30. He assures his mother that he finished most of his work during his study period today and has only some social studies questions to complete. At 6:30 his father pops his head in to tell Colby that dinner is ready. Seeing that he's playing a video game, his father asks in an impatient tone when he's going to get to his homework. Colby, in a tone matching his father's irritability, says he has only a few social studies questions to answer, and he'll take care of them after dinner. His father says nothing, not feeling like arguing tonight, but he's become more and more frustrated by the fact that Colby's grades don't match his ability. It seems to him that Colby always underestimates the amount of schoolwork he has and the time needed to complete it and always overestimates the time he has available for other activities. To Dad it's clear as day that Colby has memory and time management problems.

After dinner Colby finishes one of the social studies questions and is starting on the second when his friend calls. After half an hour, his father, exasperated, insists he get off the phone and finish his homework. Ten minutes later, he hangs up and returns to his homework. He alternates between social studies and texting and finishes the third question just before 9:00 P.M. Feeling good about the work he's done, he watches an episode of *South Park*, then reads a snowboarding magazine while in bed. Just before dropping off to sleep, he remembers the math assignment he didn't get to. He decides he can get to it tomorrow because he has lunch before math. His mother and father, having watched another night pass with their son spending time on nearly every activity but homework, wonder how his grades will look for this term.

A few weeks later Colby receives the bad news in his progress report, with grades of B–, C, C–, and D in his main subjects. He and his parents meet with his counselor and eighth-grade team leader. Although Colby has statewide achievement test scores above the 90th percentile, his counselor reports that continued poor grades will exclude Colby from honors classes in high school. Colby has a few low quiz grades from surprise quizzes when he didn't read the material, but late and missing assignments account for the bulk of his poor performance. Colby resolves to do better, but his counselor, teacher, and parents are skeptical about the benefit of these good intentions, which haven't had a major impact in the past. Colby acknowledges this and agrees to consider other options.

His parents' past attempts to monitor his work were seen by Colby as (and typically were) "nagging," which led to bickering or fights. His counselor suggests that someone else might play this role, a kind of mentor or coach. Colby is willing to try this and identifies a teacher from last year who he feels he could work with. His counselor has a plan for how coaching will work and, when approached by Colby, the teacher agrees to help. They meet for about 10 minutes at the end of each day to plan how Colby will manage his assigned work that night, and on at least two nights each week for the first 4 weeks the coach checks in with Colby via text to see if he's following the plan. Colby and his coach also get weekly updates about late and missing assignments and his current performance from his teachers through the parent and student communication platform. By the end of the semester, Colby's grades have improved to B+, B, B, and C, and he and his coach decide to set a goal of all Bs or better for the next quarter.

Intervention Steps

Step 1: Establish a Behavioral Goal

Target executive skill(s): Task initiation

Specific behavioral objective: Colby will complete his homework on time for 90% of assignments given without parental intervention or prompting.

Step 2: Design Interventions

What environmental supports will be provided to help reach the target goal?

- Colby will have a coach.
- Colby will meet with this person three times a week with additional phone contacts/emails as needed.
- Teachers will provide weekly feedback to Colby and his coach about late or missing assignments.

• • •

What specific skill will be taught, who will teach the skill, and what procedure will be used to teach it?

Skill: Task initiation on homework completion without parental reminders

Who will teach the skill? Coach

Procedure:

- Colby will choose a coach.
- Colby and the coach will establish grade objectives for next term.
- Colby, with help from the coach, will spell out any roadblocks to objectives.
- Colby and his coach will initially meet daily, and Colby will decide how much homework he has, how long it will take, and when he will do it.
- Colby and his coach will review the previous night's work as well as teachers' weekly feedback.
- Colby and the coach will talk by phone or text or through the school's communication platform at least three times a week to monitor his progress.

● ● ●

What incentives will be used to help motivate the child to use/practice the skill?

- Colby will improve his grades so that he is eligible for high school honors classes in at least two subjects.
- Colby and his parents will decrease daily arguments about homework by 75%.

Keys to Success

- *Be sure to find a coach who can work with your child and who is willing to make the brief but consistent daily contact (10 minutes and a text message) and maintain this over a period of a least a few months. At the middle school level we've seen teachers, counselors, paraprofessionals, and administrators all fill this role.*

- *Institute a system of rewards and consequences if you have a dedicated coach but your child isn't following up on commitments made. We've seen some kids actively avoid the coach or otherwise evade agreed-upon responsibilities, sometimes because their skill deficiency is severe and sometimes because no one is hovering over them when the time comes to do the work.*

- *Make sure that the coach gets feedback about how your child is doing with the plan. When a coach doesn't know that a student's performance isn't improving or is getting worse, he may not realize that he's* not being consistent enough for a long enough time to help the child gain the skill.

- *If you've tried the preceding tactics and your child is still not improving, you might consider another staff person as a coach.* Sometimes everyone is doing everything right, but the relationship between the student and coach just doesn't have that little something extra that motivates or teaches the child the necessary skill.

16

Promoting Planning and Prioritizing

The executive skill of planning/prioritizing refers to the ability to create a roadmap to reach a goal or complete a task, as well as the ability to make decisions about what's important to focus on. We adults use this skill every day for brief tasks such as preparing a meal and for longer tasks such as launching a new project at work or arranging to have an addition put on the family home. If you can't identify priorities and then stick to them or create timelines for completing multistep projects, you may be the sort of person who tends to be seen as "living in the moment." Maybe you typically rely on others who are good at planning to help you achieve goals. If so, the suggestions in Chapter 3 will help you help your child despite having the same skill weakness.

How Planning and Prioritizing Skills Develop

When kids are very young, we naturally take on the planning role for them. We set up a task as a series of steps and prompt the child to perform each step—whether it's cleaning a bedroom or helping a child pack to go on a vacation or prepare for summer camp. Smart parents let children see this planning process on paper, creating lists or checklists or pictures for their kids to follow. Even when these lists are really for us, when our kids see us creating lists to organize work tasks, we're modeling desirable behavior that they will, if we're lucky, pick up for their own use. Written lists also reinforce what planning means by giving kids the opportunity to see what a specific plan actually looks like.

Planning becomes more critical in late childhood. It comes into play most prominently in school as children are given projects or long-term assignments with multiple steps, beginning around fourth or fifth grade, if not earlier. When teachers introduce such projects, they generally break down the assignment or project into subtasks and help students create timelines, often with deadlines attached. Teachers recognize that planning doesn't come naturally to children and, if left on their own, many will leave work until the last minute. Attaching interim deadlines forces students to complete larger projects in small chunks in a sequential fashion—the essence of planning.

By the time children hit middle school, they're often expected to perform this function more independently—and by high school this expectation extends beyond school assignments to the planning required to do things like find summer jobs and meet deadlines for SAT and college applications. Of course, some teenagers are better at this than others.

The second element included in this executive skill, prioritizing, follows a similar pattern. Early in our children's lives we (and their teachers) decide what the priorities are and prompt kids to tackle the top priorities first. But beyond the high priorities that most adults would agree upon—such as doing homework before settling down in front of the TV—how much leeway parents give their kids for prioritizing the use of their time often depends more on personal values than a desire to instill good prioritizing skills in their children. Our highly competitive world is full of kids whose every "free" moment is filled with dance or music lessons, sports, art classes, or religious studies because the parents—and sometimes the children—believe it's essential that their child be an accomplished achiever.

The overall goal of enhancing your child's executive skills is to help your child become independent, and learning to plan is a big part of acquiring that independence. With young children, the decision making that goes along with free play, imaginary play, and the use of unstructured time is a nice introduction to planning. As children age, the activities they are drawn to require more detailed planning, but building these skills in the context of preferred activities is a great way to develop an executive skill that they will eventually apply to school or work tasks.

In the questionnaire on the next page, you can evaluate your child's planning skills to determine if they are developmentally typical for your child's age.

A Good Place to Start

As noted above, when teachers assign long-term projects to students, they initially do the planning *for* them. This is developmentally appropriate because it's a recognition that this is a relatively late-developing executive skill. However, it fails to take advantage of the opportunity to *teach* planning. When we're working with teachers, we often suggest that they do the planning *with* kids rather than *for* them. We suggest that parents do the same. Chapter 23 includes a template for helping a child plan a long-term project, but there are many other situations besides schoolwork where you can help your kids learn to plan. On Saturday morning you might say to your children, "OK, we have several chores and errands we need to get done today, but we also want to fit in some fun things. Let's make a plan that's logical. Any ideas where we should start?" or "These are some options. Which sounds good to you?" This will help children recognize there may be a natural sequence to things (maybe the grocery store is right near the office supply store, so you could all go grocery shopping just before or just after picking up new notebooks

How Well Developed Are Your Child's Planning Skills?

Use the following scale to rate how well your child performs each of the tasks listed. At each level, children can be expected to perform all the tasks listed fairly well to very well.

Never or rarely	Does but not well (about 25% of the time)	Does fairly well (about 75% of the time)	Does very well (always or almost always)
0	1	2	3

PRESCHOOL/KINDERGARTEN

☐ Can finish one task or activity before starting another

☐ Able to follow a brief routine or plan developed by someone else

☐ Can complete a simple art project with more than one step

LOWER ELEMENTARY (GRADES 1–3)

☐ Can carry out a two- or three-step project (e.g., arts and crafts, construction) of the child's own design

☐ Can figure out how to earn/save money for an inexpensive toy

☐ Can carry out a two- to three-step homework assignment with support (e.g., a book report)

UPPER ELEMENTARY (GRADES 4–5)

☐ Can make plans to do something special with a friend (e.g., go to the movies)

☐ Can figure out how to earn/save money for a more expensive purchase (e.g., a video game)

☐ Can carry out a long-term project for school, with most steps broken down by someone else (teacher or parent)

MIDDLE SCHOOL (GRADES 6–8)

☐ Can do research on the Internet either for school or to learn something of interest

☐ Can make plans for extracurricular activities or summer activities

☐ Can carry out a long-term project for school with some support from adults

From *Smart but Scattered, Second Edition*, by Peg Dawson, Richard Guare, and Colin Guare. Copyright © 2025 The Guilford Press. Permission to photocopy this material, or to download enlarged printable versions (*www.guilford.com/dawson4-forms*), is granted to purchasers of this book for personal use; see copyright page for details.

for school). Children can also learn that plans tend to go better when we get the "work" part of the plan done before we move on to the "fun" part—or that it may make sense to alternate between work and fun, so there's always something fun to look forward to.

Additional opportunities to guide children in the planning process present themselves as children reach the upper elementary and middle school grades. Children at this age often want to do things that involve planning and logistics. When this happens, rather than turning the child down right away or making it happen by way of your own planning skills, you could ask your child to flesh out the plan. "You want to go to the water park on Saturday. You know we have a backyard cookout planned, and we have to clean the house for our company. Can you paint me a picture of how you would fit in the trip to the water park?" Asking the child to do the planning may also be help them develop flexibility (realizing that Sunday might be a better day to go to the water park, for example).

Promoting Planning and Prioritizing in Everyday Situations

- *Create plans with your child when young.* Use the expression "Let's make a plan" and then write it out as a series of steps. Better yet, make it a checklist, so the child can check off each step as it's completed. Again, as in the paragraph above, you can either start with an open-ended question, "What comes first, then . . . ," or list some activity options and then ask about the planning sequence.

- *Involve your child as much as possible in the planning process* once you've been providing models for a while. Ask, "What do you need to do first? And then what?" and so on, and write down each step as the child dictates it to you.

- *Use things the child wants as a jumping-off point for teaching planning skills.* Children are likely more willing to make the effort to devise a plan to make a peanut butter sandwich, an ice cream sundae, or to build a tree house than they might be to plan how to clean their closets, but the same principles apply in both cases.

- *For less preferred/nonpreferred tasks, prompt prioritizing by asking your child what needs to get done first.* "What needs to happen before you can play a video game?" (maybe "Load the dishwasher") or "What needs to happen before your friend comes for a sleepover?" (possibly "Clean my room").

Timelines and Deadlines: Learning How to Plan Long-Term Projects

Max, age 13, is a good student who never had any problems with homework until the introduction of long-term projects when he was in fifth grade. At first he panicked, dreading the assignment from the day it was assigned until the day it was due. There were predictable emotional meltdowns whenever his mother brought it up and asked him what he'd done so far. As time went on, Max stopped telling his mother about the assignments at all, and she wouldn't know about it until his progress report came home or she got a note from the teacher informing her that Max had not handed in the assignment at all or that what he'd done was hopelessly incomplete. His mother noticed he did better when teachers broke down the assignment into specific tasks and required students to complete and turn in each task on a specific due date. She also found that Max tended to do everything but the assignment, and when she asked about this, he always gave some reason that made sense to him: "I have to get my math done because Mr. Jones checks it off at the beginning of the period," or "I'm having a quiz on this short story in English tomorrow, so I have to finish reading it—you don't want me to fail the quiz, do you?"

Max's mother finally decided the stumbling block was that Max actually didn't know how to plan for a long-term project. She also felt that if any given component of the project was too complicated, that became a roadblock too. She offered to help Max with the promise that if they planned right, the project wouldn't be so overwhelming to him. Using as a guide a timeline one of his teachers had put together for a project that Max finished without too much difficulty, she and Max identified the steps he needed to follow for a social studies project that was due in about 3 weeks. For each step they identified, she asked Max to estimate how difficult he thought that step was, using a scale of 1 to 10, with 1 being "a snap" and 10 being "just about impossible." They agreed that their goal was to make sure that each task felt like a 3 or less to Max. To make the whole thing a little more attractive, his mother also decided to build in incentives. Each time he completed a step on the day they had agreed upon, he would earn 3 points. If he finished the step anytime before the agreed-upon deadline, he earned 5 points. Max had been wanting to get a new video game for quite a while, but it was expensive, and he was having a hard time accumulating enough money to buy it when all he had to save was his allowance. Max and his mother agreed on how much each point was worth so that he could augment his savings and buy the video game sooner.

It took only one time through the process to be able to drop the incentive. Max's mother was pleased to see that each time they developed a plan, Max was able to do more and more of the planning himself.

Intervention Steps

Step 1: Establish a Behavioral Goal

Target executive skill(s): Planning

Specific behavioral objective: Max will learn to plan and execute long-term school assignments.

Step 2: Design Interventions

What environmental supports will be provided to help reach the target goal?

- Mother will assist in developing a plan and will supervise implementation (cueing, coaching).

• • •

What specific skill will be taught, who will teach the skill, and what procedure will be used to teach it?

Skill: To break down a long-term project into subtasks tied to a specific timeline

Who will teach the skill? Max's mother

Procedure:

- Make a list of steps required to complete the project.
- Assess how difficult each step is (using a 1–10 scale).
- Revise any step judged by Max to be more difficult than a 3 to make it easier.
- Decide on a deadline for each step.
- Prompt Max to complete each step.

• • •

What incentives will be used to help motivate the child to use/practice the skill?

- Points are given for completing each step on time (bonus points for completing it early).
- Points convert to money to help Max buy a video game he wants.

Keys to Success

- *Don't hesitate to enlist the teacher's help if you feel you don't have the skill to start this intervention or if the plan breaks down.* For this plan to succeed, you need the skill to help your child plan and to monitor the plan to make sure it's realistic and the agreed-upon timelines are followed. So here's a case where having the same weakness as your child can make success pretty elusive. You'll need the teacher's help in setting up work tasks and timelines. Sometimes teachers will feel that the project directions or rubric they've already provided is sufficient. In that case, emphasize to the teacher that this is a weak skill area and that past performance indicates your child needs more specific and short-term tasks with regular monitoring and feedback.

A Social Director in the Making:
Thinking Ahead about Getting Together with Friends

Alise is an active, social 7-year-old second grader. No kids her age live nearby, so if she's going to see friends outside of school, they have to come to her, or she has to go to them. Her mom is happy to transport her if she is not tied up with work, driving her older siblings to drama or soccer, or other responsibilities. The trouble is that Alise doesn't think ahead far enough to make sure her friends are free and her mother is available before trying to arrange a play date. She'll get up on Saturday or Sunday morning and decide that she wants to have a friend over. But often her friends are busy, or her mother has other obligations and can't drive Alise anywhere. Alise then ends up moping around the house in a bad mood, complaining that she has nothing to do. When she gets back to school on Monday, her friends will be talking about what they did with each other, and she feels left out. Mom has repeatedly told her that she needs to make plans in advance. Alise agrees but typically does not remember to do it.

Mom suggests to Alise that they try to work out a solution, and she helps Alise through the planning process with a series of questions. "Suppose you wanted Jaime to come over. What's the first thing to do?" Alise responds, "I would ask Jaime in school if she wanted to come over." "Do you need permission to do that?" "Yes, I'll ask you first," Alise says. "Suppose she says yes. Then what happens?" "She comes over." "Does she need permission?" "Yes, I forgot that she has to ask her mother." "If it's OK with her mom, what do you need to decide next?" They continue on with this until they have a planning sequence, and with Mom's help Alise makes a list for herself.

Initially her mom needs to cue Alise early in the week to think about a weekend plan, which means taking into consideration Mom's schedule as well as the activities her friends have. With practice Alise is able to plan social events and even becomes something of a "social director" with her friends.

Intervention Steps

Step 1: Establish a Behavioral Goal

Target executive skill(s): Planning

Specific behavioral objective: Alise will map out the steps to plan out-of-school activities with friends a few days in advance of the weekend.

Step 2: Design Interventions

What environmental supports will be provided to help reach the target goal?

- Parents provide questions/suggestions for activity-planning steps.

- List of steps to follow is completed.
- Mother cues Alise to start the planning process.

• • •

What specific skill will be taught, who will teach the skill, and what procedure will be used to teach it?

Skill: Planning for play dates

Who will teach skill? Mother

Procedure:

- Mom and Alise discuss steps to consider in planning a friend's visit.
- From this process, Mom helps Alise develop a written list of steps to follow.
- Mom cues Alise to begin the process before the weekend.

• • •

What incentives will be used to help motivate the child to use/practice the skill?

- Alise takes control of her social schedule and gets to have friends over.

Keys to Success

- *Figure out whether your child has reasonably good skills in task initiation and follow-through before undertaking a plan like this one. If the plan fails as written, you'll need to provide significantly more prompting and direction to help your child get started. You could also check Chapters 14 and 15 to see if you want to try some of the ideas there for boosting your child's task initiation and sustained attention skills.*

- *Make sure the problem with making play dates is not that your child is trying to make friends with a child who isn't a great match.* In our example, it's possible that some children are a better match for Alise than others. In that case, talking to the teacher could be really revealing. Ask the teacher which classmates she thinks are a good social fit for Alise and which may be less so.

- *Another option for boosting your child's social opportunities and enhancing planning at the same time is to look for regular, recurring activities on weekends.* Sports, drama, dance, and other programs can provide social opportunities in a scheduled, structured fashion that instills planning skills indirectly while ensuring that your child has predictable time with peers outside of school.

17

Fostering Organization

Organization refers to the ability to create and maintain systems for arranging and keeping track of information and materials. For us adults the benefits of organizational abilities are pretty obvious. A system for keeping track of things and an orderly home or work environment eliminate the need to spend lots of time looking for things or neatening up just to get ready to work on something. We end up much more efficient as a result of having this skill. And this makes us less stressed. There's a reason we tend to feel more comfortable when our surroundings have some degree of order and tidiness. Unfortunately in our experience, adults for whom organization is a weak executive skill (and there are many!) find it quite challenging to improve their capacity. This makes it all the more critical that parents help their children develop organizational skills beginning at a fairly early age. We've provided some tips for teaching your child to be organized when you have a similar weakness in Chapter 3.

How Organizational Skills Develop

By now this pattern should sound familiar: At first we provide our kids with organizational systems. We give them the structures they need to keep their bedrooms and playrooms neat, such as bookcases, toy boxes, and laundry hampers. We also supervise our children in maintaining tidiness. This means we neither clean our children's rooms for them nor expect them to clean their rooms on their own. Rather, parent and child work on room cleaning together, with the parent breaking the task down for the child ("OK, first we'll put all your dirty clothes in the laundry," "Now, let's put all your dolls on the doll shelf," and the like). We also establish rules such as "No eating food in the bedroom" and "Hang your coat up as soon as you come in from outdoors." But at first we don't expect kids to remember to follow the rules consistently—we assume they'll need reminders, and on those rare occasions when children remember to follow the rules without reminders, we praise them.

Gradually we can step back from the step-by-step monitoring and supervision, getting by with a prompt in the beginning and a check at the end to make sure the child followed through. And somewhere around middle school or high school, children can take over maintaining organizational systems on their own. This doesn't mean that they won't need reminders from time to time—as well as the judicious use of access to preferred activities contingent on task completion.

To assess how your child's organizational skills compare with their age group, complete the questionnaire on the next page. This builds on the brief assessment in Chapter 2, helping you take a closer look at how well your child organizes things for their age.

A Good Place to Start

Sometimes we informally survey adults in the seminars and workshops that we lead. "How many here think of themselves as being pretty organized?" Invariably somewhere between 30 and 40 percent of the audience raise their hands. We then ask, "How far back do you remember being that way?" the most common answer to that question is "Forever." We've even asked teenagers that question and gotten the same answer. We had a tenth-grade girl once say that she could remember lining up her shoes in her bedroom at the age of two!

For those who are not organized "by nature," though, this can be a slow skill to acquire. It involves recognizing there's a problem ("My bedroom is a mess, and I waste way too much time looking for things!"), figuring out an organizational system ("Where should I put everything?"), and maintaining that system over time. For children who are not naturally organized, *maintaining* an organizational system is often the most difficult piece of the whole process.

A good place to start is keeping it simple and not tackling everything all at once. This can be challenging for both parents who are highly organized and those for whom organization is not a strength. For parents who are not organized themselves, any effort to foster this skill in a child can feel daunting. Those parents might say, "Any organizational system I've ever created for myself breaks down pretty quickly. How can I get my child to use this skill?" For those parents, we suggest picking one or two tasks that they can commit to supervising. It might be always hanging up one's coat as soon as the child comes inside. Or hanging up a towel after taking a shower. If you're one of those parents, you might consider "making a deal" with your child that you'll work on some piece of organization that challenges you (such as always putting your car keys in the same place when you get home from work) if they'll work on something that feels hard to them.

Keeping it simple and starting small can also be a challenge for parents who are strong in organization. This may be because you find it uncomfortable (if not anxiety-provoking) when you see things out of place. If you see your child as very disorganized, you may need to modify your expectations—or at least your definition of "organized enough." They may never meet their parents' standard of neatness, in part because they

How Well Developed Are Your Child's Organizational Skills?

Use the following scale to rate how well your child performs each of the tasks listed. At each level, children can be expected to perform all the tasks listed fairly well to very well.

	Does but not well (about 25% of the time)	Does fairly well (about 75% of the time)	Does very well (always or almost always)
Never or rarely			
0	1	2	3

PRESCHOOL/KINDERGARTEN

☐ Hangs up coat in appropriate place (may need a reminder)

☐ Puts toys in proper locations (with reminders)

☐ Clears place setting after eating (may need a reminder)

LOWER ELEMENTARY (GRADES 1–3)

☐ Puts coat, winter gear, sports equipment in proper locations (may need reminder)

☐ Has specific places in bedroom for belongings

☐ Doesn't lose permission slips or notices from school

UPPER ELEMENTARY (GRADES 4–5)

☐ Can put belongings in appropriate places in bedroom and other locations in house

☐ Brings in toys from outdoors after use or at end of day (may need reminder)

☐ Keeps track of homework materials and assignments

MIDDLE SCHOOL (GRADES 6–8)

☐ Can maintain notebooks as required for school

☐ Doesn't lose sports equipment/personal electronics

☐ Keeps study area at home reasonably tidy

From *Smart but Scattered, Second Edition*, by Peg Dawson, Richard Guare, and Colin Guare. Copyright © 2025 The Guilford Press. Permission to photocopy this material, or to download enlarged printable versions (*www.guilford.com/dawson4-forms*), is granted to purchasers of this book for personal use; see copyright page for details.

just don't see the disorder that is painfully apparent to Mom or Dad. In one of our workshops a few years ago, a mom was lamenting how disorganized her child was. Another member of the audience (a counselor by training) turned around and said to her, "You need to lower your standards!" That's not the advice we typically give parents, but in this case we could see how this mother's (impossibly) high standards were making life difficult for both her and her child.

In one of our recent workshops, a teacher shared a mantra that she used with both her students and her own children: "Don't put it down, put it away." A quick, easy reminder that it's generally faster to put something away immediately rather than having to pick it up later.

Fostering Organization in Everyday Situations

There are two keys to helping children become better organized:

1. Put a system in place.
2. Supervise your child—probably on a daily basis—in using the system. Because this is labor intensive for adults—and because many children who have organizational problems may have parents who are organizationally challenged—we generally recommend starting very small. Identify which domains are most important and work on them one at a time. As a practical matter, the highest priorities are typically their rooms and belongings and their schoolwork, such as keeping notebooks or backpacks organized or keeping a space clean for studying.

Set up the organizational scheme carefully, involving your child as much as possible from the outset. If you and your daughter decide that keeping a desk clean is the priority, you may begin by taking her with you to an office products store and purchasing things like pencil holders, work baskets, or file cabinets and file folders. Once you and your daughter set up the desk as desired, make clearing off the desk part of the bedtime routine—initially with on-site monitoring and supervision and eventually with reminders to start and check-ins when she's finished. You may find it helpful to take a photograph of the space when you first set it up, so your child has a model to compare her work to. The last step in the process might be for your daughter to look at the photo and see how closely her desk matches it.

Controlled Chaos: Getting Kids to Put Their Belongings Where They Belong

There were three children between the ages of 9 and 14 in the Rose family, and they all had an annoying habit of leaving their belongings wherever they were used last. They shed sweatshirts and sports equipment in the kitchen, toys tended to be strewn all over the living room, and they left dirty clothes in the bathroom after they showered. The parents found that the clutter put them in a bad mood when they got home from a hectic workday and wanted to relax briefly before beginning dinner. They decided to call a family meeting to find a solution.

They began the meeting by describing the problem and the effect it had on them. The family then discussed how the kids might get in the habit of picking up after themselves. The kids suggested that there be clearly designated spaces for each of them for belongings in both "public spaces" (hall entryway, kitchen bathroom, living room) as well as their own rooms. Parents thought this was a reasonable suggestion and put cubbies and designated hooks in the entryway labeled for each child. Coats, boots, backpacks, and sports equipment could be left here. They put a single toy container in the living room for game controllers and any other toys left there. They already had bookshelves, large toy containers, and bureaus for clothes in their rooms. They each got hampers in their own rooms for dirty clothes, and the bathroom hamper was designated for dirty towels only.

The mom left a small whiteboard in the middle of the kitchen table with a reminder of the 5:00 deadline. On the whiteboard she wrote the name of each child, and as they finished their work, they were to check off their names. Mrs. Rose also placed an alarm clock next to the reminder with a recurring alarm set for 4:30. When it went off, the kids stopped whatever they were doing and tidied up. If when the parents got home there were any items left about, they called an immediate halt to whatever the children were doing to pick up any items. Parents followed the same routine 30 minutes before bedtime. On the off chance that any item was missed, the belonging would be placed in a large plastic container in the laundry room, where it would remain off limits for 24 hours. If it was something that a child needed (like homework or a piece of sports equipment), the child could "buy" it back with some of the child's weekly allowance. At the end of the week, the family would count up the money and decide how it would be spent.

Within a short time, the kids figured out they could divide up the work between them, so it went more quickly. This approach also enabled them to hold each other accountable, so they could easily identify which child was not doing their share. They also started keeping an eye out during the evening for anything out of place and reminded each other to put things away.

Intervention Steps

Step 1: Establish a Behavioral Goal

Target executive skill(s): Organization

Specific behavioral objective: Children will put away belongings in their appropriate places.

Step 2: Design Interventions

What environmental supports will be provided to help reach the target goal?

- There will be a daily reminder and alarm clock on kitchen table when children get home from school.

• • •

What specific skill will be taught, who will teach the skill, and what procedure will be used to teach it?

Skill: Organization

Who will teach the skill? Parents

Procedure:

- Set a recurring alarm clock for 4:30.
- Cleanup process begins at 4:30 every day.
- Children work until the house is tidy, then check off their names on the whiteboard.

• • •

What incentives/penalties will be used to help motivate the children to use/practice the skill?

- Any activities children are engaged in will be halted until pickup is complete.
- Children will lose access to the belonging for 24 hours (with an opportunity to buy back the item using allowance).
- Kids mutually assist each other.

Keys to Success

- *The children maintain responsibility for pickup and give up their own time until the job is complete.* In the event that something slips by, it is the responsibility of the child to decide whether to buy it back or leave it.

- *Make this a joint project if you're organizationally challenged too.* For example, agree that you'll clear off your kitchen counters or your own desk when your child is doing the same thing.

A United—and Organized—Front:
Helping an Older Child Fulfill His Potential

Devon is a bright 14-year-old middle school student. For as long as he can remember, he has had difficulty organizing himself and routinely misplaces or loses things. Since entering middle school, the problem has gotten worse. He has more things to keep track of in and out of school, and his parents and teachers expect him to manage his belongings more independently. Therefore they're less willing than they were in the past to get him organized, search for his things, or replace them when he can't find them.

Until recently, his parents and teachers had adopted the approach of letting him suffer the consequences of his disorganization. If he lost his sports equipment, he couldn't play; if he lost his homework, he got a failing grade; if he lost some belonging, he had to earn the money to replace it. While they saw occasional improvements, these natural consequences did not resolve the problem. Devon's grades declined, his coaches got upset, and he lost some items he valued, such as his phone. Devon became increasingly discouraged and felt more and more incompetent. His parents finally acknowledged that Devon clearly did not know how to solve the problem and it was time to offer some other kind of help.

They quickly realized this was a major undertaking and was going to take additional work by Devon, his parents, and teachers. They decided to take on two areas: his homework because this was impacting grades and his room because he needed some consistent space to maintain any organization. For homework, they wanted a fairly simple system. His homeroom teacher agreed to check in with him in the morning to see if he had brought in his homework and in the afternoon to see if he had his assignments recorded and the materials he needed. His parents provided the teacher with a checklist that she would have Devon use and she would initial (see below). Devon was typically conscientious about completing his homework, so all his parents needed to see was that Devon had put his homework in the homework folder and put the folder in his backpack.

Subject	Homework handed in	Assignment written down	Materials in backpack
English			
Social Studies			
Science			
Math			
Spanish			

Room cleaning was more complicated. It had been Devon's decision to work on this because he felt that if he could get his room organized and could keep it that way to some extent, he could better track his belongings. While he and his parents had worked on room cleaning from time to time in the past, they never made a systematic or long-term plan or made the same commitment to making it happen.

Devon and his parents agreed that rather than following their suggestions or schemes, it would be best if he came up with his own plan, getting assistance from them when he was stuck. He first took an inventory of his room and decided what categories each item fit into (shirts, pants, sports equipment, and so on). They then looked at what they had available for storage for different categories and what else Devon would need to organize everything and bought the various supplies. Although Devon agreed about the benefits of labeling these storage bins, he didn't want his friends to see the labels if they came over. So they compromised by making removable labels using Velcro.

Devon put in storage things that he didn't currently need but was unwilling to throw out, and his parents worked with him initially to help him get his room organized. He made up a checklist sequence he could follow to pick up his room and took pictures to serve as a model to compare the current state at any point with the ideal.

Devon realized that staying ahead of the clutter was critical. His parents initially agreed to remind him, but then he had the idea to place a cue on his computer that would remind him at least once a day to pick up. The real key to success, however, was a check-in by his parents every other day either after school or within an hour of waking on weekends to determine if he needed to pick anything up. If so, this would happen before he began to use his computer or phone.

As might be expected, over the course of months, while Devon did not maintain his original standard of organization, his room was significantly neater than prior to the system, and his parents were able to decrease cueing to once a week. The homework system also improved markedly, but everyone agreed that the afternoon teacher check-ins and the home check by the parents needed to continue.

Intervention Steps

Step 1: Establish a Behavioral Goal

Target executive skill(s): Organization

Specific behavioral objectives: Devon will keep track of work handed out by his teacher, materials needed, and homework to be handed in. Devon will arrange his room according to categories of objects.

Step 2: Design Interventions

What environmental supports will be provided to help reach the target goal?

- Homework folders
- Checklist of assignments and materials

- Monitoring by parents and teacher
- Pictures of model room
- Storage bins with labels
- Cleaning sequence checklist
- Cueing by parents and computer

• • •

What specific skill will be taught, who will teach the skill, and what procedure will be used to teach it?

Skill: Organizing homework and room

Who will teach the skill? Teacher and parents

Procedure:

- Teacher checks for assignments recorded, materials needed, and assignments returned in folder.
- Parents check folder for presence of homework.
- Materials in room are categorized.
- Storage spaces are made available and labeled.
- Checklist for cleaning is developed and used.
- Parents monitor/cue and computer cues.

• • •

What incentives will be used to help motivate the child to use/practice the skill?

- Improved grades with on-time completion of work
- Retention of and ready access to belongings

Keys to Success

- *To increase the likelihood of success, begin with just one task.* We wrote the Devon story to show that different settings/tasks may be affected by weak organization and to demonstrate how strategies might be designed to address them. But realistically, addressing all of these at the same time would be labor intensive for your child, for you, and for your child's teacher(s). So consider picking one area—such as homework organization—getting that system up and running, and after a month or two moving on to another task.

18

Instilling Time Management

Time management is the capacity to estimate how much time one has, how to allocate it, and how to stay within time limits and deadlines. It also involves a sense that time is important. You probably know some adults who are great at time management and some who aren't. Adults for whom this is a strength are on time for obligations, can estimate how long it takes to do something, and can pace their work depending on the time available (speeding up as needed). They tend not to overextend themselves, in part because they have a realistic sense of what they can accomplish. Adults who are weak at time management have difficulty sticking to a schedule, chronically "run late," and miscalculate when determining how long it takes to do anything. If you have these problems, see the suggestions in Chapter 3 for helping your child with a shared weakness.

How Time Management Develops

Children develop a rudimentary sense of time by sequence of events at around 4 to 5 years old, but a more fully developed sense of time comes at age 9 to 11. Because we know young children can't manage time, we do it for them. We prompt them to get ready for school or daycare, for example, allowing what we think will be enough time to complete the tasks at hand. Or we let them know what time they need to start getting ready for bed to have enough time to read a story after they've put on their pajamas, brushed their teeth, and washed up. If a special event is planned, we estimate how long it will take to get ready and cue children to do what they need to do so the family is ready on time. We notice that children work at different speeds, and we adjust our plans and prompts accordingly.

Gradually we give over the responsibility for this to our children. Once they've learned to tell time (somewhere around second grade), we can remind them to check the clock as they become more autonomous. When the day has predictable events built in, such as sports practice or favorite TV shows, we help children plan their time around those events. When we insist that children finish their homework or chores before going to a sports practice or before watching a television program, we're helping them learn to plan their time.

Sometimes kids hit a snag around middle school because the demands on their time increase just as we tend to cut back on monitoring and supervision. And the number of obligations increases right as the number of distracting activities also increases. How can you fit in homework when you want to play video games, text, surf favorite websites, listen to newly discovered music, text on cell phones with friends, and watch favorite TV shows? No wonder today's young people attempt to multitask! For some, the temptations are just too great, in which case we have to step back in and help them manage their time more effectively.

By high school, many young people have become more adept at juggling options and obligations and planning their time more effectively. If your children have not achieved this, it may be a cause of increasing friction between parents and teenagers because they are at an age where they resist direction and directives from parents. Chapter 3 includes pointers for parents on how to handle that friction, especially when it arises in part due to parents and kids having different profiles of executive skill strengths and challenges.

You can use the questionnaire on the facing page to assess how well developed your child's executive skills are and how they might compare with what is typical for a child of that age.

A Good Place to Start

Time management incorporates a number of executive skills, including task initiation, sustained attention, and planning. But in addition to these skills, a component that is unique to time management is *time estimation*—the ability to estimate how long it takes to do things. In our experience it is this component that people with weak time management skills struggle with. It is not uncommon for children with weak time estimation skills to *underestimate* how long an effortful task will take, and then they leave it until the last minute or run out of time before the deadline is upon them. However, we also see children who do the opposite: they *overestimate* how long a task will take, and then they don't want to start it because in their minds the task is going to take *forever*.

In either case, the place to start is to teach time estimation. And luckily parents have many opportunities to help children practice this. Have your children estimate how long it will take them to make their beds in the morning, or get ready for school, or load the dishwasher or complete their science homework. Write down the start time and the stop time and do the subtraction with them. Were their time estimates correct? With this kind of practice, the ability to calibrate time improves.

When your child's time estimate is not accurate, talk with them about why they were off. Did they not have a clear sense of how long the task should take? Did they forget that some aspect of the task required them to do some additional work that they

How Good Are Your Child's Time Management Skills?

Use the following scale to rate how well your child performs each of the tasks listed. At each level, children can be expected to perform all the tasks listed fairly well to very well.

Never or rarely	Does but not well (about 25% of the time)	Does fairly well (about 75% of the time)	Does very well (always or almost always)
0	1	2	3

PRESCHOOL/KINDERGARTEN

☐ Can complete daily routines without dawdling (with some cues/reminders)

☐ Can speed up and finish something more quickly when given a reason to do so

☐ Can finish a small chore within time limits (e.g., pick up toys before turning on the TV)

LOWER ELEMENTARY (GRADES 1–3)

☐ Can complete a short task within time limits set by an adult

☐ Can build in an appropriate amount of time to complete a chore before a deadline (may need assistance)

☐ Can complete a morning routine within time limits (may need practice)

UPPER ELEMENTARY (GRADES 4–5)

☐ Can complete daily routines within reasonable time limits without assistance

☐ Can adjust a homework schedule to allow for other activities (e.g., starting early if there's an evening Scout meeting)

☐ Can start long-term projects far enough in advance to reduce any time crunch (may need help with this)

MIDDLE SCHOOL (GRADES 6–8)

☐ Can usually finish homework before bedtime

☐ Can make good decisions about priorities when time is limited (e.g., coming home after school to finish a project rather than playing with friends)

☐ Can spread out a long-term project over several days

From *Smart but Scattered, Second Edition*, by Peg Dawson, Richard Guare, and Colin Guare. Copyright © 2025 The Guilford Press. Permission to photocopy this material, or to download enlarged printable versions (*www.guilford.com/dawson4-forms*), is granted to purchasers of this book for personal use; see copyright page for details.

didn't factor in? Did they get distracted along the way, which led the task to take longer than their estimate? If they routinely underestimate how long a task should take, you might help them build in a "fudge" factor for future time estimates. If a child routinely thinks they can finish their math homework in 15 minutes but it takes 30 minutes, then they should multiply their initial estimate by two to plan their time more accurately.

This can lead to other interesting conversations about time. Have they noticed that they tend to be more accurate in estimating time when it involves something they like to do compared to something they don't like to do? Do they notice their attention flags with tasks that take a long time? If so, can they make an adjustment for this, such as building in short breaks or breaking the task down to shorter segments spread out over hours or days?

While talking with children about time from an early age is helpful (see the suggestions below), it is unrealistic to assume that very young children can manage time on their own. No parent of a 7-year-old would tell them, "You can go to bed whenever you want; just make sure you get enough sleep." As noted, middle school often poses challenges for kids because their schedules tend to get more complicated and the expectation is that they can manage those more complicated time demands on their own. While we think this may be unrealistic, if we start having conversations with children about how to manage time before they reach middle school, that transition may go more smoothly.

A friend of ours who acknowledges that she has ADHD told us that she learned to estimate time by setting a timer for 5 minutes and asking herself, "I wonder how much I can get done in 5 minutes." When the timer rang, she assessed her work and set the timer for another 5 minutes, posing the same question. Over time, she had a better sense both of how long 5 minutes is and how much she could typically accomplish in that time. This might be a good approach to use with children who struggle with this skill.

Instilling Time Management in Everyday Situations

• *Without going overboard, maintain a predictable daily routine in your family.* When children get up and go to bed at around the same time every day, and meals occur on a fairly set schedule, they grow up with a sense of time being an orderly progression from one event to another. This makes it easier for them to plan their time in between scheduled events (such as meals and bedtime).

• *Talk to your children about how long it takes to do things,* such as chores, picking up their rooms, or completing a homework assignment. This is the beginning of developing time estimation skills—a critical component of time management.

• *Plan an activity for a weekend or vacation day that involves several steps.* When you work with your child on planning skills, you're also working on time management because planning involves developing timelines for task completion. When you talk with your child about "the plan for the day" and discuss how long it will take to complete the activity, your child is learning about time and the relationship between time and tasks. Doing this type of planning can actually be fun if you choose a fun activity, like spending the day with a friend. Ask the child to figure out how long it should take to have lunch, go to the park or beach, stop for ice cream on the way home, and so forth. The lessons learned will be especially meaningful to your child if he realizes that he and his friend got to pack the day with everything they wanted to do only because they blocked out their time in advance.

- *Use calendars and schedules yourself and encourage your child to do the same.* Some families post a large calendar in a central location where individual and family activities are posted. This has the effect of making time visible to your child.

- *Purchase a commercially available clock,* available from Time Timer (*www.timetimer.com*), that can be set to show visually how much time a child has left to work. This device can also be downloaded for free as a smart phone app or purchased in wristwatch form.

- *Consider apps that help children follow daily routines.* One of our favorites is Choiceworks because the app enables you to program both the steps in the routine as well as a time estimate for how long each step should be expected to take. This app also allows you to import photographs of the child doing each step in the routine (although it also provides a picture bank to choose from). Common Sense Media also has a list of apps that offer similar options.

Out of the House on Time: Managing Morning Routines

Seven-year-old Tarik is the youngest in a family of four boys and has always desperately wanted to keep up with his older brothers. He wants to be independent, and when he was younger his favorite line was "I do it myself." Tarik seems to understand the concept of time. He can tell time to the quarter hour and has a pretty fair idea of when his favorite shows are on TV. However, he often seems to lose track of time, and he has little sense of time urgency. This has led to problems at home and at school. At home, getting ready to go anywhere can be a major chore. Although the situation can be worse if the destination is a place that Tarik doesn't want to go (for example, a doctor's appointment), he is slow getting ready even for preferred activities (for example, going to a water park). To get or keep him moving his parents or one of his siblings routinely cue or nag him. While this usually works eventually, it's a source of growing frustration for family members. Tarik doesn't struggle academically or exhibit any learning problems, but he's often the last to finish his work. His teacher has noticed that he can be more efficient when he needs to finish a task to get to a preferred activity such as recess.

His parents decide that Tarik is old enough to begin to learn some basic skills in time management. They reason that if Tarik is to learn how to finish tasks within a certain amount of time, he first needs to know what tasks are expected of him. Because leaving the house has been the issue, they decide to concentrate on the tasks he might need to complete to leave the house. This could range from the full-blown morning routine (wake up, get dressed, eat breakfast, brush teeth, and so on) to something as simple as getting his shoes on. Because the morning routine includes most of the "getting ready" tasks and he is slow in the morning, they decide to begin with this.

To take advantage of Tarik's desire to be a "big boy" and be independent, they talk with him about a schedule of jobs in the morning. They try to sell the plan by telling him that if he can do his jobs on time, they won't have to nag him. Tarik isn't particularly interested until they tell him that when he is finished, he can use whatever time is left for one of his preferred activities. He has fun making up the schedule, which consists of pictures and words, because he gets to "act" each scene (getting up, eating breakfast, brushing his teeth, and so on). His parents basically let him decide the order of the tasks on the schedule. They create a Velcro strip so that the order of the pictures can be changed and they can be removed. The plan is that as each job is finished, Tarik will move that picture and put it in the "done" pocket attached to the bottom of the schedule. Rather than giving him a set time to begin with, over two mornings they agree that they will time him and use the result to decide how long he needs to finish. With him, they also create a short list of preferred activities that he can choose from when he completes his schedule. To increase his chances of success, his parents agree that for the first week or two they will check with him twice during the schedule as a reminder. His parents, after discussing it with Tarik and clearing it with the school, also add that if he is slow in getting through his schedule and late for school as a result, he will make up the time either during recess or after school.

Using this system, Tarik becomes more efficient and independent in the morning. For other "getting ready" times, his parents use a mini-version of this plan involving one or two pictures, the timer, and preferred activities.

Intervention Steps

Step 1: Establish a Behavioral Goal

Target executive skill(s): Time management

Specific behavioral objective: Tarik will complete his morning routine tasks within a specific amount of time.

Step 2: Design Interventions

What environmental supports will be provided to help reach the target goal?
- Picture/written schedule with removable pictures
- Timer

- Cues from parents two times during the schedule
- Teacher support of the plan if he is late for school

• • •

What specific skill will be taught, who will teach the skill, and what procedure will be used to teach it?

Skill: Time management

Who will teach the skill? Parents/teacher

Procedure:

- Tarik and his parents make up a visual/written schedule.
- Tarik arranges activities in his preferred order.
- Parents set a timer in the morning.
- Parents check with Tarik twice during his schedule.
- Tarik removes a picture as each activity is completed.
- Tarik chooses from the prize box if he gets through his schedule within the agreed-upon time.
- If Tarik is late for school, he makes up missed work during free time.

• • •

What incentives will be used to help motivate the child to use/practice the skill?

- Tarik can choose an inexpensive treat from the prize box if he completes tasks on time.

Keys to Success

- *Keep a rough count of the number of cues you provide and how close you need to be (in the doorway versus at the bottom of the stairs, for example) to make your reminders effective. Twice during the schedule may prove not to be enough. You may need to issue more reminders to get your child used to getting the assigned tasks done during the allotted time. Although it can be somewhat annoying to keep this kind of record, it will allow you to see progress and appreciate the pace needed to wean your child from these supports. Without having this sense of progress, parents often feel the system isn't working and go back to nagging.*

Time Warp: Learning to Estimate How Long a Task Will Take

Nathan's parents have always appreciated the eighth grader's mellow nature, which contrasts so sharply with his sister, who panics every time she has a test to study for. But ever since he entered middle school, his parents have become increasingly concerned about his tendency to put off homework until too close to bedtime, which means he rushes through it or may not finish it all. Problems are compounded when he has long-term projects because he often leaves them until the day before they are due. Over time his mother has realized that part of the problem is that Nathan has no idea how long things take to do. A paper he thinks he can write in half an hour may take him 2 hours, and a project he thinks he can put together in a couple of hours may take 5 or 6. His parents have tried repeatedly to get Nathan to understand that his ability to estimate time is weak, but even when he acknowledges the fact that the last time he wrote a paper it took him 2 hours, this time, because he knows what he wants to write about and has a rough outline in his head, he's sure he can whip it out in an hour max.

After one too many arguments when his parents pointed out yet again that he was no judge of time and Nathan told them in no uncertain terms to "Get off my case!" his parents decided they had to figure out another way to handle the problem. They took Nathan out to dinner on a Saturday night when he wasn't doing anything with friends. They discussed a few different options, and Nathan decided that each day when he got home from school, he would make a list of the homework assignments he had to do that night and estimate how long each assignment would take. He would then decide at what time he was going to start his homework based on his estimates, with the understanding that he would be done by no later than 9:00. If he was off by more than 20 minutes, then the next day he would start his homework at 4:30. If his estimates were accurate, he could determine what time he would start his homework the next day. They also agreed he had to build in time to study for tests and do a little work on long-term projects at least two to three nights a week unless his daily homework took more than 2 hours. Nathan agreed to this plan because he thought it would give him a chance to prove his parents wrong and was the best option to let him manage on his own—he even spent an hour on the computer when he got home, happily creating a spreadsheet he could use to keep his data. He told his mom he would email the spreadsheet to her as soon as he filled out his daily plan. They agreed that she would check the plan and check in with him at the time he said he would be done with his homework, at which point he would show her all the assignments he had completed.

For the first couple of weeks his mom needed to remind Nathan to make the plan and email it to her. Nathan quickly learned that he wasn't as good at estimating as he thought he was. But because he hated starting his homework so soon after he got home from school, he gradually improved his ability to estimate how long homework would take. A couple of times when he showed his parents his work, they saw that he'd done a rather sloppy job, apparently in an effort to get it done on time. They talked about introducing a penalty for sloppiness, and with a warning that this would happen if sloppiness became an issue, Nathan cleaned up his act—at least enough so that his parents decided not to push the issue.

Intervention Steps

Step 1: Establish a Behavioral Goal

Target executive skill(s): Time management

Specific behavioral objective: Nathan will learn to accurately estimate the time needed to complete homework by a specific time each night.

Step 2: Design Interventions

What environmental supports will be provided to help reach the target goal?

- Start and stop times for homework
- Spreadsheet for estimated work times
- Check-ins with mother

• • •

What specific skill will be taught, who will teach the skill, and what procedure will be used to teach it?

Skill: Time management

Who will teach the skill? Parents/Nathan

Procedure:

- Nathan will make a list of homework assignments and the estimated time needed to complete them, put this on a spreadsheet, and send it to his mother.
- Based on these estimates, he will decide what time to begin homework.
- Work will be completed by 9:00 P.M., and if his estimate is off by 20 or more minutes, he will start work earlier the next day.
- Nathan will build in time to study for tests and will commit to work on long-term projects two to three nights per week.

• • •

What incentives will be used to help motivate the child to use/practice the skill?

- Nathan can manage his own time without interference or nagging from his parents.

Keys to Success

- *Vigilance from you is critical in the early stages of the intervention because most kids will find that some elements of the plan require a lot of effort and will therefore forget or avoid them.*

- *Have the child's teachers independently verify the amount and quality of work completed by the child. As designed, this plan requires accurate reports from the child. In our experience the most effective way to prevent breakdown of the plan is to have the teachers offer feedback, through whatever communication platform the school uses. Reports should come to you, with a copy to your child.*

19

Increasing
Goal-Directed Persistence

Goal-directed persistence refers to setting a goal and working toward it without being sidetracked by competing interests. Anytime we keep striving to reach a long-term goal, we're exhibiting this skill. A 25-year-old who decides to run a marathon and trains for a year to do that shows good goal-directed persistence. A store clerk who wants to become a manager and volunteers for additional jobs at work to demonstrate the motivation to work their way up also has goal-directed persistence. And when couples cut back on recreational and entertainment expenses to save up enough money for a down payment on a house, they too are showing goal-directed persistence. If you find yourself changing your goals a lot in response to new interests that arise or you don't consider improving your performance over time important, you may have a skill deficit in goal-directed persistence and can use the suggestions in Chapter 3 for making the most of your efforts to help your child when you share your child's weakness.

How Goal-Directed Persistence Develops

Although goal-directed persistence is one of the last executive skills to mature, from the time your child was quite young you've been encouraging the development of this skill—even if you've never recognized it as such. Whether it's helping your toddler put together a puzzle or helping your 5-year-old learn to ride a bike, every time you've encouraged your child to keep trying even when something is hard, you've given their goal-directed persistence a nudge forward. Likewise, when you impress upon your child that mastering new skills takes time, practice, and effort, and you praise your child for sticking with something tough, you've helped the child value goal-directed persistence. Most notably, children learn the idea of persistence through sports or learning a musical instrument, but you also teach persistence by assigning tasks such as chores. In the beginning chores are kept brief and contained within a small space (like putting away one's toothbrush or hanging up one's coat). As your child has gotten older, you've naturally recognized that they could handle longer chores or those that demand working in larger spaces (cleaning their room, raking leaves, walking the dog, and the like).

Giving your child an allowance and helping him learn to save money for desired objects is another way you help your child develop goal-directed persistence. By third grade most children have learned to save at least a little money toward something they want to buy. By the time they reach middle school, a majority of children have learned the concept of goal-directed persistence at least well enough to practice a sport or a musical instrument or to make choices about how they spend their time so they can earn good grades in school. By early high school youngsters are beginning to understand that their daily performance in school can affect outcomes such as college choices, and by late sophomore year or the beginning of their junior year, they may be taking bigger steps to alter their behavior to achieve desired long-term goals.

To assess how your child's goal-directed persistence compares with her age group, complete the questionnaire on the facing page, which builds on the simpler assessment you did in Chapter 2.

A Good Place to Start

Just as time management incorporates earlier-developing skills such as task initiation and sustained attention, goal-directed persistence is not a single skill. You can't just set a goal—you have to remember it, which requires working memory. You need a plan for achieving the goal, which requires planning. Then you need to start and finish the plan, which involves task initiation and sustained attention. You also have to resist the temptation to do all those other fun things you'd rather be doing than working toward your goal, so you need response inhibition. And finally, if that's irritating or annoying to you, you also have to manage your emotions, so you need emotional control.

Although we think that all 11 executive skills are critically important, if children develop goal-directed persistence, they can use that executive skill to overcome other executive skill challenges. Children may not be great at task initiation, but if the goal is important to them, they will get started on it. And sustained attention may be challenging for them, but with strong goal-directed persistence, they will persist with the task, even though they may feel themselves running out of steam.

We sometimes describe goal-directed persistence as the "killer skill" for parents of middle school students. So many parents expect their kids to have this skill by middle school, but, in our experience, many kids this age don't quite have it yet. So their expectations for their kids end up dead on arrival. Many parents kill any chance their middle schoolers have of meeting these expectations by focusing on goal-directed persistence primarily through academic performance. This was the mistake I made (Peg talking) when my sons were that age. I was leaning on them to bring their grades up or even make the honor roll, but that wasn't particularly important to either of them at the time.

How Good Is Your Child at Goal-Directed Persistence?

Use the following scale to rate how well your child performs each of the tasks listed. At each level, children can be expected to perform all the tasks listed fairly well to very well.

Never or rarely	Does but not well (about 25% of the time)	Does fairly well (about 75% of the time)	Does very well (always or almost always)
0	1	2	3

PRESCHOOL/KINDERGARTEN

[ ] Will direct other children in play or pretend play activities

[ ] Will seek assistance in conflict resolution for a desired item

[ ] Will try more than one solution to get to a simple goal

LOWER ELEMENTARY (GRADES 1–3)

[ ] Will stick with a challenging task to achieve the desired goal, such as building a difficult LEGO construct

[ ] Will come back to a task later if interrupted

[ ] Will work on a desired project for several hours or over several days

UPPER ELEMENTARY (GRADES 4–5)

[ ] Can save up allowance for 3–4 weeks to make a desired purchase

[ ] Can follow a practice schedule to get better at a desired skill (sport, instrument)—may need reminders

[ ] Can maintain a hobby over several months

MIDDLE SCHOOL (GRADES 6–8)

[ ] Able to increase effort to improve performance (e.g., work harder to get a higher grade on a test or a report card)

[ ] Willing to engage in effortful tasks to earn money

[ ] Willing to practice without reminders to improve a skill

From *Smart but Scattered, Second Edition*, by Peg Dawson, Richard Guare, and Colin Guare. Copyright © 2025 The Guilford Press. Permission to photocopy this material, or to download enlarged printable versions (*www.guilford.com/dawson4-forms*), is granted to purchasers of this book for personal use; see copyright page for details.

So here are three pieces of advice for parents of children as they reach the middle school years:

1. *Focus on goals that are important to your children rather than the ones that are important to you.* If they're into sports, see if they'd like to set a sports goal. Maybe they want to be rock stars and are bound and determined to learn to play the electric guitar. Encourage them in that pursuit even as you may be skeptical of the likelihood of their becoming a member of the next Rolling Stones.

With younger children, you might encourage them to save up money for something they want that costs more than their weekly allowance. That means you can talk with them about how they're going to earn the money they need, how they will *save* that money, and how they will resist the temptation to spend smaller amounts of money on a sudden desire rather than sticking with their original goal.

2. *Be patient.* We often tell our parent audiences that the child standing in front of you at 15 will not be the same person at 25. Since we have watched our own children grow from infancy to adulthood and watched how they changed—and pretty dramatically well into their 20s—we can assure you of this with some confidence.

3. *Model goal-directed persistence for your kids.* I survived my sons' middle school years (Peg talking again) by assuring myself that my kids had two parents with strong goal-directed persistence and that at the point where they discovered their passions they would channel that executive skill strength. And that's what happened—on two very different timetables because my sons were so different, but when they found their calling, they threw themselves into the work with all their energy.

Increasing Goal-Directed Persistence in Everyday Situations

While this skill is one of the last executive skills to develop fully, there are steps you can take beginning when your child is quite young to help them develop goal-directed persistence:

- *Start very early, beginning with very brief tasks where the goal is within sight* (in terms of time and space). Offer to help your child complete the task and praise her for getting the task done. For instance, one of the earliest toys children enjoy is puzzles. Begin with puzzles with very few pieces, and if the child gets stuck, give her cues or assistance (for example, point to the piece the child needs and the place it needs to go and have the child put the piece in place).

- *As you help your child stretch and reach more distant goals, begin with ones that the child wants to work on.* Your son will likely be more interested in persisting with a task such as building a more complicated LEGO structure than he is in cleaning up his bedroom floor. Encourage him, provide small cues, hints, and assistance as needed (the minimal help necessary for the child to be on a path to success), and then praise him for sticking with it.

• *Give your child something to look forward to doing when the chore is finished.* This will encourage your child to persist with tasks that aren't so much fun, such as chores. If your child's stamina is pretty low, divide the task into parts with short breaks in between. As they practice, each part becomes less effortful, and you can gradually increase the length of each step and reduce the number of breaks.

• *Gradually build up the time needed to reach goals.* At first the goals should be reachable within a few minutes or in less than an hour. The amount of time can be increased, and eventually your child will be able to go longer before achieving the goal or reaching the preferred activity. To help her learn to delay gratification from minutes to hours to days, build in concrete feedback about her progress toward the goal. Younger kids can visually self-monitor by coloring footsteps on a path or putting Velcro stars on a chart to represent progress. For older kids, coloring steps on a thermometer and drawing graphs are good self-monitoring strategies, and self-monitoring enhances skill acquisition and motivation.

• *Help the child remember what he is working toward.* If he's saving money for a toy or a game, take a picture of the desired object, laminate it, and cut it into pieces. Each piece can represent a certain amount of money, and as the child earns that sum, he can Velcro a piece until the object is complete. Visual reminders are more effective than verbal reminders, and verbal reminders are often interpreted as nagging by kids!

• *Use technology to provide the reminders.* One example is the sticky notes that appear on the desktop when the computer screen is turned on. Youngsters who have smart phones can use reminder programs, and there is a wide variety of goal-tracking apps available for both computers and cell phones. When selecting any app, personal preference is important. A goal-tracking app that looks "perfect" to a parent may hold no appeal at all to their child.

• *Make sure a reward you use as incentive for goal-directed persistence is one your child really wants and doesn't have free access to.* A child who loves video games, for instance, and has three different game systems and two dozen games and can play them whenever she wants is not going to be motivated to delay gratification and persist toward any goal to get video games or game time.

Quitters Never Win Self-Confidence: How to Help a Child Stick with Work and Play

Five-year-old Chen is a curious kindergartner who likes to try new things, but he seems quick to abandon every activity, either from loss of interest or because it's too hard. He gives up on "work" tasks such as simple chores and school activities but also on the fun stuff, like video games and athletics (hitting/catching a ball, riding a bike). Chen's

3-year-old sister is a "bulldog" who will persist until she achieves whatever she set out for, which makes Chen's parents worry even more about their son. Will his lack of persistence make him more passive and less open to new activities? He already seems less confident than he was when he was younger.

Chen's parents want to help him, but neither encouragement during an activity nor insistence that he finish has had a lasting impact. They would like to make a plan with Chen, but they need some additional information. When Chen starts an activity, are his expectations too high? Once he starts, does his goal seem too far off? After talking with Chen about some activities that he has put aside, they realize both factors can come into play. With baseball he wanted to hit a "home run" (off the tee and out of the yard) when he batted. After a few failures he thought he'd never get there, so he stopped.

Chen's dad offers to help him with hitting if Chen agrees on shorter, easier goals (such as any contact with the ball) and a short time limit for practice (5–10 minutes). Chen is OK with this, and they make a chart on the computer to keep track of the number of swings and the number of hits for each day of practice. Chen plots the data. He seems to like this plan, and his parents see him sometimes go out on his own to practice. He gets confident enough about hitting to play T-ball in the rec program with his friends.

Chen's parents try a similar plan for a chore: putting the dishes in the dishwasher. Because he dislikes this chore, his parents initially keep the demand small (only his dish and glass) and set it up to be a "first—then" where once he completes the task, he can do a preferred activity. Until he completes the task, access to a preferred activity or free time is on hold. They increase the demand very gradually, so the end and his preferred activity are in sight. Over the course of a month, he is putting the rest of the family dishes in and regularly getting to his free time. His parents adopt these approaches as a general strategy to teach Chen effort and persistence whenever he seems to struggle with an activity or task.

Intervention Steps

Step 1: Establish a Behavioral Goal

Target executive skill(s): Goal-directed persistence

Specific behavioral objective: Chen will improve his task persistence for preferred and less preferred tasks.

Step 2: Design Interventions

What environmental supports will be provided to help reach the target goal?

- Keep demands easy and establish easily achievable, short goals.

- Track progress on a simple chart.
- Provide parent support to build the skill.

• • •

What specific skill will be taught, who will teach the skill, and what procedure will be used to teach it?

Skill: Chen will achieve a goal or complete a task demand through the successful completion of small task steps.

Who will teach the skill? Chen's parents will help teach the skill, and Chen will begin to practice on his own.

Procedure:

- Chen's parents work with him to set achievable goals and task demands.
- Chen agrees to a practice schedule and criteria.

• • •

What incentives will be used to help motivate the child to use/practice the skill?

- Positive feedback indicating that performance objectives are being met
- Charting to make progress visible and concrete
- His preferred free-time activity for job completion

Keys to Success

- *If your child avoids the activity because they don't succeed quickly enough, position the task before a more preferred task.* It's not hard to see that having Chen do the dishes before he can have computer or TV time might provide an added incentive to do the dishes. But the same may go even for something like practicing batting. The fact that it's a recreational activity doesn't mean practice will seem like fun to a child who has trouble persisting toward a goal. These kids lose their patience quite easily.

Saving Money

From her parents' perspective, 9-year-old Amani is a "here-and-now" type of kid. She doesn't have a lot of patience for waiting and is easily frustrated when she has to work toward a goal or wait for something she wants. For example, she expects to be as good at soccer as her best friend, even though she started later and doesn't practice as much on her own. Saving the money she gets for allowance or for things like birthdays is especially tough, and as soon as she has money, she wants to go to the store to spend it. As a result she is often broke and routinely asks her parents to either buy her something she wants or to "lend" her the money until she gets her allowance. Getting her to pay the money back can be very difficult, so her parents have adopted a "no loan" policy except in unusual cases. They want to see her learn to follow a plan to get to a future goal, even if it's relatively short-term.

Amani wants a video game system. In the past her parents have told her she can have one if she saves the money for it. Although she has tried, she hasn't made it past a week or so before she decides to spend her savings on something more immediate. While her parents have concerns about having video games at home, they also see Amani's desire as a means to teach her about getting to a goal. They see Amani potentially working for the system and for the various games she will want. If a savings plan is to work, Amani has to see progress toward her goal fairly quickly. Simply saving the $5 per week that she gets for allowance is not likely to be fast enough. Because her birthday is coming up, the money she gets from her parents, other relatives, and friends can help to "jump start" this fund. Still, her parents know that she needs to see visible progress toward her game system.

Her parents decide they will help her develop a plan to buy her game system if she is definitely interested. Talking with her demonstrates that she is. They propose that if Amani is willing to devote all her birthday money toward the game, she could probably buy it in as little as 5 or 6 weeks by adding in her allowance money. Amani is a little uncomfortable with this because it means she will get no presents at her birthday party. She suggests that the four friends she is having over bring birthday presents, and she will use the birthday money she gets from her parents and relatives toward the game and then add the rest from allowance. Her parents still worry that she will lose sight of the goal. They discuss getting a picture of the game system and laminating it. They will then cut it up into pieces like a puzzle and make each piece correspond to a $5 payment. With her birthday money Amani will get a good start on completing a large part of the puzzle, and then each week another piece will be added with her allowance. Ten weeks after her birthday Amani completes the puzzle and happily buys her game system. She and her parents like this system and are able to use it for other, longer-term goals.

Intervention Steps

Step 1: Establish a Behavioral Goal

Target executive skill(s): Goal-directed persistence

Specific behavioral objective: Amani will successfully save the money needed for her video game system within 10 weeks of her birthday.

Step 2: Design Interventions

What environmental supports will be provided to help reach the target goal?

- Amani and her parents will construct a picture puzzle that when completed means she has achieved her goal of buying a video game system.
- Amani's parents will remind Amani that each time she gets $5 she can buy another puzzle piece.
- Each week Amani and her parents will review how much of the puzzle is completed.

• • •

What specific skill will be taught, who will teach the skill, and what procedure will be used to teach it?

Skill: Achievement of a short-term goal through planning and saving

Who will teach the skill? Parents

Procedure:

- Amani and her parents will establish a concrete objective using a picture puzzle.
- Amani's parents will help her set a timeline so that the end is in sight.
- Amani will begin the plan at a time (her birthday) that allows her to get a good jump start on the goal.
- Amani and her parents will formally check the puzzle progress weekly, and her parents will be cheerleaders, encouraging her each time she buys another piece of the puzzle.
- At least every 2 weeks her parents will take Amani to the store to play the demo model of the game, so she is in close contact with her goal.

• • •

What incentives will be used to help motivate the child to use/practice the skill?

- Amani will have a video game of her own that she otherwise would not have at all.
- Parents will use a similar system for purchase of the games that Amani wants to play.

Keys to Success

- *Remember that a child's time horizon is much shorter than yours.* For a plan like this to succeed, the end always has to be in sight *for the child*. So don't get too ambitious in teaching this skill. Expectations that the child will save for months or put all her resources into savings are unrealistic.

- *Remember that learning to save requires ongoing and long-term practice.* Be prepared to use savings systems over an extended period.

20

Cultivating Metacognition

Metacognition refers to the ability to stand back and take a bird's-eye view of oneself in a situation. It's an ability to observe how you problem solve. It also includes self-monitoring and self-evaluating your performance—asking yourself, "How am I doing?" or "How did I do?" Adults who have this skill can size up a problem situation, take into account multiple pieces of information, including past experience, and make good decisions about how to proceed. They can also evaluate afterward how they did and decide to do things differently in the future if need be. Adults who struggle with this skill may miss or ignore important information (particularly social cues) and tend to make decisions based on "what feels right" rather than careful analysis of the facts. If you feel like you put your foot in your mouth a lot, make decisions you regret, and can't always get a handle on how well you're doing in your endeavors, follow the procedure suggested in Chapter 3 for helping your child learn a skill that isn't your strong suit either.

How Metacognition Develops

Metacognition is a complex set of skills that begins developing during the first year of life as infants work to organize their experiences, by sorting and classifying and by starting to recognize cause–effect relationships. These skills get extended during toddlerhood, when order, routine, and ritual—all mechanisms whereby they can control their experiences—become important to kids. By later preschool and kindergarten, children begin to recognize that other people have different perceptual experiences, and they begin to identify emotions in others and to be able to role-play. Shortly after that, between the ages of 5 and 7, children begin to recognize that others have different thoughts and feelings, and they start being able to make rudimentary interpretations of intent (such as whether someone hurt them on purpose or by accident). By middle childhood, the metacognitive vista widens dramatically. Children at this age not only have a deeper understanding of their own thoughts, feelings, and intentions, but they understand that their thoughts, feelings, and intentions can be the object of the thinking of others. This is why youngsters in middle school develop such self-consciousness about their own actions and why conformity becomes such a priority for many. They have not yet learned that just because other people *can* think about them in a way that may seem intrusive doesn't mean they are! By high school they can step back and put things in a little more perspective, as the building blocks of metacognition accumulate and fall into place.

To assess how your child's metacognitive skills compare with his age group, complete the questionnaire on the facing page, which builds on the assessment you did of your child in Chapter 2.

A Good Place to Start

Of all the executive skills in our model, metacognition tends to be the most confusing. The most common definition of metacognition is that it is "thinking about thinking." We think that's too vague to be of much use. Here's a refinement of that definition that we think is more helpful: *metacognition is the awareness that you have thoughts and that you can use those thoughts as tools to understand the world and yourself, solve problems, and make sense out of things.*

Now obviously children have thoughts from a very early age. When they first learn to talk, all their thinking is out loud. It eventually goes "underground"—we call that *internalized speech*. But it takes a long time for children to realize that they can use their thoughts as "tools." Once this happens, there tends to be a bump in their other executive skills, particularly the more advanced skills, because now they can use their thoughts to plan and prioritize, to create organizational systems, to manage their time, and to set goals.

Of course parents and teachers can encourage metacognitive thinking from the time children are very young (see the suggestions in the following section). Teaching kids to reflect on and evaluate their performance is a great way to do this. Parents and teachers often focus on self-reflection when things go wrong. "You got sent in from recess again," a teacher might say to an elementary-school-age child who struggles with response inhibition and emotional control. "What went wrong? And what can you do differently to make sure that doesn't happen again?" Young children may not know what to do. If that's the case, brainstorm with them and offer options they can choose from. Write down the two or three options they choose and, just prior to the next recess, review the options with them. When they come in from recess, ask them what, if any, option they used and how it went. This is a process that can be used across a variety of problem situations, and children learn a strategy that builds metacognition.

We recommend that an emphasis be placed on reflections following successes. "You went 3 whole days without getting sent in from recess. Great job! What strategies were you using to pull that off?"

How Well Developed Are Your Child's Metacognitive Skills?

Use the following scale to rate how well your child performs each of the tasks listed. At each level, children can be expected to perform all the tasks listed fairly well to very well.

Never or rarely	Does but not well (about 25% of the time)	Does fairly well (about 75% of the time)	Does very well (always or almost always)
0	1	2	3

PRESCHOOL/KINDERGARTEN

☐ Can make minor adjustments in a construction project or puzzle task when a first attempt fails

☐ Can come up with a novel (but simple) use of a tool to solve a problem

☐ Makes suggestions to another child for how to fix something

LOWER ELEMENTARY (GRADES 1–3)

☐ Can adjust behavior in response to feedback from a parent or teacher

☐ Can watch what happens to others and change behavior appropriately

☐ Can verbalize more than one solution to a problem and make the best choice

UPPER ELEMENTARY (GRADES 4–5)

☐ Can anticipate the result of a course of action and make adjustments accordingly (e.g., to avoid getting in trouble)

☐ Can articulate several solutions to problems and explain the best one

☐ Enjoys the problem-solving component of school assignments or video games

MIDDLE SCHOOL (GRADES 6–8)

☐ Can accurately evaluate their own performance (e.g., in a sports event or school assignment)

☐ Can see the impact of their behavior on peers and make adjustments (e.g., to fit in with the group or avoid being teased)

☐ Can perform tasks requiring more abstract reasoning

From *Smart but Scattered, Second Edition*, by Peg Dawson, Richard Guare, and Colin Guare. Copyright © 2025 The Guilford Press. Permission to photocopy this material, or to download enlarged printable versions (*www.guilford.com/dawson4-forms*), is granted to purchasers of this book for personal use; see copyright page for details.

That one question—*What strategies were you using?*—is a great one to encourage metacognition. Until an adult uses the word *strategy* to label what the child did, that child may not be aware that is what they were doing. Young children may need help recognizing that what they did qualifies as a strategy and may need an adult to help them make that connection. "It looks like you found someone else to play with when Alex was doing something else. That's a great strategy."

With older kids, metacognition can be strengthened by letting kids make decisions for themselves. One of our favorite books, *The Self-Driven Child* by William Stixrud and Ned Johnson, has a chapter titled "It's Your Call," which gives parents great advice for identifying when and how kids can make their own choices.

Cultivating Metacognitive Skills in Everyday Situations

There are two sets of metacognitive skills that you can help your child develop. One set involves the child's ability to evaluate her performance on a task, such as a chore or a homework assignment, and to make changes based on that evaluation. The second set involves the child's ability to evaluate social situations—both her own behavior and others' reactions and the behavior of others.

To help your child develop skills related to task performance, try the following:

● *Provide specific praise for key elements of task performance.* For instance, if you want to encourage your child to be thorough in completing a task, praise him for that: "I like the way you put every single block back in the box" or "I like the way you looked under your bed to see if there were any dirty clothes there."

● *Work with your child to evaluate their own performance on a task.* After finishing spelling homework where the assignment was to write each spelling word in a sentence, you might ask, "How do you think you did? Did you follow the directions? Do you like the way the paper looks?" You can also offer brief, specific suggestions for improvement, preferably starting with a positive: "You wrote really good sentences, but your words sometimes run together on the page. You might try putting your finger on the page at the end of every word and leaving that much space between one word and the next." In providing feedback and suggestions, suspend judgment because criticism always muddies the water.

● *Have the child identify what finished looks like.* If your son's job is to empty the dishwasher, get him to describe what that means (no more dishes in the dishwasher, everything put away in drawers or cupboards). You may want to write this down and post it prominently to help the child remember.

● *Teach a set of questions children can ask themselves when confronted with problem situations.* These might include "What is the problem I need to solve?" "What is my plan?" "Am I following my plan?" or "How did I do?"

To help your child learn to read social situations, try the following:

• *Play a guessing game to teach your child to read facial expressions.* Many youngsters who have problems with this skill do not know how to read facial expressions or interpret feelings. One way to teach this skill is to turn it into a guessing game where both parents and children make facial expressions, and each has to guess what feeling the other person is trying to convey. Another way is to watch a television show with the sound off and guess the person's feelings based on facial expression and body language (you may want to record the show so that you can rewind and watch segments with the sound on again to check your hypotheses).

• *Help children begin to recognize how tone of voice changes the meaning of what is being said.* It is said that 55% of communication is facial expression, 38% is tone of voice, and only 7% is the actual words spoken. Give your child labels for different tones of voice (teasing, sarcastic, whining, angry) and then ask your child to use them to identify the tones of voice the child uses to communicate as well as those used by others.

• *Talk about the clues to someone's feelings that can be spotted, even when the person is trying to hide their feelings.* Are there subtle signs (a tightening of the mouth to signify anger, fiddling with things to denote anxiety)? Turn it into a detective game.

• *Ask your child to identify how their actions might make someone feel.* This teaches the language of feelings and cause–effect relationships.

No More Know-It-All:
Helping Your Child Learn to Listen

Eleven-year-old Yoshi is the oldest of three children in her family. She is a fairly conscientious student. Yoshi has always had a good memory and has always liked to read and watch informative shows on TV like those on the Discovery Channel and Animal Planet. As a result of her skills and her interests, Yoshi has stored a lot of information and has become something of a "junior expert" on a variety of subjects. Her parents and relatives have encouraged this and continue to look to her for information at times. Yoshi likes to share her wealth of information with others, enjoying the role of expert and the praise she sometimes gets from adults. But she doesn't know where to draw the line. She often corrects others or dismisses what they have to say, dominating the conversation. At home this has become a major source of conflict with her two younger siblings. Her parents now see that Yoshi's volunteering the knowledge she's gained is a problem at times. Yoshi's closest friends are tiring of her being a know-it-all, and in school this behavior has caused conflicts in the classroom. For her part, Yoshi is sometimes aware of people's reactions to her comments or corrections, but she tends to see it as their issue, not hers. Yoshi's parents are concerned about the rift her behavior is creating in the family and between their daughter and her peers.

When her parents initially approach her, Yoshi insists that she isn't doing anything "wrong" and that she is trying to be helpful to other people. But as they talk more, Yoshi admits that she is worried because sometimes she feels that people don't like her.

Helping Yoshi is complicated because talking about what she knows is so automatic. Yoshi suggests that maybe they can start working on this at home because it happens often with her siblings, especially at family meals. Her parents suggest and she agrees that the first step is to think about being a listener rather than a talker. The second step, for now, is accepting what people say and not correcting them.

To start the plan, Yoshi agrees to practice being a "listener" by being the last person at the table to speak, after her siblings and parents have spoken. When she does speak, she can ask them for more information about their topic and/or compliment them. She also can talk about her activities and interests. Yoshi and her parents have worked out a cueing system so that if she begins to correct or "lecture," they can signal her. Before starting, the family gets together, and Yoshi explains how she is trying to change and what she will do.

At first Yoshi finds it difficult to follow the plan and often sits through meals silently. Over time, however, with her parents modeling compliments and questions, she is able to do this herself and interact without giving corrections or advice. She begins using the same strategies with her friends and with peers in school. She is comfortable enough to tell her teacher about her plan, and her teacher agrees to cue her if she begins to dominate a discussion or criticize others. Because she is not always being a know-it-all, adults and peers are more inclined to ask her for opinions and information.

Intervention Steps

Step 1: Establish a Behavioral Goal

Target executive skill(s): Metacognition

Specific behavioral objective: Yoshi will increase listening and decrease lecturing and correcting others in conversations.

Step 2: Design Interventions

What environmental supports will be provided to help reach the target goal?

- Other people in the family will speak first.
- Parents/teacher will cue Yoshi if she begins to lecture or correct.
- Parents/teacher model listening and acceptable conversation behaviors.

• • •

What specific skill will be taught, who will teach the skill, and what procedure will be used to teach it?

Skill: In a social interaction, listening before speaking and demonstrating interest in what others have to say

Who will teach the skill? Parents/teacher/friends

Procedure:

- Yoshi is the last person to speak at family meals.
- Yoshi's comments are directed at getting additional information from the listener or complimenting what the listener says.
- Parents (and teachers) cue lecturing or correcting.
- Yoshi models parents' verbal behavior.
- Yoshi tries these techniques at school and with friends.

• • •

What incentives will be used to help motivate the child to use/practice the skill?

- Parents and teacher compliment Yoshi on her listening skills.
- Friends welcome Yoshi into the group, and negative comments stop.

Keys to Success

- *Because you can't always be on hand to monitor your child's behavior, you'll need an alternative to keep track of progress.* One possibility is to have your child keep track (even informally) of situations when she has listened to her siblings or friends without interrupting or correcting and report back to you, giving a few specific examples. Another possibility is for the child to arrange with one trusted friend to give her a subtle cue if she starts to dominate.

- *When helping your child evaluate his performance, keep in mind that what's important to you is not always important to your child.* The best way to handle this may be to agree to meet in the middle. The standard to be working toward should not be perfection, but a degree of quality that the child can feel good about. Just as adults will choose to put more time and effort into some tasks than others, children need to be allowed to do this as well—not every homework assignment will be a masterpiece, not every social interaction a triumph.

Learning to Evaluate Performance

Cory is 14, an eighth grader with a 10-year-old sister. The two live primarily with their mother and see their father one night during the week and on alternate weekends. Mom works full time, and the children are expected to share chores around the house. In addition, Cory takes care of his sister some days after school. He plays the trumpet in the band and works about 10 hours a week in a local grocery store, retrieving grocery carts.

Cory sees himself as motivated and fairly hard working, but he's an average student. Since entering middle school he's been increasingly frustrated about what he feels is a lack of payoff for the amount of work he puts in. In school his grades don't seem to reflect the fact that he does his homework without needing to be reminded or prodded and studies for tests. At work he is reliable, but he hasn't had a raise since he started, and his manager sometimes says he needs to be more attentive. At home he carries out his chores and is more than willing to help out. Since he was young, however, his mother has always had to check on his work and at times have him complete or redo a task that he thought he had finished.

Cory's weakness has always been in checking his work. When he was young this was less of an issue because his parents or teachers were there to monitor him closely. But now that he's older he's expected to review his work more independently. Cory's mother gives him concrete examples of where his inconsistency affects the quality of his work, from spotty vacuuming to failing to edit essays assigned at school. Cory has always been willing to accept such feedback and correct his work, so what he needs to do is figure out in advance what needs to be checked, so he can monitor rather than waiting for other people to tell him his work hasn't measured up after he's completed it.

Using vacuuming as an example, his mother asks Cory to think about the task and create a "start to finish" list for what would be a thorough job. When he is done, they look at the list together, and his mother suggests one additional step. This becomes Cory's list for this chore. Understanding the idea, Cory goes to his manager and asks how he could improve his performance on his specific job. His manager is happy to oblige, and Cory arranges to check back with him in 2 weeks to see if he has it right.

School is a little more complicated because of the number of subjects and the variety of work. Cory and his mother first meet with his teaching team, and he explains what he wants to work on. Together they review his report cards and progress reports to see if there are specific areas where the problem is more likely to come up. From this information the teachers see that writing assignments are the primary problem. His English teacher suggests they meet because this is her area. She provides a task list (rubric) for his writing assignments, and she agrees to review this with Cory prior to his starting an assignment and also to look at Cory's first draft to determine how well he has monitored his work and followed the rubric. Having the lists in these different areas, reviewing them beforehand, and having someone (teacher, manager, or the like) evaluate his monitoring helps Cory improve his work. From this process he realizes that when he gets feedback that he needs to be more careful or thorough, he will need to follow a similar plan for the task or job.

Intervention Steps

Step 1: Establish a Behavioral Goal

Target executive skill(s): Metacognition

Specific behavioral objective: During specific tasks, Cory will evaluate his performance against a standard given for that task and work to meet the standard.

Step 2: Design Interventions

What environmental supports will be provided to help reach the target goal?

- Parent/manager/teacher provide standards (in list form) for selected tasks in each of their areas.
- Parent/manager/teacher provide feedback about performance to Cory.

• • •

What specific skill will be taught, who will teach the skill, and what procedure will be used to teach it?

Skill: Cory will learn to evaluate and, where needed, correct his performance so that it meets a standard given for that task.

Who will teach the skill? Parent/manager/teacher will provide standard and performance feedback.

Procedure:

- Cory, together with adults, chooses a set of tasks for monitoring and improvement.
- Adults provide an acceptable performance standard for these tasks.
- Cory reviews expectations before beginning the task.
- Cory performs tasks and monitors performance, and adults provide feedback on how well the standard was met.
- Cory corrects his performance as needed.

• • •

What incentives will be used to help motivate the child to use/practice the skill?

- Positive feedback from adults about performance
- Improved grades in school and improved job performance leading to raises

Keys to Success

- *Don't try to tackle too many different behaviors at once.* Limit the intervention to one or two in the beginning. It's probably also best to address only one domain at a time, such as home or school, not both.

- *Give your child very specific feedback about very specific behaviors to be changed.* This plan has a good chance of succeeding if your child is motivated and can accept feedback from others, but even then it's doomed to fail if you say things like "You need to be more careful," your child's teacher says, "Spend more time studying," or the child's boss says, "Pay attention when you're working." Your child needs concrete directions such as "Check all six rows between the cars for shopping carts as well as the return areas."

21

When What You Do Is Not Enough

For children with significant executive skill weaknesses, what you can do on your own to resolve the problem may not meet your expectations or prove sufficient. If you've tried the strategies and suggestions presented so far in this book with only limited success, and the troubleshooting advice offered in Chapters 10–20 hasn't helped, you need to look a little more closely at what's going on.

When a home plan is not working, we suggest you take a close look at the intervention to make sure the key elements necessary for success are in place. As we've said, and hopefully demonstrated, you *can* improve your child's executive skills. As we have also said, doing so involves effort and attention to detail, especially on the front end of the plan. Although it may seem simplistic, it is important to quickly review each step of the plan.

If you came to us, these are the questions we would ask:

What is the specific problem you've attempted to tackle? For example, does your child get upset with any change in plans? Does she have to spend money as soon as she gets it? Does he lose or misplace belongings on a daily basis?

Have you stated the problem definition with enough specificity to enable you to judge success or failure? The description of the behavior needs to be precise enough so that you, your child, and anyone else involved has no doubt about whether the behavior has occurred. Descriptions that include the words *always, never, everything, all the time,* and so forth are likely to be too general. For example, "Kim is constantly losing her belongings," "Javi is late for everything," "Mikey cries at the drop of a hat," "Amy is late all the time," and "Taylor can't follow directions" do not provide sufficient information either to address the problem or to evaluate the success of the plan. Specifying what (for example, what does the child lose?), when (at what times is the behavior most likely or does it pose the biggest problem?), and where (in what situations does it happen most?)

helps better define the problem. Even if the behavior happens across more situations, the key is to pick a specific starting point (remember, "baby steps").

What is your standard for judging that the problem has improved, and what behavior can you live with? Wholesale behavior change is not only hard to elicit but may be well-nigh impossible, at least in the short term, so we encourage you to be realistic in your expectations for improvement. List two or three specific situations where the problem occurs now, state how you want things to go in those situations, and state what you would like your child to do. Some examples: voices displeasure with change but accepts it without tantrum; saves at least 30% of any money earned; requires your help to find missing materials no more than twice a week. It's important to start with small improvements and build on these rather than expecting that the problem will be completely resolved. Baby steps toward the goal should be considered a success.

Given your child's age, current skills, and the amount of effort needed from your child to accomplish what you want, are your expectations realistic? Watch how you answer this question. If you find yourself saying, with some exasperation, "When I was her age, I certainly didn't have this problem" or "Every other kid his age can handle this situation without falling apart," you may be reaching too high. Go back to the previous question: What can you live with as evidence of improvement?

What environmental supports have you put in place? Have you simplified the initial task demand so that the effort required is small? Do you have a visual cue to signal that a change in plans is coming? When your child receives money, is a place to store it immediately available? Do storage spaces for belongings have specific pictures or written labels?

What specific skill are you trying to teach? As with the problem definition, you need to be clear about the behavior you are trying to teach. Although we've encouraged you to begin by identifying the executive skill involved, these skills are taught in the context of more specific behaviors. In the examples above, you may be teaching your child to recognize and react acceptably to a change symbol, to take the money she's earned and immediately put it in her bank, or to place toys in a specific storage area.

Who is responsible for teaching the skill, what is the procedure, and how often is it done/practiced? Particularly in the beginning stages of helping your child improve executive skills, the work is as much on the person teaching the skill as it is on the child. Our job as parents would be so much easier if what psychologists call *one-trial learning* worked for the skills we wanted our kids to acquire. In reality most of the important behaviors we expect children to master by the time they leave our homes require practice over a long period of time. Have you built that into your plan?

What motivators are being used to help your child learn the new skill/behavior and practice it when the situation arises? As we've said, your attention and recognition of your child's efforts using process praise are powerful motivators. The same is true for visual representations of progress such as simple graphs. If these aren't sufficient, a "first—then" where access to a preferred activity is contingent on task completion is the next option. In our experience, these interventions are sufficient in most cases. The last option is some type of reward system. If you decide to use this, it is important that the reward be time-limited and/or for a specific, new task demand. The objective is to incentivize the child to start the task and then to fade the incentive as the child becomes proficient.

If you believe you've addressed these issues and developed a reasonable, specific plan with supports and incentives, there are still a few other factors to consider when a plan is not working.

• *The consistency with which the plan is followed.* We're all busy, and it's not always easy or convenient to make sure your child has been cued about a schedule change or monitored to ensure that money or belongings are stored away. Recognition for your child's efforts or ensuring that first—then sequences are followed are not always remembered. Occasional slipups are bound to happen, and they will not cause a plan to fail. On the other hand, if the plan is followed only intermittently, it *will* fail. You'll see that your child is not changing, and therefore there is little incentive for you to work at the plan. Your child will see that the plan is not important to you and hence will make less effort, returning instead to old behaviors. For these reasons, plans and incentives should be relatively simple and fit within the time frames that you reliably have available.

• *Consistency among adults using the plan.* Another parent, an older sibling, or a teacher who is supposed to use the plan or some part of it must adhere to the key elements or the plan is likely to fail. A mother we know wanted to implement a savings plan using allowance, but her husband initially resisted because he hadn't received an allowance as a child and did not think his children should. The mother put the plan on hold until she sold him on the benefits of their child learning to save for a future goal. Had she implemented the plan without him, problems were likely. If several people share child care/management responsibilities, they should discuss the plan and agree on the role each will play from the beginning. If the plan involves homework or school materials (books and so on), parents and teachers should be clear about what is expected from each, the frequency of communication and how this will occur, and in most cases, the method of communication should not involve the child, since children are not always reliable informants.

• *The time that the plan is in place.* There are no hard-and-fast rules about how long a plan should be tried. If the plan is reasonable—that is, it meets most of the preceding criteria—try it for 14–21 days. This may not seem long, but in our experience parents typically try a plan for 4–5 days and then become inconsistent. You too may fall prey to this temptation, for two reasons: If you don't see any change, the lack of immediate payoff may make it difficult to sustain the necessary effort. On the other hand, you may see an almost immediate improvement, feel like you've accomplished what you hoped for, and slack off. In this case, the change does not last, and within a few weeks the old pattern returns. To keep yourself honest, you may want to take time at the end of each day the plan is in place to rate how well you stuck to the plan, using a 5-point scale (1, *I didn't follow the plan today*, to 5, *I stuck to the plan 100%!*).

How do I know whether my child can't or won't? Maybe she is just lazy! In all our years of professional practice, we have met very few children we would call lazy. We've met children who are discouraged, who doubt their abilities, who feel it is more punishing to try and fail than not try at all, or who prefer to spend time doing things they find fun rather than things they find tedious or difficult. The critical issue is not whether children can't or won't, but what it would take to help them overcome whatever obstacle is preventing them from acquiring proficiency at tasks or completing tasks that are currently not getting done. The way to help them overcome obstacles usually involves a combination of modifying the task, so it doesn't seem so daunting, teaching them the steps to follow to complete the task and supervising them as they do it, and building in an incentive to make it worth their while to engage in work that feels effortful to them. If you do all this, they can be smart but not scattered.

Seeking Professional Help

So you've done the best you can, and you're still not seeing much improvement. Now what? It's certainly true that some children have more challenging executive skill problems than parents can handle easily on their own. If you decide your child is one of these children, you can look for help from a licensed clinician such as a psychologist, social worker, or mental health counselor. The title of the professional is less important than the orientation of the clinician's practice. We recommend finding a specialist who uses either a behavioral or a cognitive-behavioral approach and is experienced in parent training.

Clinicians who use a behavioral approach focus on identifying the specific environmental triggers that contribute to the problem behavior (called *antecedents*) as well as the way the behavior is responded to (called *consequences*). They then help parents alter either the antecedents or the consequences or both. Cognitive-behavioral therapists may use a similar approach, but they also address how children and their parents *think* about the problem situations and teach them to think differently (for example, by giving them coping strategies such as self-talk, relaxation strategies, and thought-stopping techniques). For skill acquisition we do not recommend traditional talk therapy or relationship therapy because we believe that children and their parents benefit from learning specific skills and strategies for handling problems caused by weak executive skills challenges.

When Testing Might Be Warranted

Parents of children with more severe executive skill problems often ask us if they should have their child tested. Psychological tests designed to assess executive skills in a controlled situation are different from the real-world demands on executive skills, and results do not necessarily reflect real-world situations. If the assessment is specifically for executive skills, the evaluation should include parent, teacher, and child interviews and behavior checklists and ideally behavior observations. There are other considerations in which testing may be useful:

- If you think your child will need additional support in school, for which an evaluation might provide the necessary documentation that there is a problem that needs to be addressed.
- If you think there may be additional learning problems (such as a learning disability or an attention disorder) that an evaluation could help clarify.
- If you think there may be other explanations for the behavior of concern that may suggest different treatment options. Psychological disorders such as bipolar, anxiety, depression, posttraumatic stress, and obsessive–compulsive disorders all have an impact on executive skills. Treatments have been developed to address disorders such as these (including medication and specific therapeutic approaches), and an accurate diagnosis would be helpful in pointing you in the direction of an appropriate intervention.

If you decide to seek an evaluation that would include an assessment of your child's executive skill strengths and weaknesses, the professionals who typically do this kind of assessment include psychologists, neuropsychologists, and school psychologists. If the problems are significant enough to cause school failure, then schools are obligated to provide this kind of evaluation. (See Chapter 23 for further clarification about what constitutes school failure.)

In addition to whatever "tests" the evaluator might use (such as IQ tests or achievement tests), the specialist should use rating scales designed to assess executive skills (such as the Behavior Rating Inventory of Executive Function, or BRIEF) as well as collect information, usually through a detailed interview, from parents about how the executive skill problems show up in the everyday life of the child. The benefit of collecting this kind of information is that it leads naturally to the development of interventions, which is, after all, the primary purpose of an evaluation.

Thoughts on Medication

Medications are used to treat psychological disorders/biologically based disorders such as ADHD, anxiety disorders, and obsessive–compulsive disorders. These medications may result in improvement in executive functioning, but they were not designed specifically for that purpose.

Stimulant medications have been shown in many studies conducted over many years to be very effective in controlling a number of the symptoms associated with ADHD, including distractibility, difficulty completing work, overactivity, and impulse control. Because children with ADHD can work more efficiently and persist longer with tasks when they take stimulants, improvements with time management and goal-directed persistence may be seen. Medications for anxiety disorders can address problems with emotional control when those problems are due to underlying anxiety.

The parents we see in our clinical practice usually prefer to try nonmedical interventions first, and we support this approach. The use of medication may lead parents and teachers to believe that this intervention alone is sufficient, and we believe the effectiveness of medication can be enhanced when it is combined with behavioral or psychosocial interventions. Furthermore, some research studies suggest that when medication is combined with other interventions, lower dosages can be prescribed. For these reasons, we recommend using approaches such as environmental modifications, home-school report cards, and incentive systems prior to considering medication.

There may be times, however, when medication use is warranted. For children with ADHD, there are a number of warning signs parents may look for that signal that a trial of stimulant medication might be worth considering. These include:

- *When the attention disorder (especially impulsivity and motor activity level) is having an impact on a child's ability to make or keep friends.* The ability to form social relationships in childhood is a strong predictor of good adjustment throughout life, and if attention problems prevent this from happening, medication may be warranted.

- *When the attention disorder begins to affect self-esteem.* Children with even milder forms of ADHD become aware that their attention problems are making them stand out in school (for example, the teacher is always prompting them to pay attention) or are preventing them from achieving success in schoolwork (for example, by leading them to make many careless mistakes). When children start making negative comments about themselves, the attention disorder is likely having an impact on self-esteem that may be reduced through the use of medication.

- *When the attention disorder interferes directly with the child's ability to learn.* This can happen in several ways: (1) they have difficulty sustaining attention in class and therefore miss instruction or fail to complete seatwork; (2) they become so easily frustrated that they give up and learning becomes short-circuited; or (3) they lack the patience to plan and execute tasks that can't be done quickly. This is seen either in a child's difficulty *slowing down* when tasks require this for success or in an inability to handle multistep problems because they lack the capacity to think through the steps involved to achieve success.

• *When the amount of effort required on the part of the child to control distractibility, impulsivity, or motor activity is great enough to affect their overall level of emotional adjustment.* We often see children in our clinical practice who appear to be managing well because their grades are satisfactory and they're passing tests, producing quality work, and handing in homework on time. But when we talk to the child and parents, we learn that they are under a great deal of stress, are staying up too late at night because their distractibility makes it hard to focus or work efficiently, or are engaging in unhelpful or risky behaviors designed to relieve stress. When we delve further into what is going on, we decide that the symptoms of their attention disorder are making school (and life in general) much more difficult than it needs to be. Medication to relieve or mitigate their ADHD symptoms can have a significant positive impact on both productivity and well-being.

For youngsters for whom emotional control is problematic, due to either depression or anxiety, parents should consider the severity of the problem when making medication decisions. Research with adults suggests that cognitive-behavioral therapy may be just as effective in treating anxiety and depression as is medication, but when this kind of therapy is unavailable, and the child's depression or anxiety is pervasive enough to significantly affect quality of life, medication is worth considering.

22

A Brief Look at Technology

Over our years of practice working with families, we have fielded a variety of questions from parents about the impact of technology on their children. In the past these questions revolved around TV and video games. How much should they watch or play? What's safe and what's not? How does it impact their brains and executive skills? How do we manage the conflicts that arise when we try to set limits? We still hear these questions and others. But now they come with a new sense of urgency. Why?

Because there is a key difference between past generations and the present, particularly when it comes to children. That difference is information technology, and its reach extends far beyond stationary TVs and game consoles. We now have a global network, an internet, of connected devices—smart phones, tablets, computers—that operate at speeds allowing almost instantaneous connection with any person or piece of information that is part of that network. It is estimated that worldwide nearly 5 billion people are active internet users.

And there is a second key difference for this generation—the development and proliferation of smart phones. According to Common Sense Media, 42 percent of children through age 10 have a cell phone. This jumps to 71 percent by age 12 and 91 percent by age 14. That means that adults and an increasing number of their children can have 24/7 unfiltered access to people, information, and games.

There are undeniable benefits from technology—learning, acquisition of knowledge and skills, communication with family and friends, information access, entertainment, shopping, directions, emergency contacts, tracking apps, and more. There are also undeniable risks—increased distraction, decreased inhibition, cyberstalking and bullying, pornography, images of violence, misinformation, social isolation, poor nutrition, sleep deprivation, compulsive use, and so on. The statistics indicate that it is no longer a simple question of whether kids should have access or not. Short of draconian measures, your children are going to access technology, if not at home, then at school, at the library, via their friends, or elsewhere. The issue for parents now comes down to how to manage access to technology in a way that maximizes the benefits and minimizes the risks. We want to be clear here. When it comes to technology use for you and your children, there is no one size fits all. Hence our objective here is to provide you with a set of considerations and guidelines to use in deciding what is the best fit for your family.

Where do we start? As with just about everything else we've discussed in this book, we start with you. Why? Because your children want to be like you. They are keen observers of your behavior, want your attention, and imitate what they have seen when they are with you. The next time you go to a family restaurant, look around. Are parents interacting with their children or with their phones? Ditto for playgrounds, children's museums, kids' sporting events, swimming lessons, plays, musical concerts. Kids watch their parents in these situations to see if they are paying attention. In the context of parent–child interactions, the term *technoference* refers to the disruption in parent–child communication and attention that results when parents are attending to personal technology devices. Research indicates that when technology interferes with parental attention, children engage in increased disruptive and aggressive behavior, activity levels, and emotional reactivity, all of which involve executive skills. Other effects include anxiety and withdrawal. Children also react with frustration when attention is suddenly withdrawn for attention to a mobile device, especially if they don't know why. Researchers additionally note less conversation and more hostile parent reactions when children solicit parent attention while parents are absorbed in mobile devices. We're not suggesting that you never use a mobile device while with your children, rather that you be judicious in your use and that when engaged in parent–child activities, your children be the primary recipients of your attention. If incoming mobile information demands your attention, explain to your child why and try to keep it brief.

Executive Skills and Lifestyle

We've chosen lifestyle factors as a focus for the impact of technology for two reasons. The first is that executive skills and the lifestyle behaviors of children go hand in hand, and lifestyle factors can either enhance or undermine the development of executive skills. The second is that if you are concerned about whether technology is having an adverse impact on your children, changes in lifestyle factors are an important early indicator that it is. For purposes of this chapter, we include the following as lifestyle factors:

- Nutrition
- Sleep
- Physical activities
- Socialization
- Exploration of interests and hobbies

We'll consider two issues in our discussion. The first involves research about the impact of each factor on executive skills, and the second relates to the impact that technology can have on these factors.

Nutrition. It should come as no surprise that healthy nutrition plays a key role in brain growth and development and in the development of cognitive functions including executive skills. Conversely, a diet of processed foods containing high fat and sugar content contributes to overweight and obesity in children, and these factors are related to reductions in executive skills. Research in children's health confirms that a greater amount of sedentary digital media is associated with an increased likelihood of obesity. Food consumed is also affected, with children showing a preference for sweets and fast food as opposed to more nutritional choices such as fruit and vegetables and eating greater amounts of these foods. These effects are that much more evident when children are engaged with digital media during mealtimes.

Sleep. Recent research indicates that good sleep quality serves as a protective factor for cognitive maturation and executive skills during childhood development. Evening use of electronic media is associated with reduced sleep quality and delayed onset of bedtime. There are also associations between electronic media use and problems with sleep initiation as well as an association between poor sleep quality and social media use. Sleep disruption in children has an adverse effect on executive skills, in particular on working memory, response inhibition, and attention.

Physical Activity. Physical activity, and in particular aerobic activity, has a direct, positive effect on the development of executive skills in children. The Centers for Disease Control and Prevention's guidelines for children recommended at least 60 minutes per day of moderate to vigorous physical activity. Not surprisingly, increased digital media time results in decreased physical activity with further adverse effects on weight. Physical activity counterbalances the effects of sedentary digital media activities and can help mitigate potential adverse effects on nutrition and sleep.

Socialization. Executive skills develop and are enhanced in the context of social relationships and interpersonal interactions. Social skills involve sustained attention, response inhibition, emotional control, flexibility, and metacognition and are part and parcel of successful social interaction. These skills both enhance and are enhanced by social interactions. With the proliferation of smart phones, these interactions increasingly take place via texting and social media (Facebook/Meta, X, Instagram, Snapchat, YouTube, and others). Although there are definite benefits to this type of communication, when compared to being physically present in social interactions, something is lost in translation. Nonverbal communication involves eye contact, facial expressions, vocal intonation, gestures, posture and interpersonal space, and the like and is an essential component of social interaction. These nonverbal cues are considerably stronger in the context of in-person as opposed to digital interactions.

Exploration of Interests and Hobbies. As we noted in Chapter 6, learning opportunities that are self-directed, experiential in a hands-on way, and rich in content are known to enhance executive skills in children. That means that children's museums, nature centers, science museums, aquariums, libraries, and zoos, especially those that offer hands-on opportunities, are ideal environments for children to expand their interests and test out their skills. Music, dance, and sports, although somewhat more structured, offer similar opportunities. Equally significant in these settings is the ready availability of peers who present opportunities for social interaction as well as learning new skills by observing and modeling the actions of other children.

School and Homework. While we don't consider school a lifestyle factor in the vein of those above, school and homework have a reciprocal role in executive skills. On the one hand executive skills—particularly sustained attention, response inhibition, task initiation, and time management—are necessary for successful school and homework performance. At the same time school and homework play a key role in the ongoing development of these executive skills. Our focus here is on homework since that is where you as parents have influence. The available research indicates that excessive use of technology can have a detrimental effect on homework and hence school performance. Thus, as with lifestyle factors, it is important to monitor the amount of technology use to mitigate its potential adverse effects on your children's executive skill development.

To summarize, at the end of the day technology is in many ways not so different from other aspects of kids' lives. We note examples of when technology can interfere with specific things, like mealtime, or sleep, or homework, and the executive skills associated with these factors. When it comes to the effects on executive skills of specific types of technology—video games, social media, TV, and others—current research offers no clear answers. Whether the effects are beneficial or harmful depends on the child, their age, and the content and context of use. The research indicates that the larger issue is time; use of technology takes up time, and everyone, whether a kid or an adult, only has so many hours in a day. Where kids' executive skills are most impacted by technology is *not* by harmful impacts of the technology itself, but the *time* spent using it, which is time taken away from . . . well, just about anything else. Think about this in terms of opportunity costs. If your children are spending much of their free time on technology, what are they *not* doing that might be better? Technology doesn't seem to be inherently good or bad for us, but at this moment in society it does seem particularly good at unbalancing our lives. So we'd encourage parents to think about it less in terms of the active "harm" that technology causes and more in terms of time and balance.

Content and Context

If you are concerned about your children's use of digital media, the content of the media and the context in which it is being used are important considerations in understanding what is important to your child and what is acceptable to you. The landscape of digital media is changing constantly. Given that, our best option is to provide you with access to information that is regularly updated to reflect those changes. In the Resources at the end of the book, we have provided links to four organizations designed to help you and your children decide the content and context of digital media that best suits your needs. These organizations provide detailed information about the benefits and risks of digital media, up-to-date research, guidelines for use, content reviews, examples of how to discuss digital media issues with your children, and how to create family plans for media use including planning templates.

Steps You Can Take

There is a general consensus in the literature about the steps that parents can take to help manage technology use with children. The following summarize some of those steps, and more detail can be found in the Resources at the end of the book.

- *Take an active role in educating your children about technology from a young age.* Explain that digital media devices—TVs, tablets, computers, smart phones—are tools rather than toys and, like other tools, need to be handled carefully. These are ongoing discussions that will change as your child ages and their exposure to technology increases.

- *Do your best to keep up with the ever-evolving array of technology and digital media that children are exposed to.* The Family Online Safety Institute and Common Sense Media are valuable resources to assist you with this.

- *Discuss the benefits and risks of technology.* Emphasize the importance of their privacy, protecting personal information and not sharing their information online. This includes downloading unfamiliar programs, clicking on suspicious links, and being very careful about knowing *who* is on the other end of the screen. The guideline here is "If you see something, say something." This applies to responding to messages from strangers or content that involves threats, cyberbullying, misinformation, or inappropriate content.

- *Pay attention to what your kids are doing and using via digital media.* This is comparatively easy with younger children since you have an active role in what's available to them. With older children this means access to their passwords, checking history or usage, using timers or scheduled access settings. If there is content that is off-limits, know what filters or software are available for you to block access.

- *When they are old enough, have an open and honest discussion about technology with your children:* what they like and don't like, what technology and media sites are important to them and why, their opinion about your technology use, and what they think your role in their technology management should be. Explain your view of technology, what your role is, and why.

- *Make a technology plan.* For a younger child, this is your decision about when, where, what, and how much. We recommend that you be clear in your own mind about limits and rules and communicate these to your child in language they can understand.

Doing this proactively helps avoid conflicts and tantrums that can occur and that we've seen even with toddlers. For older children, the plan comes as an outcome of your discussions with your child. It's preferable to have the plan in writing with the understanding that it will evolve over time. The objective is to minimize proactively the conflicts that otherwise can result when you and your child disagree about technology use. (See specifically Common Sense Media for suggestions and guidelines.)

Throughout this book, we have highlighted a collaborative approach to problem solving with your children as the most effective means to promoting increasing independence in decision making, cooperation, and executive skills. Our approach to decisions about technology is the same. That said, as with everything else we have discussed involving your child's well-being, the final decision about technology management is your call.

23

The Role of Schools
in Executive Skill Development

A second grade teacher we know was trying to figure out how to explain executive skills to second graders and came up with this definition: they're the skills you need to get things done. That's a perfect explanation in the simplest of terms for the skills that kids need to be successful in school—and that all people need to be successful in life.

Without executive skills, all the "smarts" in the world won't get you very far. In fact research shows that executive skills are a better predictor of school performance than IQ. So you'd think that schools would build executive skills into their curricula. Sadly that's not done. When the Common Core Curriculum—the closest the United States has come to agreeing on a common set of learning standards—came out a few years ago, we pored through it looking for explicit references to executive skills. There weren't any. This led us to referring to executive skills as the "hidden curriculum"—they're a set of skills that are absolutely critical to school success, and yet no one is charged with teaching them. And if no one is charged with teaching them, then whether or not kids acquire these skills is "hit or miss."

Some kids are lucky. They have both genetics and environmental supports on their side, and in this case these skills may develop fairly naturally. But a child who is missing one or both of those key ingredients is disadvantaged in school. And the longer they stay in school, the more disadvantaged they are because by the time they reach middle school, virtually everything they're asked to learn and do not only requires executive skills, but advanced executive skills built on the foundational skills that develop first.

What Schools Do Now
to Support Executive Skill Development

We're not saying that teachers don't do things to support executive skill development. They just aren't explicit about how classroom and school structures support the development of these key skills. Right from the start, teachers make accommodations to support children whose executive skills are just emerging or yet to emerge. This is particularly evident in preschool and lower elementary classrooms. Teachers set up physical classrooms to make them easy for young children to navigate. Good preschool teachers, for instance, will tell you they avoid classrooms with wide open spaces between furniture—because those are runways and preschool children like to run. What executive skills are they accommodating in this way? Response inhibition of course. Preschool children are more likely to control their impulse to run indoors if they can't run very far before running into a piece of furniture.

Preschool teachers also arrange materials so that they are accessible in a way that makes sense to young children. These classrooms are often designed around "centers" that encourage specific activities, with the relevant materials at hand. This classroom design models organization and facilitates working memory because children quickly learn where to find what they need for their center activities.

Teachers of young children also build in routines and impose rules to make the day flow smoothly and help children learn to function in social groups. Routines and classroom rules support emotional control, response inhibition, and planning, and when teachers review the rules and how the day will go at the beginning of the school day, they are helping children strengthen their working memory.

Preschool and lower elementary teachers also understand that children at this age have limited attention spans, do not retain lengthy instructions, and often need to be prompted to initiate tasks that seem effortful. Thus, they provide cues to support working memory, sustained attention, and task initiation. Children at this age do not have a strong sense of time or how long it takes to do things, so teachers take responsibility for time management.

Good teachers also understand that executive skills have room to grow when children are given opportunities for free play, both indoors and out. In these settings, children learn to manage emotions and impulses and they learn to solve problems and resolve conflicts as they arise. Free play and more loosely structured small group activities are fertile grounds for supporting response inhibition, emotional control, planning, metacognition, and even goal-directed persistence—all in a developmentally appropriate fashion.

As children continue through elementary school, teachers change their expectations to adjust for gradually developing executive skills. They ask students to sustain attention longer, they may give them a list of things they expect children to accomplish by morning recess or lunch time, they ask students to remember to bring home books and homework and bring them back the next day. By asking children to do homework, they are helping them learn to initiate or sustain attention more independently (although many children at this age will need prompting by their parents to do their homework and to put it in their backpacks when they have finished).

Once children reach middle school, the demands on executive skills increase dramatically—and, we would argue, in many cases unrealistically. As we said in Chapter 1, a rapid period of brain development begins at around age 11 or 12—the beginning of middle school in most school systems. In the early stages development is uneven and unpredictable. That means more support, rather than less, is critical. Think about how children learn to ride a bike. At the point where training wheels are removed, they need more guidance, encouragement, and support from parents than they did when they were riding around with training wheels. The onset of adolescence, and the brain growth that accompanies this stage, requires the same thing.

For most children, middle school is the first time when they have multiple teachers, each with their own set of expectations regarding how work is formatted, notebooks are organized, projects are managed, and assignments are handed in. Demands on working memory, planning, organization, and time management increase accordingly. And the complexity has only increased since many schools use web-based platforms and electronic tools for accessing assignments and completing work. At an age when many students are just beginning to figure out how to keep track of information and materials and when they are still novices at planning and managing their time, too often there is the expectation (from both parents and teachers) that they should be proficient in these executive skills. The fact that they aren't can be a source of considerable frustration to parents and teachers—and ultimately to the students themselves.

At the middle school level, students are expected to manage a variety of "systems" just to get through their day. Here's a list of those systems, along with the executive skills students need to draw on to manage those systems (you may be able to think of others):

1. A system or routine for writing down assignments consistently (working memory, planning)
2. A system for keeping track of assignments—like notebooks, folders, a laptop, and the like (working memory, organization)
3. A system for knowing which materials need to be brought home or taken to school every day (working memory, planning, organization)
4. A system for planning how the student will organize study time, both daily assignments as well as studying for tests and completing long-term assignments (planning, time management)
5. A system for planning and monitoring long-term assignments, including breaking them down into subtasks and timelines (planning, time management)
6. A system for keeping track of how to locate necessary information when every teacher may use a different platform or use the same platform differently (working memory, organization)
7. A system for keeping track of other belongings—pencils, pens, calculators,

assignment books, gym clothes, lunch money, permission slips, and so on (working memory, organization)

8. A system for dealing with changing classes, including the problems associated with having to take different materials to different classes and having teachers with different organizational styles and expectations—not to mention block scheduling with schedules that change from day to day or week to week (working memory, planning, organization)

9. A system for managing after-school schedules, including extracurricular activities, play dates, changing parent work schedules or living in two homes (working memory, time management)

This list should make it clear how much we're expecting middle school students to keep track of at their age. To further emphasize this, a few years ago we presented this list to a group of middle school teachers and asked them to generate a checklist that a student might use to get through one day of middle school. The checklist had 92 items on it! And we get annoyed with our kids when they forget something?!

What can parents do about this? It's tempting to pull back on supervision and homework monitoring at this age—in part because children are beginning to look for more independence and freedom from parental scrutiny. While some children's executive skill development allows for a high level of self-management, many are not there yet. You'll know which category your children fall into—but if they fall into the "not there yet" category, then checking in with them daily about homework, helping them keep in mind long-term assignments (for example, by posting them on a calendar located in a prominent place in the house), and asking them how they plan to study for tests may be advised.

What More Could Schools Be Doing to Support the Development of Executive Skills?

Most teachers don't write their lesson plans specifically with executive skill development in mind. Teachers and parents inherently understand, at least roughly, what they can expect from kids at different ages and set the bar accordingly. We think, however, that if teachers understood the role executive skills play in fostering independent and self-regulated learning—and how much they are already doing to encourage the development of executive skills—they might do even more. They might infuse their instruction with questions and prompts designed to enhance executive skill development. We've written a book, *Executive Skills in Children and Adolescents*, for educators and other professionals such as school psychologists that describes how to do this (see the Resources at the end of the book).

We are sometimes asked by schools to recommend an executive skills curriculum. We've also been asked by schools to help them develop their own curriculum to teach executive skills. Similarly, parents will sometimes contact us asking about summer camps or programs they could send their kids to that would teach them the executive skills they need to be better students.

While a curriculum that focuses on teaching executive skills may be beneficial, we think there are a number of problems with conceptualizing executive skills as a set of lessons to be taught. A major limitation is that these are skills that are hard for students to master when they are taught in isolation. Imagine a summer camp that decided to teach students planning, organization, and time management, for instance—three of the skills that middle schools expect students to be good at. Is it realistic to think that in July you can teach a student how to plan and in October they'll be able to apply what they've learned when a science teacher assigns a long-term project? Or can you teach "time management" in the summer when students have all the time in the world and expect them to apply what they've learned toward the end of the marking period when due dates and exams pile up?

There are also dangers to teaching these skills in discrete lessons in the classroom. Planning an English essay is a very different process from the planning required to build a robot for science class or planning how one will study for a final exam in Spanish. Executive skills look different in different contexts, and how does a lesson on planning take that into account?

Not only do these skills look different in every class, but every student is different and therefore the needs are different. One student may be challenged by a long-term project assignment because they can't think of a topic (*flexibility, metacognition*), while another may know how to do the research but can't figure out how to organize all the information they've collected (*planning, organization*). A third student may have no idea how long it will take to do the project (*time management*), and another thinks the project is pointless (*goal-directed persistence*).

In the work we've done with schools, we've had the most success in integrating executive skills into the work teachers do with kids when the focus of professional development is on helping teachers:

1. Understand what executive skills are and how they impact learning and school performance.
2. Make a connection between student behavior and specific executive skills, so they know what it looks like in the classroom (and so they stop using words like *lazy* or *disruptive*).
3. Learn how to give this information to students—so that students understand what executive skills are and can look at their own skill set and identify strengths and challenges.
4. Work with students to help them recognize the obstacles that are getting in the way of their using executive skills successfully and to find just the right strategies that will work for them to help them overcome those obstacles.

We think this process looks less like a curriculum and more like a conversation. And a conversation that changes from year to year and student to student depending on the developmental level of the child and where that child is on her own path toward executive skill mastery.

What Can Parents Do to Encourage Schools to More Explicitly Support Executive Skills?

Reading this book may have given you a greater understanding of how important executive skills are to school success, and you may be eager to share this insight with your child's teachers. You may be tempted to barge into your child's classroom and insist that her teacher focus on helping your child develop these skills. This is understandable—but not likely to meet with the outcome you are hoping for. The classroom is the purview of teachers, and teaching is their expertise. They may not take kindly to a suggestion from you that they should be doing their jobs differently.

If you participate in your child's PTA or if your school district offers other avenues for parents to be involved, such as a parent advisory group, you may be able to plant seeds. We have been asked to do presentations for parents at the invitation of PTAs that have the effect of introducing executive skills to both parents and teachers and beginning a conversation between parents and teachers about how they can support each other as they work to build executive skills in their children.

Parents are most concerned about their own children, and what's frustrating for many of the parents we work with is that they can work really hard at home to address the problems, but they have no control over the school environment and the problems that arise there. This book would not be complete if it didn't offer advice and guidance on how to work with schools.

Here's what we've learned from years of working on executive skill problems with parents, teachers, and students: for genuine improvement to occur, *everybody has to work harder*. Teachers have to do more for children with executive skill challenges than for other students, parents need to provide more supervision and monitoring than a typical child would need, and children with executive skill challenges will have to work harder than they would have to if all their executive skills were developing normally. We have found that tensions, conflict, and unhappiness are most likely to occur if any one of these three parties is not pulling their own weight.

Tactically, a nonadversarial approach usually works better than blame or accusations in persuading teachers to change how they handle a child. Working from the premise that everyone has to work harder, we generally recommend that you start the conversation with your child's teacher by laying out the problem as you see it and saying, "Here's what we can do, and here's what we're prepared to ask our child to do." Follow this with an open-ended question, such as "What do you think would help?" For example, for a child who has trouble getting all his homework done and remembering to hand it in, you might say, "We're willing to check his assignment book every night, make a homework plan with him, and supervise him to make sure he's put his homework in a homework folder and the homework folder in his backpack. What else can be done to make sure the homework actually gets handed in?" If your child's teacher doesn't feel that it's their responsibility to provide any individual support to address the problem, you may want to refer the teacher to this book or the one we wrote specifically for educators (*Executive Skills in Children and Adolescents: A Practical Guide to Assessment and Intervention*). This will give the teacher a better understanding of executive skills and ideas for how to address the problem in the classroom.

Some Thoughts about Homework

Of all the challenges parents face as they guide their children through school, homework is, for many, the most daunting. Both parents and children often look forward to summer vacation each year because it means a truce in the homework wars. And they dread the return to school in the fall because they fear the battle will be joined where it left off in June. Sure there are some youngsters who tackle homework with the same energy and enthusiasm that they bring to school each day. But in our experience, children with executive skill challenges do not fall into that category!

Homework has been around as long as public schools have, and over the years considerable research has been conducted regarding the effectiveness of homework practices. While the results are not uniform—and this kind of research is difficult to do because so many nonhomework variables can impact results—in general results suggest that there is little consistent positive impact of homework on school achievement at the elementary level. Researchers speculate that elementary-school-age children have less effective study habits and have more difficulty sustaining attention to homework than older children. There's also some evidence to suggest that elementary school teachers may assign homework to strengthen nonacademic skills, such as time management, rather than assigning homework for the purpose of enhancing academic achievement.

By middle school the relationship between homework and school achievement is a little more clear-cut, and by high school there is consensus that students who do homework learn more (as measured by standardized achievement tests) than those who don't. It cannot be said, however, that the more time students spend on homework the better they do—in part because students with attention disorders and learning disabilities tend to spend more time getting through homework than do students without those learning challenges.

One of the benefits of homework is that it offers the opportunity for children to improve their executive skills. When we interview the parents of children we've been asked to evaluate, a key question we ask them is "How does your child handle homework?" Just by the answers parents give, we can begin to identify executive skill challenges. Here are some examples:

- "My child leaves his homework until just before bedtime." This suggests problems with *task initiation*.
- "My child starts her homework, but then she runs out of steam before it's done

[*sustained attention*] or gets distracted and never gets back to it [*response inhibition*]."

- "My child has a meltdown because they can't remember how to do the math homework and they tell me the teacher showed them a different way than the way I suggest." When we hear this, we hypothesize that this child struggles with *working memory* and *emotional control*—and maybe *flexibility* as well.

- "My child has the hardest time with long-term projects—he can't figure out where to start, and he always thinks it's going to take way less time than it does." This is a child who's struggling with *planning/prioritizing* and *time management*.

What role should parents play in homework management? On the one hand we want our children to become independent with tasks such as homework completion—and more adept at using the executive skills this kind of independence requires. On the other hand executive skills develop slowly—and more slowly in some kids than others. This suggests there is a role for parents to play in homework support, at least through middle school if not longer.

So it's a balancing act, isn't it? Principle 7 from Chapter 4 captures that: *Provide just enough support for the child to be on a path toward success.* In fact, the research on homework supports this approach. A large-scale study done in Finland a few years ago looked at how mothers of over 2,000 children handled homework supervision, and it found that children whose mothers provided *direct instruction* with homework showed smaller achievement gains than children whose mothers took an approach that communicated clear expectations for homework but that supported their children's autonomy. Another study looked at fifth- and sixth-grade students in Mexico and found that although parental approach (control versus autonomy) did not have a direct effect on academic achievement, focusing on encouraging autonomy in their children's approach to homework led to increases in academic self-efficacy and self-regulated learning in their children. In other words, an approach that encouraged self-expression and self-engagement helped students develop executive skills.

Here are some steps you can take to communicate the expectation that homework will be done while at the same time encouraging your child to make good choices and take ownership over doing the work:

1. ***Find a location in the house where homework is to be done.*** The right location will depend on the child and the culture of the family. Some children do best at a desk in their bedroom. It is a quiet location, away from the hubbub of family noise. Other children become too distracted by the toys, video games, or televisions they have in their bedroom and do better at a place removed from those distractions, like the dining room table. Some families create a common work time for both children and adults in a common location. While kids are doing homework at the dining room table, parents are doing paperwork, such as paying bills or planning home projects.

2. *Make sure your child has the necessary materials to do homework easily accessible*—pens, pencils, erasers, calculators, paper, colored markers. Each child may have their own portable bin or tub to hold these materials.

3. *Make a written homework plan with your child.* This may be as simple as asking your child, "What are you going to do, and when are you going to do it?" (as Peg did with one of her sons), or it could be having your child make a written plan. A template for this is on the facing page. At a minimum the child should list what assignments they have to do that night, when they plan on starting each assignment, and where they plan on working. They should also estimate how long they think each assignment will take. This kind of planning shouldn't take more than 5 minutes, and we recommend that the child complete the plan as soon as they get home from school.

4. *Ask your child what help they think they might need.* Many kids feel they need parents with them while they work—and many parents report that their kids don't do the work unless a parent is by their side. Since the goal is increasing their autonomy, parents should work to fade their presence. This might mean initially being present throughout the homework session and working toward helping your child get started on each assignment and then telling them, "I'll be back in a bit to see how you're doing." Some common challenges that students face with homework are completing long-term projects, writing essays, and studying for tests. If your child is willing to accept help from you with these homework challenges, we include templates and instructions for use at the end of this chapter.

5. *For some children, especially those at the upper elementary and middle school level, doing all their work in one sitting is unrealistic.* Parents may ask kids, "How long can you go before you need a break?" and then work with them to stretch out the work sessions slowly over time. It's also helpful for parents to talk with their children about what they plan to do during their break and to ask them whether they need a cue to tell them the break time is over.

6. *One of the most powerful motivators to help kids get through homework is identifying something that they want to do as soon as their homework is finished.* We often recommend that parents have this conversation with their kids, but we recently asked groups of middle school kids, "How do you get through homework when there are more fun things to do?" They offered a variety of strategies, but the one that came up more than any other was this one: "I just keep thinking about that fun thing I want to do as soon as I finish my homework."

When should you talk to your child's teacher about homework issues? We know that some kids fight homework more than others, and this means parents need to adapt their approach to each child. Some kids may need more supervision than others. Here are some situations where it makes sense to alert the teacher to the problems your child is encountering:

Homework Plan

Date: _____

Task	How long will it take?	When will you start?	Where will you work?	Actual start/ stop times		Done (✓)

From *Smart but Scattered, Second Edition*, by Peg Dawson, Richard Guare, and Colin Guare. Copyright © 2025 The Guilford Press. Permission to photocopy this material, or to download enlarged printable versions (*www.guilford.com/dawson4-forms*), is granted to purchasers of this book for personal use; see copyright page for details.

• *On a fairly consistent basis your child needs supervision because they don't understand the lesson.* It is not the job of parents to teach their children. If you find yourself doing this a lot, then a conversation with your child's teacher is warranted. Additional instruction or support at school may be needed—or it may be that the teacher can check in with the child to make sure they understand the assignment.

• *Your child is spending an unhealthy amount of time on homework.* Some kids work exceptionally slowly, and by the time they hit middle school they are spending almost every waking minute either in school or doing homework. For these students, adjustments in homework load are reasonable requests. Homework load adjustments may also be justified for children with ADHD, especially in cases where the disorder is being treated with medication and the medication wears off at the end of the day.

• *Conflicts about homework are having a significant impact on family adjustment.* While we believe in holding children accountable, children who struggle mightily with emotional control often have trouble tolerating homework. Sometimes these are children who work exceptionally hard to keep their emotions in check during school because they don't want to get in trouble or embarrass themselves in front of their peers. As a result, by the time they get home their psychic reserves are so depleted that they have nothing left to get them through homework.

In all these cases, we should note, we are not arguing for no homework (unless that's the school's policy for all students). But a little may go a long way. And giving kids choices about the kinds of homework they do can also make the task more palatable.

Frequently Asked Questions

Here are some of the school-related issues that frequently arise in our work with parents:

My daughter's teacher clearly thinks that if my daughter were on medication, everyone would be a lot happier. I'd prefer to try other things first. How can I handle this? Our response to this question is straightforward: Medication should never be a school decision. Rather, medication decisions are exclusively an issue between you and your child's physician (see Chapter 21 for a discussion about medication). It may be easier for teachers or other educators to accept your response to their raising medication as a possibility if you couch it in terms of your hesitation about medication. You might say, "I'm nervous about my child taking medication. I know there can be side effects, and that worries me. Here's what I would like to try. . . . " If you let teachers know you're willing to try harder, they may be more willing to try harder, too.

My child's teacher says he'll make accommodations for my child's executive skill problems (like checking in with him at the end of the day to make sure he has everything he needs for homework or sending home a weekly progress report so I can find out about missing assignments), but then he forgets to do it and my son fails assignments as a result. What can I do about this? If the teacher is well intentioned (but perhaps has executive skill challenges of his own), you should be sympathetic. "I know you're busy at the end of the day. Is there something I could do to help?" Some teachers only grudgingly agree to provide increased cueing, monitoring, or supervision, however, and when they fall short, the truth comes out. "I think your child should be doing this himself," they may say when pressed. The response to this kind of comment is "We've tried that before, and it hasn't been effective. We need to do something more than hold him accountable to do this all on his own." There are things you can do to make it easier for teachers, though. We often recommend that parents email teachers on a weekly basis to find out about missing homework assignments. Because it's easier to reply to an email than to generate one, this reduces the burden on the teacher and may make the communication task more manageable. Contacting teachers through the school portal rather than emailing them directly can also make communication with teachers easier. We've also known mothers who have happily come to their child's school once a week to help clean out desks or lockers. In neither case are parents or teachers letting the child "off the hook." Rather, they're putting in place systems that help hold children accountable while supervising them at the same time.

What is reasonable to expect classroom teachers to do to help my child develop more effective executive skills? We've found that those teachers who are most effective in supporting the development of executive skills are ones who create whole-class routines that help children develop skills such as organization, planning, working memory, and time management. They also embed instruction in executive skills into subject matter teaching. They teach children how to break down long-term assignments into subtasks and to develop timelines for subtask completion. They build in homework routines to ensure that students remember to hand in their homework and end-of-day routines to help children learn to check their assignment books and put in their backpacks everything they need for homework. They develop classroom rules for behavior that help children control impulses and manage their emotions, and they review the rules regularly and at opportune times (for example, just before a guest is about to address the class or just before recess).

Again, because teachers like everyone else have executive skill strengths and challenges, some of them incorporate these kinds of activities more than others. If your child has a teacher who doesn't do this well, it's reasonable to look for resources other than the teacher to help—a classroom aide, guidance counselor, principal, assistant principal, or the like. Many schools offer Teacher Assistance Teams where classroom teachers, administrators, and specialists meet regularly to discuss how to address learning or behavior problems of specific students. You can ask that your child be put on that agenda and meet with the team to brainstorm solutions to the problem.

When are executive skill problems severe enough to warrant additional services, such as a Section 504 Plan or special education? How do I access those services? The general rule of thumb we subscribe to is that when a child's executive skill challenges interfere with that child's ability to succeed in school, additional services are warranted. Certainly failing grades would be evidence of school failure. But we would also argue that grades that don't reflect a child's potential when those poor grades attributed to executive skill challenges also signal a need for additional supports. These supports might be provided informally (as implied in the answer to the previous question), but they also may be provided more formally, either through a Section 504 Plan or through special education.

Section 504 Plans and special education are governed by laws and regulations that specify who is eligible for services and for what kinds of services. Section 504 is a civil rights law that prohibits discrimination against individuals with disabilities. It's designed to ensure that children with disabilities have access to the same education that children without disabilities have access to. The services provided under this law are typically accommodations and modifications provided in the regular classroom and designed to enable the child to benefit from classroom instruction. Examples of these include allowing extended time on tests or alternative test methods, modified home-work assignments, allowing for breaks (so a child with ADHD, for instance, can get up and move around or leave the classroom temporarily), and modified grading procedures (for example, weighing daily work higher than tests if the student tests poorly).

Special education is intended for children with an educational disability that adversely affects educational performance and that requires specialized instruction to correct. Children with executive skill deficits may qualify for a 504 Plan to build appro-priate modifications or accommodations into the classroom, or they may qualify for special education when direct instruction is needed. Helping a student learn to become organized, to manage time effectively, or to do the planning required to complete long-term projects or to juggle multiple assignments at once very often requires individual-ized instruction that would warrant special education. In either case begin with your child's teacher and ask how to contact the 504 Plan coordinator or special education coordinator for the school. Request that a meeting be set up where your child's problems can be discussed and steps can be taken to determine whether the child is eligible for either special education or a 504 Plan.

Special education has traditionally involved a comprehensive evaluation to deter-mine whether the child has an educational disability that would qualify him for special education services. The most common disabilities are learning disabilities, emotional or behavioral disorders, a speech/language handicap, mental impairment or intellectual disability, or another health impairment (referred to as OHI, or other health impaired), such as ADHD or another medical condition that might affect learning. However, in the most recent revision of the federal special education laws, states and local schools now have the option of using a response-to-intervention model, or RTI, sometimes referred to as MTSS (multi-tiered system of support). This is an assessment–intervention model that begins with high-quality instruction and behavioral supports in the regular class-room. When children struggle in that setting, a series of interventions are put in place to address the problem, beginning with fine-tuning classroom-based interventions, and increasing in intensity as necessary to address the problem. This model emphasizes high-quality instruction as well as data-based decision making so that there will be no question of the success of any intervention attempted.

We think this approach lends itself well to the needs of children with executive skill deficits. For instance, let's say Kevin, age 15, is failing geometry because he is handing in only 50% of his homework assignments. His test grades are good, in part because he actually does most of his homework, but he loses it or forgets to hand it in about half the time. The obvious first step to help Kevin (who clearly has problems with organization and working memory!) is to design systems to prevent him from losing his homework and to cue him in class to help him remember to hand in his homework. Under the traditional special education framework, Kevin's parents—or even his math teacher—might refer him to special education for an evaluation to determine whether he has a disability. With an RTI/MTSS model, Kevin and his parents and teacher could meet and design an intervention they think will work. Using the principle that *everyone has to work harder,* Kevin's parents could agree to check in with Kevin each night before he goes to bed to make sure he has put his geometry homework in a folder designated for that purpose (Kevin decides a fluorescent green folder picked up from a local office supply store will do nicely). If he has remembered to put the assignment in his folder without a reminder from his parents, he'll earn points from his parents, which he can use to save up for a video game he wants to purchase. His geometry teacher agrees to institute a procedure whereby he collects the homework assignments from each student individually as soon as the class has finished the homework review. If these steps are successful in resolving the problem, and there's no reason to believe they won't be, assuming each person involved in the intervention plays her part consistently, then there's no need to go further in the special education process.

For another student, however, who fails to hand in his homework because he doesn't understand the material, a different intervention will need to be designed, and this one may lead to the need for special education services.

I think my child needs to be on an IEP (individualized education program). How would you write an IEP for someone with executive skill challenges? Based on the most recent revision of the federal special education laws (the Individuals with Disabilities Education Improvement Act, or IDEIA), IEPs must include measurable annual goals and a statement about how progress will be measured. For a student with executive skill deficits, an IEP should include a description of the specific skill to be addressed as well as how it manifests itself in the classroom or on specific academic tasks. The method of measurement is tied to the functional behavior and should be as objective as possible. Progress can be measured by (1) counting behaviors (for example, the number of times a child gets in a fight on the playground); (2) calculating a percentage (for example, percent of homework handed in on time); (3) rating performance using a rating scale with each point on the rating scale carefully defined; or (4) using naturally occurring data such as test or quiz scores, absences from class, number of discipline referrals, and so on.

Sometimes schools draft IEP goals that address executive skills in general. We do not believe this provides enough specificity, both in terms of defining the executive skill challenge and in defining a desired outcome. A formula for writing an executive skills IEP goal that can be tailored to whatever executive skill the goal needs to address might begin with the sentence "The student will exhibit [specific executive skill] by [specific behavioral descriptor]." Here are a few examples:

- The student will demonstrate response inhibition by waiting his turn in a conversation, game, or any other activity that involves turn taking.
- The student will demonstrate emotional control by playing with other students at recess without engaging in verbal or physical aggression or unsafe behavior.
- The student will demonstrate sustained attention by accurately completing classwork within the time allotted or within suggested time frames.

We offer numerous examples of IEP goals for all 11 executive skills in our book *Executive Skills in Children and Adolescence, Third Edition.*

IEP goals should also identify the time frame involved, the setting in which the goal will be measured, how progress will be measured, the accuracy level expected, and the kinds of supports the students may receive. Thus, a complete IEP goal might read, "By the end of second grade, the student will demonstrate sustained attention by completing 80 percent of classwork with a minimum of 80 percent accuracy within the time allotted in the classroom, with no more than two cues from the teacher to stay on task."

My child has an IEP (or 504 Plan) with executive skill goals, but the school is not following it. What can I do to get them to do what they say they will do? The first step is to make sure that the goals and measurement procedures are defined precisely. This includes stating the IEP goal in measurable terms and defining *how* the goal will be measured. If this is in place, you can then ask the IEP team to share the data with you whenever they collect the data or on a regular basis (for example, weekly, biweekly, monthly). As much as possible, we recommend that data be kept on a computer (such as on a spreadsheet) so that results can be emailed easily to you. You may want to ask your child's case manager if it would be easier for them to remember to share the data with you if you sent email reminders at the appropriate times.

As we stated earlier, you're likely to get more cooperation, and therefore better results, when you take a nonadversarial approach with schools. However, if despite your best efforts you hit a dead end in your efforts to collaborate with your child's teacher or special education team, you may have no recourse but to hire an advocate or a lawyer to help you get the services your child needs.

Templates for Specific Homework Issues

Long-Term Projects

Executive skills addressed: Task initiation (Chapter 15), sustained attention (Chapter 14), planning /prioritizing (Chapter 16), time management (Chapter 18), metacognition (Chapter 20)

Ages: 8–14; kids as young as 7 might be assigned such a project, but it will probably involve a simpler process, meaning this intervention should be simplified too.

1. With your child, look at the description of the assignment to make sure you both understand what is expected. If the assignment allows your child a choice of topic, topic selection is the first step. Many children have trouble thinking up topics, and if this is the case with your child, you should brainstorm topic ideas, providing lots of suggestions, starting with topics that are related to your child's areas of interests.

2. Using the Long-Term Project-Planning Sheet (pages 304–305), write down the possible topics. After you have three to five, go back and ask your child what they like and don't like about each choice.

3. Help your child make a final selection. In addition to thinking about what topic is of greatest interest, things to think about in making a final selection are (a) choosing a topic that is neither too broad nor too narrow; (b) how difficult it will be to track down references and resources; and (c) whether there is an interesting "twist" to the topic that will either make it fun to work on or appealing for the teacher.

4. Using the Project-Planning Sheet, decide what materials or resources will be needed, where the child will get them, and when (you may want to fill in the last column after completing the next step). Possible resources include websites, library books, things that may need to be ordered (for example, travel brochures), people who might be interviewed, or places to visit (for example, museums, historical sites, and so on). Also consider any construction or art materials that will be needed if the project involves building something.

5. Using the Project-Planning Sheet, list all the steps that will need to be done to carry out the project and then develop a timeline so your child knows when each step will be done. It may be helpful at this point to transfer this information onto a monthly calendar that can be hung on the wall or a bulletin board near your child's desk to make it easier to keep track of what needs to be done when.

6. Cue your child to follow the timeline. Before the child begins each step, you may want to discuss what exactly is involved in completing the step—this may mean making a list of things to be done for each step. Planning for the next step could be done as each step is completed so that your child has some idea what's coming next and to make it easier to get the next step started.

Fading the Supervision

Children who have problems with planning and with the metacognitive skills required to do open-ended tasks often require lots of support for a long time. Using the Long-Term Project-Planning Sheet as a guide, you can gradually hand over the responsibility of having your child complete the sheet more and more on their own. As you sense your child's ability to do more of the work independently, sit down with the planning sheet and have the child indicate which pieces they think they can do alone and which pieces

Long-Term Project-Planning Sheet

STEP 1: SELECT TOPIC

What are possible topics?	What I like about this choice:	What I don't like:
1.		
2.		
3.		
4.		
5.		

Final Topic Choice:

STEP 2: IDENTIFY NECESSARY MATERIALS

What materials or resources do you need?	Where will you get them?	When will you get them?
1.		
2.		
3.		
4.		
5.		

(continued)

From *Executive Skills in Children and Adolescents, Third Edition,* by Peg Dawson and Richard Guare. Copyright © 2018 The Guilford Press. Reprinted in *Smart but Scattered, Second Edition* (The Guilford Press, 2025). Permission to photocopy this material, or to download enlarged printable versions (*www.guilford.com/dawson4-forms*), is granted to purchasers of this book for personal use; see copyright page for details.

STEP 3: IDENTIFY PROJECT TASKS AND DUE DATES

What do you need to do? (List each step in order)	When will you do it?	Check off when done
Step 1:		
Step 2:		
Step 3:		
Step 4:		
Step 5:		
Step 6:		
Step 7:		
Step 8:		
Step 9:		
Step 10:		

Reminder List

Include here any additional tasks or details you need to keep in mind as you work on the project. Cross out or check off each one as it is taken care of.

1. _____
2. _____
3. _____
4. _____
5. _____
6. _____
7. _____
8. _____
9. _____
10. _____

they will need help with. It is likely that you will continue to need to remind your child to complete each step in the timeline for a long time before the child can be independent in this part of the process.

Modifications/Adjustments

Use reinforcers as necessary for meeting timeline goals and for completing the project by the deadline; you can award bonus points for completion without reminders (or with a minimum, agreed-upon number of reminders).

Writing a Paper

Executive skills addressed: Task initiation (Chapter 15), sustained attention (Chapter 14), planning/prioritizing (Chapter 16), organization (Chapter 17), time management (Chapter 18), metacognition (Chapter 20)

Ages: 8–14; children don't usually start writing papers until third grade, and they are typically shorter than five paragraphs for the youngest kids in this age range, so if your child is only 8, you may have to shorten the form accordingly.

Step 1: Brainstorm Topics

If your child has to come up with a topic to write about, make sure you understand the exact assignment requirements before beginning. This may necessitate a phone call to the teacher or a friend of your child to clarify directions. The rules of brainstorming are that any idea is accepted and written down in the first stage—the wilder and crazier, the better because wild and crazy ideas often lead to good, usable ideas. No criticism by either parent or child is allowed at this point. If your child has trouble thinking of ideas on their own, throw out some ideas of your own to "grease the wheels." Once you and your child run out of topic ideas, read over your list and circle the most promising ones. Your child may know right away what he wants to write about. If not, talk about what he likes and dislikes about each idea to make it easier to zero in on a good choice.

Step 2: Brainstorm Content

Once a topic has been selected, the brainstorming process begins again. Say to your child, "Tell me everything you know or would like to know about this topic." Again, write down any idea or question—the crazier, the better at this point.

Step 3: Organize the Content

Now look at all the ideas or questions you've written down. Together with your child, decide whether the material can be grouped together in any way. If the assignment is to do a report on aardvarks, for instance, you might find the information clusters into categories such as what they look like, where they live, what they eat, who their enemies are, how they protect themselves. Create topic headings and then write the details under each topic heading. Some parents find that it's helpful to use sticky notes for this process. During the brainstorming phase, each individual idea or question is written on a separate note. The sticky notes can then be organized on a table under topic headings to form an outline of the paper. The paper can then be written (or dictated) from this outline.

Step 4: Write the Opening Paragraph

This is often the hardest part of the paper to write. The opening paragraph, at its most basic level, describes very succinctly what the paper will be about. For instance, an opening paragraph on a report about aardvarks might read:

> *This paper is about a strange animal called an aardvark. By the time you finish reading it, you will know what they look like, where they live, what they eat, who their enemies are, and how they protect themselves.*

The one other thing that the opening paragraph should try to do is "grab the reader"—give the reader an interesting piece of information to tease his or her curiosity. At the end of the paragraph above, for instance, two more sentences might be added:

> *The reader will also learn the meaning of the word* aardvark *and what language it comes from. And if that hasn't grabbed your interest, I will also tell you why the aardvark has a sticky tongue—although you may not want to know this!*

Children with writing problems will have trouble writing the opening paragraph by themselves and may need your help. You may be able to help by asking general questions, such as "What do you want people to know after they read your paper?" or "Why do you think people might be interested in reading this?" If they need more help than that, you may want to give them a model to work from. You could write an opening paragraph on a topic similar to the one your child is working on, or you could use the paragraph here as an example. If your child needs more guided help writing this paragraph, provide it. Then see if the child can continue without the need for as much support. Remember, the first paragraph is often the hardest part of the paper to write.

Step 5: Write the Rest of the Paper

To give your child just a little more guidance, suggest that the rest of the paper be divided into sections with a heading for each section (sort of the way this book is written). Help the child make a list of the headings and then see if they can continue with the writing task alone. Each paragraph should begin with a main or topic sentence that makes one main point. Following the topic sentence should be three to five sentences that expand or explain the main point. It's helpful to use connecting words to link sentences or paragraphs. Examples of simple linking words are *and, because, also, instead, but,* and *so.* Examples of more complex linking words are *although, moreover, on the other hand, therefore, as a result, finally,* and *in conclusion.*

In the early stages of learning to write, children with writing problems need a great deal of help. You may feel like you're writing half the paper in the early stages. It should get better with time, especially if you end each writing session by giving your child some positive feedback about something done well. Note in particular any improvement since the last writing assignment. You might say, "I really like the way you were able to come up with the headings on your own this time, with no help from me."

If you don't see progress over time—or if you feel you lack the time or skills to teach your child to do this kind of writing, talk with your child's teacher to see if additional support can be provided in school. Even if you're willing to help out in this way, you may want to ask for more help in school if you believe your child's writing skills are significantly delayed compared to other children of the same age.

The form on pages 309–310 is a template for writing a paper or essay, with the sections of the template corresponding to the steps described above.

Studying for Tests

Executive skills addressed: Task initiation (Chapter 15), sustained attention (Chapter 14), planning/prioritizing (Chapter 16), time management (Chapter 18), metacognition (Chapter 20)

Ages: 10–14; children usually don't have tests until fourth grade, and even then the teacher is likely to tell them what to study, so this routine probably won't be of much use to you until your child is in at least fifth grade.

1. Keep a monthly calendar with your child on which any upcoming tests are written.

2. From 5 days to a week before the test, make a study plan with your child. The form on page 311 outlines the process for making a study plan and evaluating the results.

3. Using the Menu of Study Strategies in the Tools for Studying form (page 311), have your child decide which strategies to use to study for the test.

4. Have your child make a plan for studying that starts 4 days before the test. Psychological research over many years shows that when new material is learned, *distributed practice is more effective than massed practice.* In other words, if you plan to spend 2 hours studying for a test, it is better to break the time down into smaller segments (such as 30 minutes a night for 4 nights) than to spend the full 2 hours studying the night before the test. Research also shows that learning is consolidated through sleep, so getting a good night's sleep the night before an exam is more beneficial than "cramming" the night before.

Writing Template for a Five-Paragraph Essay

INTRODUCTORY PARAGRAPH

Sentence 1 summarizes what your essay is about:

Sentence 2 focuses in on the main point you want to make:

Sentence 3 adds more detail or explains why the topic is important:

BODY PARAGRAPHS

Paragraph 1, topic sentence:

    Supporting detail 1:

    Supporting detail 2:

    Supporting detail 3:

Paragraph 2, topic sentence:

    Supporting detail 1:

    Supporting detail 2:

    Supporting detail 3:

(continued)

From *Executive Skills in Children and Adolescents, Third Edition*, by Peg Dawson and Richard Guare. Copyright © 2018 The Guilford Press. Reprinted in *Smart but Scattered, Second Edition* (The Guilford Press, 2025). Permission to photocopy this material, or to download enlarged printable versions (*www.guilford.com/dawson4-forms*), is granted to purchasers of this book for personal use; see copyright page for details.

Paragraph 3, topic sentence:

    Supporting detail 1:

    Supporting detail 2:

    Supporting detail 3:

CONCLUDING PARAGRAPH

Restate the most important point from the paper you want to make (what the reader should go away understanding):

Tools for Studying

A. MENU OF STUDY STRATEGIES

Check off the ones you will use.

Passive strategies (use sparingly)	Active strategies (better)	Active strategies with feedback (best)
☐ 1. Reread text	☐ 7. Make study guide	☐ 13. Quiz myself with Quizlet/ study guide/flash cards
☐ 2. Reread notes	☐ 8. Make flashcards/ Quizlet	☐ 14. Take practice test (check answers)
☐ 3. Highlight notes/text	☐ 9. Make concept maps	☐ 15. Redo old tests or homework (check answers)
☐ 4. Ready study guide	☐ 10. Organize notes	☐ 16. Have someone else quiz me
☐ 5. Rewrite notes	☐ 11. Complete review packet (no answers)	☐ 17. Complete review packet (check answers)
☐ 6. Read/watch Spark Notes, Khan Academy, and so on.	☐ 12. Attend review session or study group	☐ 18. Meet 1:1 with teacher
		☐ 19. Other:_____

B. STUDY PLAN

Date	Day	Which strategies will I use? (write #)	How much time for each strategy?
	4 days before test	1. 2. 3.	1. 2. 3.
	3 days before test	1. 2. 3.	1. 2. 3.
	2 days before test	1. 2. 3.	1. 2. 3.
	1 day before test	1. 2. 3.	1. 2. 3.

C. POSTTEST EVALUATION

How did your studying work out? Answer the following questions:

1. What strategies worked best?
2. What strategies were not so helpful?
3. Did you spend enough time studying?   Yes   No
4. If no, what more should you have done?
5. What will you do differently next time?

From *Executive Skills in Children and Adolescents, Third Edition*, by Peg Dawson and Richard Guare. Copyright © 2018 The Guilford Press. Reprinted in *Smart but Scattered, Second Edition* (The Guilford Press, 2025). Permission to photocopy this material, or to download enlarged printable versions (*www.guilford.com/dawson4-forms*), is granted to purchasers of this book for personal use; see copyright page for details.

5. For children who have problems with sustained attention, using several strategies each for a short amount of time may be easier than using one strategy for the full study period. You can set a kitchen timer for the length of time for each strategy, and when the bell rings, your child can move on to the next strategy (unless the child likes the one being used and wants to continue it).

Fading the Supervision

Depending on your child's level of independence, they may need help making the study plan, may need prompting to follow the plan, and may need supervision while following the plan. You can gradually fade this support, first by having your child check in with you after finishing each strategy but keeping all the other supports in place. Cueing to make the study plan and prompting to start studying will likely be the last supports you can fade.

Modifications/Adjustments

1. After your child takes the test or after the graded test is returned, ask your child to evaluate how the study plan went. Which strategies seemed to work the best? Which ones were less helpful? Are there other strategies he or she might try the next time? How about the time devoted to studying? Was it enough? Make some notes on the study plan to help your child when it's time to plan for the next test.

2. If your child felt he or she studied adequately but still did poorly, check with his or her teacher for feedback about what might have been done differently. Did your child study the wrong material—or study it in the wrong way? Consider asking your child's teacher to prepare a study guide if that hasn't been done already.

3. If your child consistently does poorly on tests despite studying long and hard, consider asking his or her teacher for testing modifications (for example, extended time, the chance to retake tests, the chance to do extra credit work to make up for poor test grades, alternatives to tests, or allowing your child to prepare a cheat sheet or take open-book exams). This may require that your child be evaluated to determine whether he or she qualifies for special education services or a 504 Plan.

4. Add an incentive system—rewards for good grades on tests.

Parting Thoughts

If you read this book from cover to cover, your head may be reeling. That texting acronym, TMI, comes to mind—Too Much Information! At least too much to absorb easily.

So let us leave you with two messages that may help you decompress. The first is to remind you of our "perfect intervention" to support executive skill development that we shared in the Introduction. Remember it? The perfect intervention to support executive skill development is one that (1) takes no more than 5 or 10 minutes a day, and (2) you're willing to do forever (or as long as it takes).

Here's the second message—one that we build into every parent presentation we do: The nice thing about being a parent of a child with executive skill challenges is that you get the longitudinal perspective. You get to see what these kids look like when they grow up. And both from following our own children and talking to parents of kids who were once "smart but scattered," what we've learned is this: *Most of these kids turn out fine.* When we give people this message, we often see the audience visibly relax. And sometimes people share their stories afterwards.

One mom told us that a school administrator had told her when her son was in middle school that he would likely end up in jail. She said (*so proudly*), "He's 25 years old, he's in a master's degree program, and he has a wife and child." How wrong that administrator was!

Another mom, Lisa Howe, who is also a social worker and Certified Peaceful Parenting Coach, wrote us recently after attending a virtual parent presentation: "I've read *Smart but Scattered* multiples times and use it daily in my work for myself, my own 11-year-old daughter with ADHD, and to guide the parents I work with. I frequently get discouraged and worry we aren't doing enough to help our daughter. I worry she won't be able to do well in middle school, or will struggle with life. My husband is much more chill than I am, so that's a good balance. But what I wanted to share was that every single time I read your work and hear you speak, I feel my shoulders drop, and usually cry with relief. She IS already doing OK. We ARE doing all the things we should be doing."

We can't think of a better message to leave you with at the end of this book.

Resources

Executive Skills Development

These articles and books relate to the development of executive skills, their underlying brain structures, and the factors that can enhance or inhibit their progress.

Beuriat, P. A., Cristofori, I., Gordon, B., & Grafman, J. (2022). The shifting role of the cerebellum in executive, emotional and social processing across the lifespan. *Behavioral and Brain Functions, 18*(6), 1–11.

Blair, C., & Raver, C. C. (2016). Poverty, stress, and brain development: New directions for prevention and intervention. *Academic Pediatrics, 16*(3), S30–S36.

Buffalmann, F., & Karbach, J. (2017). Development and plasticity of cognitive flexibility in early and middle childhood. *Frontiers in Psychology, 8*(1040), 1–6.

Dehaene, S. (2020). *How we learn: Why brains learn better than any machine . . . for now.* New York: Penguin Books.

Fiske, A., & Holmboe, K. (2019). Neural substrates of early executive function development. *Developmental Review, 52,* 42–62.

Friedman, N. P., & Miyake, A. (2017). Unity and diversity of executive functions: Individual differences as a window on cognitive structure. *Cortex, 86,* 186–204.

Kao, K., Nayak, S., Doan, S. N., & Tarullo, A. R. (2018). Relations between parent EF and child EF: The role of socioeconomic status and parenting on executive functioning in early childhood. *Translational Issues in Psychological Science, 4*(2), 122–137.

Luerssen, A., Gyurak, A., Ayduk, O., Wendelken, C., & Bunge, S. A. (2015). Delay of gratification in childhood linked to cortical interactions with the nucleus accumbens. *Social cognitive and affective neuroscience, 10*(12), 1769–1776.

Lunkenheimer, E., Panlilio, C., Lobo, F. M., Olson, S. L., & Hamby, C. M. (2019). Preschoolers' self-regulation in context: Task persistence profiles with mothers and fathers and later attention problems in kindergarten. *Journal of Abnormal Child Psychology, 47*(6), 947–960.

Reynolds, G. D., & Romano, A. C. (2016). The development of attention systems and working memory in infancy. *Frontiers in Systems Neuroscience, 10*(15).

Ryan, R. M., & Deci, E. L. (2017). *Self-determination theory: Basic psychological needs in motivation, development, and wellness.* New York: Guilford Press.

Simpson, A., & Carroll, D. J. (2019). Understanding early inhibitory development: Distinguishing two ways that children use inhibitory control. *Child Development, 90*(5), 1459–1473.

Smortchkova, J., & Shea, N. (2020). Metacognitive development and conceptual change in children. *Review of Philosophy and Psychology, 11*, 745–763.

Society for Neuroscience. (2018). *Brain facts: A primer on the brain and nervous system* (8th ed.). Author.

Parenting Resources

Barkley, R. A. (2015). *Attention-deficit hyperactivity disorder: A handbook of diagnosis and treatment* (4th ed.). New York: Guilford Press.—This book is fairly technical but provides a good description of executive skills within a developmental framework and argues that executive skills are at the core of ADHD. Russell Barkley has written a number of other books that parents may find helpful, especially parents of defiant children or those with ADHD. These include:

- *Taking charge of ADHD: The complete authoritative guide for parents* (4th ed.). New York: Guilford Press, 2020.
- *Your defiant child: Eight steps to better behavior* (2nd ed.; coauthored by Christine Benton). New York: Guilford Press, 2013.
- *Your defiant teen: 10 steps to resolve conflict and rebuild your relationship* (coauthored by Arthur Robin). New York: Guilford Press, 2008.

Braaten, E. (2023). *Bright kids who couldn't care less: How to rekindle your child's motivation.* New York: Guilford Press.

Dawson, P., & Guare, R. (2018). *Executive skills in children and adolescents: A practical guide to assessment and intervention* (3rd ed.). New York: Guilford Press.—This book, written primarily for educators and school psychologists, describes how executive skills are assessed but also provides descriptions of school-based interventions for executive skill challenges following the same framework that we describe in this volume.

Dawson, P., & Guare, R. (2023). *Coaching students with executive skills challenges* (2nd ed.). New York: Guilford Press.—This practical manual presents an evidence-based coaching model for helping students whose academic performance is suffering because of deficits in executive skills, including time and task management, planning, organization, impulse control, and emotional regulation.

Gordon, R. M. (2008). *Thinking organized for parents and children: Helping kids get organized for home, school, and play.* Silver Spring, MD: Thinking Organized Press.—A book and workbook providing strategies and step-by-step instructions that parents can use to help children develop executive skills, particularly in the context of school-related tasks such as reading comprehension and writing, as well as strategies for enhancing working memory, time management, study skills, and organization.

Greene, R. W. (2021). *The explosive child: A new approach for understanding and parenting easily frustrated, chronically inflexible children* (6th ed.). New York: HarperCollins.—This very readable book is a source of comfort to parents of inflexible children, as it describes the causes of inflexibility as well as ways to treat the problem in clear, straightforward language.

Kenworthy, L., Anthony, L. G., Alexander, K. C., Werner, M. A., Cannon, L., & Greenman, L. (2014). *Solving executive function challenges.* Baltimore: Brookes.—This book particularly targets children on the autism spectrum, but the strategies described would be helpful for parents of all children with executive function challenges, particularly those who struggle with flexibility.

Kurcinka, M. S. (2015). *Raising your spirited child* (3rd ed.). New York: Harper.—The author describes spirited children as "intense, sensitive, perceptive, persistent, and energetic." The book helps parents understand the role of temperament in the behavior of their children and offers advice for how to handle common problems of daily living with children who have problems with emotional control and response inhibition.

Shapiro, D. (2016). *Parent child journey: An individualized approach to raising your challenging child.* North Charleston, SC: CreateSpace Independent Publishing.—For parents of a challenging child, this book provides a detailed guide in the use of behavioral strategies, including implementation of rewards and consequences.

Stixrud, W., & Johnson, N. *The self-driven child: The science and sense of giving your kids more control over their lives.* New York: Penguin Books.—Written by a neuropsychologist and college counselor, this book offers advice for parents on how to work collaboratively with their children to develop the skills they need to make autonomous decisions and become resilient in the face of stress.

Wallace, J. B. (2023). *Never enough: When achievement culture becomes toxic and what we can do about it.* New York: Portfolio/Penguin.—The author offers an antidote to what she describes as a "toxic achievement culture" that leads kids to believe that self-worth is measured by external achievements.

Wood, C. (2018). *Yardsticks: Child and adolescent development ages 4–14* (4th ed.). Turners Falls, MA: Center for Responsive Schools.—This is a primer on developmental milestones to help parents understand what children are capable of doing at each age from early childhood to early adolescence.

Magazines

ADDitude is a magazine for families affected by ADHD (*www.additudemag.com*).

Attention! is the official publication of CHADD (Children and Adults with Attention-Deficit/Hyperactivity Disorder) (*www.chadd.org*).

Parents magazine offers general advice on child development and parenting issue (*www.parents.com*).

Websites Offering Guidance on Handling Technology and Social Media

American Academy of Pediatrics (*www.aap.org*). Guidelines regarding social media use can be found here: *www.aap.org/en/search/?k=social%20media*

Boston Children's Digital Wellness Lab (*https://digitalwellnesslab.org*)

Common Sense Media (*www.commonsensemedia.org*)

Family Online Safety Institute (*www.fosi.org*)

Other Helpful Websites

American Academy of Pediatrics (*www.aap.org*). The official website of the American Academy of Pediatrics is an excellent source of information about all aspects of children's health.

Center on the Developing Child, Harvard University. This organization is devoted to science-based policy and practice that supports children facing adversity. They have a significant focus on executive skills. Here are specific links that are helpful:

- https://developingchild.harvard.edu/resources/5-steps-for-brain-building-serve-and-return
- https://developingchild.harvard.edu/resources/activities-guide-enhancing-and-practicing-executive-function-skills-with-children-from-infancy-to-adolescence
- https://developingchild.harvard.edu/science/key-concepts/serve-and-return
- https://developingchild.harvard.edu/resourcetag/executive-function

Centers for Disease Control and Prevention (CDC) (*www.cdc.gov*). Part of the U.S. Department of Health and Human Services, this is the primary federal agency for conducting and supporting public health activities in the United States. The site contains links to research studies on executive skills/functions in children as well as comprehensive information on disorders associated with executive skill deficits, including autism and ADHD.

CHADD (*www.chadd.org*). This organization is dedicated to providing advocacy, education, and support for individuals with ADHD. The website is an excellent source of information for individuals, parents, and professionals about topics related to ADHD.

Neuroscience for Kids (*https://faculty.washington.edu/chudler/newslet.html*). Eric Chudler produces a monthly online newsletter with links to neuroscience news that might be of interest to kids. It includes stories in the news as well as contests for kids and other activities that might be of interest to students.

PBS (*www.pbs.org*) has provided and continues to provide excellent, scientifically based programming on child health and development, including brain–behavior relationships.

Smart but Scattered Kids (*www.smartbutscatteredkids.com*). This is the authors' website, which includes resources and videos as well as links to professional development opportunities.

Zero to Three (*www.zerotothree.org*) provides authoritative information on a host of topics (brain development, nutrition, child rearing) for adults who influence the lives of infants and toddlers.

Resources for Toys, Games, and the Benefits of Play

Childswork/Childsplay (*www.childswork.com*) is a catalog of games and activities primarily designed for guidance counselors and therapists to help children learn to recognize and manage their feelings. Most of the materials are not restricted to professionals and may be helpful for parents who want to work on emotional control with their children.

The Genius of Play (*www.thegeniusofplay.org*). This website describes the benefits of play and offers advice for parents as well as suggestions for toys and play activities.

Learning Works for Kids (*http://learningworksforkids.com*) helps parents identify video games designed to help children develop specific executive skills. The website was created on the principle that popular video games and other digital media, when used mindfully and responsibly, can be powerful tools for sharpening and improving children's academic performance and cognitive skills.

Mindware (*www.mindware.orientaltrading.com*), a catalog of "brainy toys for kids of all ages," offers a wide variety of toys designed to build creativity and problem solving (that is, metacognitive skills).

Apps and Websites with Tools to Support Executive Skills

Choiceworks (*https://apps.apple.com/us/app/choiceworks/id486210964*). This is an app that helps children complete daily routines, learn to wait, and manage emotions. Available for iPhone in their App store.

Goblin Tools (*https://goblin.tools*). To quote their website, "goblin.tools is a collection of small, simple, single-task tools, mostly designed to help neurodivergent people with tasks they find overwhelming or difficult." They include an app for estimating time as well as other apps supported by simple artificial intelligence.

The Original Beeper App (*https://originalbeeperapp.com*). An app that sounds tones at random intervals to prompt the user to catch "mind wandering" and bring them back to task. Available for both iPhone and Android.

Time Timer (*www.timetimer.com*), available in a desktop or computer version, helps children understand time by providing a graphic depiction of time passing. Its use can help children learn to monitor work production and build time management skills.

Picture Books/Read-Alouds

Response Inhibition

Goldilocks and the Three Dinosaurs (Mo Willems)
If You Ever Wanted to Bring an Alligator to School, Don't (Elise Parsley)
Interrupting Chicken (David Ezra Stein)
Ricky Sticky Fingers (Julia Cook)
Waiting Is Not Easy (Mo Willems)
What If Everybody Did That? (Ellen Javernick)
What Were You Thinking? (Bryan Smith)

Working Memory

How Do I Remember All That? (Bryan Smith)

Emotional Control

Alphabreaths (Christopher Willard and Daniel Rechtschaffen)
Mindful Kids (Whitney Stewart and Mina Braun)
My Mouth Is a Volcano (Julia Cook)
Of Course It's a Big Deal (Bryan Smith)
What's Your Choice? (Bryan Smith)
Wilma Jean the Worry Machine (Julia Cook)

Flexibility

The Girl Who Never Made Mistakes (Mark Petty and Gary Rubenstein)
Ish (Peter Reynolds)
My Day Is Ruined (Bryan Smith)
Stuck (Oliver Jeffers)

Task Initiation

The Best Story (Eileen Spinelli)
Poppy's Best Paper (Susan Eaddy)
Time to Get Started (Bryan Smith)

Sustained Attention

Are You Working Hard or Hardly Working? (Bryan Smith)
Fix It with Focus (Bryan Smith)
Interrupting Chicken (David Ezra Stein)
Quiet (Tomie DePaola)
Whole Body Listening Larry at School! (Elizabeth Stauter, Kristen Wilson, and Eric Hutchinson)

Planning/Prioritizing

I'll Never Get All of That Done (Bryan Smith)
Planning Isn't My Priority (Julia Cook)

Organization

I Can't Find My Whatchamacallit (Julia Cook)
It Was Just Right Here (Bryan Smith)

Time Management

We can find no picture books on this topic, in part because it's not a skill that we expect children who are at the picture book stage to master.

Goal-Directed Persistence

The Most Magnificent Thing (Ashley Spires)

Metacognition

You Are a Social Detective (Michelle Garcia Winner)
What's the Problem? (Bryan Smith)

For Older Elementary-School-Age Students

The Day Frankie Left His Frontal Lobes at Home (Laurie McCloskey and George McCloskey)

Index

Note. *f* or *t* following a page number indicates a figure or table.

About the Authors

Peg Dawson, EdD, is a psychologist who provides professional development training on executive skills for schools and organizations nationally and internationally. She was previously on the staff of the Center for Learning and Attention Disorders at Seacoast Mental Health Center in Portsmouth, New Hampshire. Dr. Dawson is a past president of the New Hampshire Association of School Psychologists, the National Association of School Psychologists (NASP), and the International School Psychology Association, and a recipient of the Lifetime Achievement Award from NASP. She is coauthor of bestselling books for general readers, including *Smart but Scattered Teens; Smart but Scattered—and Stalled* (with a focus on emerging adults); and *The Smart but Scattered Guide to Success* (with a focus on adults). Dr. Dawson is also coauthor of *The Work-Smart Academic Planner, Revised Edition,* and books for professionals including *Executive Skills in Children and Adolescents, Third Edition.*

Richard Guare, PhD, BCBA-D, is a neuropsychologist and board-certified behavior analyst who frequently consults to schools and agencies on attention and executive skills difficulties. He is former Director of the Center for Learning and Attention Disorders at Seacoast Mental Health Center in Portsmouth, New Hampshire. Dr. Guare is coauthor of bestselling books for general readers, including *Smart but Scattered Teens; Smart but Scattered—and Stalled* (with a focus on emerging adults); and *The Smart but Scattered Guide to Success* (with a focus on adults). He is also coauthor of *The Work-Smart Academic Planner, Revised Edition,* and books for professionals including *Executive Skills in Children and Adolescents, Third Edition.*

Colin Guare, MS, is a Rhode Island–based behavior analyst and writer. He is coauthor of bestselling books for general readers, including *Smart but Scattered Teens* and *Smart but Scattered—and Stalled* (with a focus on emerging adults). Mr. Guare currently works with schools, organizations, parents, and kids of all ages. He has a special interest in motivation and behavior change and has worked on several projects developing new techniques to help adults seek and achieve their long-term career and personal goals.